Foreword

We need to build a health political science

The challenge for health promotion at the beginning of the 21st century is to reinvent itself and address the key determinants of health. But in order to do so it needs a new mental map and another type of theoretical base. In this book Clavier and de Leeuw call for a new field of study which has been sorely missing in health research—*health political science*. In the first and last chapters they set out the contours for such a political science paradigm for health promotion based on a rigorous, argued application of political theory.

I have long worried about this glaring political theory gap in public health and health promotion. I have argued that we must add the political and commercial determinants to our list of economic, social, and environmental determinants of health, and in order to analyse them well we need a theoretical base (Kickbusch, 2012). We clearly need to prioritize the analysis of the political determinants of health at this point in time because health has moved up in the political agenda in countries, in development policies, and in global agreements. This is not only because of its consequence to the economy but also because of its relevance to power, legitimacy, and the expectations of citizens—witness the recent events in Brazil or Greece. Health is of a highly political and symbolic nature. It boils down to the central question: is health and wellbeing something that 'we collectively strive to pursue' (Sandel, 2009) with a concern for equity and social justice, or something we want to buy in the marketplace like any other private good?

I would argue that the current health debate is fundamentally about the common good and the role of the state, the market, and the community in a world of globalization, commercialization, and individualization. Dr Margaret Chan, the Director-General of the World Health Organization (WHO), has rightly pointed out that the globalization of lifestyles is by no means just a technical issue for public health: it is just as much a political issue, a trade issue, and an issue for foreign affairs (2013). In the health society the political nature of health again becomes visible, as it does in periods of major change and crisis. Structural adjustment in the 1980s, just as austerity policies in the 2010s, are the result of political configurations and decisions—not of an evidence-based technical decision-making process. Challenging the tobacco industry in a landmark case at the World Trade Organization—as done by Australia—is the result of a deeply political process, related not only to evidence but also to values.

Health is, has been, always will be, political—and of course there have always been authors that have drawn attention to this deeply political nature of health and health policy decisions: for example, Navarro, Mechanic, Levin, Katz, and Kahn or

Director-Generals of WHO such as Halfdan Mahler or Gro Harlem Brundtland. But strangely enough much of the health promotion literature has approached policy-making as if it could be considered an objective and neutral undertaking that we just need to learn to do better. Political will—encompassing a wide range of ideological positions, value judgments, and sociopolitical contextual alignment—has been approached as if it were just another technical component of the policy process rather than the ingredient that shapes most of the decisions taken.

The early health promotion literature—including the Ottawa Charter with its call for healthy public policies—was very aware of the political and social nature of health. But somewhere along the line the language became more technocratic and more careful. It became a health promotion mantra to call for a move from 'theory to practice' rather than to ask if the field was working from the right theoretical base. Sadly, the wealth of theory development in the political sciences has only very scantily been applied to health promotion policy issues, with perhaps the exception of global health issues. The call for more knowledge on 'how' to better implement health promotion or health in all policies was essentially interpreted as a recipe type of approach rather than applying theory to understand not just *that* something happens, but *how* it happens—so that we can change it. Indeed on the whole, despite its foundations in some of the best social and political theory of its day—Foucault, Illich, Giddens, Bateson, Beck—health promotion has been very theory averse. This has been to its detriment and has weakened the field.

This must change. This book can be an important step in the new direction. And I hope the editors are already planning a second edition with further applications—also from low- and middle-income countries.

Ilona Kickbusch
Director, Global Health Programme,
The Graduate Institute for International
and Development studies

References

Chan, M. (2013).*Opening address at the 8th Global Conference on Health Promotion, Helsinki, Finland, 10 June 2013*. Geneva, World Health Organization. Available at: <http://www.who.int/dg/speeches/2013/health_promotion_20130610/en/> (accessed 15 July 2013).

Kickbusch, I. (2012). Addressing the interface of the political and commercial determinants of health. *Health Promotion International*, **27**(4), 427–8.

Sandel, M. (2009). *Justice: what's the right thing to do?* New York: Farrar, Straus and Giroux.

Acknowledgements

This book is a collective achievement and we would like to thank all those who have supported and inspired us in the process: all the contributors of this book for their enthusiasm and dedication to this project, ever since they agreed to meet at a workshop during the 20th IUHPE World conference on health promotion in Geneva in 2010; Louise Potvin, for organizing an impromptu lunch between Carole and Evelyne back in 2009—this is when the idea for this book emerged; the Chair on Community Approaches and Inequalities in Health (CACIS) and the Montreal Public Health Directorate, where Carole worked respectively as a postdoctoral fellow and a researcher at the time of writing; Deakin University for awarding an Outside Studies Programme grant to Evelyne, and the Lea-Roback Centre on social inequalities in health for welcoming her in Montreal during that time; the Quebec Population Health Research Network of the Fonds de la recherche en santé du Québec (FRSQ) for its financial contribution towards the publication of this book; Susan Lempriere for her finest linguistic revision of the chapters authored by non-native English speakers; the doctoral students from the health promotion programme at the Université de Montréal for their astute comments on the introductory chapter; Patrick Vachon for his encouragement and inspiration every day of the development of this book; and Lynne Adamson for always being there (whether in Geelong, le Plateau-Mont-Royal, or in the Cloud).

Contents

Contributors

Karim Abu-Omar
Institute of Sports Sciences and Sport, Friedrich-Alexander University, Erlangen-Nürnberg, Germany

Fran Baum
South Australian Community Health Research Unit, Southgate Institute for Health, Society and Equity, Flinders University, Adelaide, Australia

Pierre Bergeron
INSPQ Institut National de Santé Publique du Québec, Quebec, Canada

Éric Breton
INPES Health Promotion Chair, EHESP School of Public Health, Rennes, France

Toba Bryant
Faculty of Health Sciences, University of Ontario Institute of Technology, Toronto, Canada

Carole Clavier
Department of Political Science, UQAM Université du Québec à Montréal, Montreal, Canada

Evelyne de Leeuw
Community Health Systems & Policy, Faculty of Health, Deakin University, Geelong, Australia

France Gagnon
School of Administration Sciences, TELUQ, Université du Québec, Quebec, Canada

Peter Gelius
Institute of Sports Sciences and Sport, Friedrich-Alexander University, Erlangen-Nürnberg, Germany

Marjan Hoeijmakers
Academic Collaborative Centre for Public Health Limburg, Regional Public Health Service, Geleen, the Netherlands

David Hunter
Fuse Centre for Translational Research and Wolfson Research Institute, Durham University, Durham, UK

Marie Jacques
Agence de la santé et des services sociaux de Montréal, Montreal, Canada

Catherine M. Jones
Department of Social and Preventive Medicine, Université de Montréal, Montreal, Canada

Michael Keizer
Independent Consultant in Logistics for Global Health and Aid

Angela Lawless
South Australian Community Health Research Unit, Southgate Institute for Health, Society and Equity, Flinders University, Adelaide, Australia

Erik Martin
School of Medicine, Deakin University, Geelong, Australia

Louise Potvin
Department of Social and Preventive Medicine, Université de Montréal, Montreal, Canada

Lucie Richard
Faculty of Nursing Science and IRSPUM Public Health Research Institute, Université de Montréal, Montreal, Canada

Alfred Rütten
Institute of Sports Sciences and Sport, Friedrich-Alexander University, Erlangen-Nürnberg, Germany

Belinda Townsend
School of International and Political Studies, Deakin University, Burwood, Australia

Carmel Williams
Health in All Policies Unit, Department of Health and Ageing, Adelaide, Australia

Chapter 1

Framing public policy in health promotion: ubiquitous, yet elusive

Carole Clavier and Evelyne de Leeuw

Introduction

For the past 25 years the health promotion field has been emphasizing the importance of public policy in effectively addressing the macro-level determinants of health. However, translating this need into action has proven challenging. This book aims to provide health promoters with a range of tools and experiences that will help them make inroads into the field of public policy. These tools and experiences have not been selected randomly: rather, they are rooted in theories of the policy process. We argue that such theories represent very practical tools for understanding, appraising, and developing health promotion action on the determinants of health at the societal level.

This introductory chapter pursues two distinct goals. The first is to set the stage for the work presented in this book through a close examination of the nature of public policy and the policy process, and their implications for health promotion. We examine the unique characteristics of public policy and the policy process that explain why the health promotion community has been struggling with the call, from within its own ranks, for the development of policies that will support integrated efforts to achieve human health. We show how public policy processes are complex and iterative, and how they obey a rationality all their own, and hence require specific analyses.

The second goal is to present the chapters that comprise this book and to underline their distinctive contributions to this field of knowledge and practice. The work presented in these chapters serves to situate public policy within theories from the health promotion literature and to show how such theories are powerful allies in understanding not only *whether* public policies work, but mostly *how* they work, thus providing invaluable practical and critical knowledge to health promoters.

Elusive public policy

The Commission on Social Determinants of Health underlined several different ways in which governments could, and should, use public policies to create more health and more equity in health (CSDH, 2008). Indeed, public policies are ubiquitous: they are present in most aspects of our daily lives that have an impact on health, from structures that regulate society like welfare programmes to physical constructs like roads and bike lanes. They shape the form of urban neighbourhoods, whether densely populated new suburban developments or run-down housing projects. They are everywhere in the school system: they are responsible for the content of curricula, for healthy cafeteria menus, for how admission lotteries for charter schools are run. Public policies are pervasive in the workplace: they shape the career opportunities of women, the safety of workers, and what happens to domestic industries in dire straits. They are embedded in and drive trade agreements between countries and continents. They determine the tolls paid by cars entering major cities and the origin of food in our local supermarket, as well as when, how, and in what form our health care is delivered.

Not surprisingly, because of their far-reaching influence on society, public policies have been identified as a major determinant of human health for decades. The pioneering work of Thomas McKeown first showed that the reduction in mortality and morbidity that occurred in 19th-century England and Wales owed more to improvements in living conditions than to improvements in therapeutic techniques (McKeown and Record, 1962). Although his research methods have been the object of considerable debate (Colgrove, 2002), a number of authors have reinforced his conclusions (Illich, 1976; Link and Phelan, 2002) and demonstrated how much social determinants affect inequalities in health (Navarro, 2002; Wilkinson, 1996).

In the early 1980s, Nancy Milio gathered impressive data on how agriculture, revenue, and social policy influence the health of populations (Milio, 1981). She also suggested that other sector policies—for example in industry, transportation, or culture rather than simply health care—would make a significant contribution to health by taking into account the effects of their actions on health. She coined the term 'healthy public policy' for the idea that health is the product of social and political forces, many of which are under the control of political action in various policy sectors.

The year before the World Health Organization (WHO) adopted the Ottawa Charter for Health Promotion (1986), Trevor Hancock also proposed a distinction between 'public health policy', which is concerned with the 'sick-care system' and the prevention of ill health, and 'healthy public policy' (Hancock, 1985). He argued that healthy public policy should embrace a holistic approach to health, question the impact of existing policies and institutions on health, and deal 'both with the health problems of the individuals and the great global issues of the day, such as energy, food production, pollution and unemployment' (Hancock, 1985: 10).

Building on these ideas, the health promotion community has proclaimed that creating healthy public policy is a highly effective course of action when attempting to alleviate health problems and health inequalities. In fact, it has done a remarkable job of advertising the importance of public policies for health, first with the 1986 Ottawa Charter, then with the 1988 Adelaide Recommendations on Healthy Public Policy, and continuing with the 8th Global Conference on Health Promotion, held in Helsinki in June 2013, which focused on governance and the theme 'Health in All Policies'. Since Adelaide, healthy public policy has been seen as 'characterized by an explicit concern for health and equity in all areas of policy and by an accountability for health impact' (WHO, 1988).

It has brought the concepts of equity, impact, accountability, and cross-sector action to the forefront. These concepts were reiterated, most notably, in the 1991 Sundsvall Statement on Supportive Environments for Health and the 2005 Bangkok Charter for Health Promotion in a Globalized World, and they are still at the heart of healthy public policy-making today (WHO and Government of South Australia, 2010).

From an idea(l) asserted in political declarations by the health promotion community, healthy public policy has transformed into a strategy supported by methods, governmental commitment, and resources. Health impact assessments, the principal method used to identify the effects of certain policies or projects on health, have been the first instruments used to put health on the agenda of other sector policies or projects (Kemm, 2001; Lock, 2000; Lock and McKee, 2005). Political authorities in a number of jurisdictions have elected to use them when making policy decisions, including the European Union, the Province of Quebec (Canada), and regional authorities in Switzerland (Gagnon et al., 2008; Koivusalo, 2010; Simos, 2006). The rationale underlying the promotion of health impact assessments is that producing knowledge about the effects of policy decisions sparks changes leading to the improved health of populations. Such changes, however, depend on several factors, including the constraining power of legal requirements around health impact assessments, the strength of advocacy surrounding a particular project or policy under assessment (Veerman et al., 2006), and possible conflicts between the numerous requirements for impact assessments on not only health issues but also the environment, the economy, and so forth (Smith et al., 2010).

Healthy public policy has also gained political purchase from the perspective of governance. The Health in All Policies concept and whole-of-government strategies have emphasized the importance of situating healthy public policy within the governance structures of political authorities (Bacigalupe et al., 2010; Kickbusch and Buckett, 2010; Kickbusch et al., 2008; Ritsatakis and Järvisalo, 2006). The common underlying argument is that governments, when making any policy decision, need to adopt an integrated strategy—and a matching governance structure—that considers not only the impact of other sector policies on health but also the contribution of improved health and well-being to other sector policies. Joined-up ministerial action is proposed as a way to counter the enduring 'conflation of health with health care' (Joffe and Mindell, 2004: 968) and to involve the responsibility of the whole government. In this respect, the 2006 Finnish presidency of the European Union has done a great deal towards placing the Health in All Policies approach, including health impact assessments, on the agenda of several governments (Ståhl et al., 2006). The current government of South Australia is adopting some of the most cutting-edge innovations in healthy public policy-making (see Baum et al., Chapter 10 in this volume).

Yet public policies are also elusive. Despite the demonstrated impact of public policies on health, awareness that influencing public policy is a legitimate and promising course of action to improve the health of populations is still in its infancy. Health promotion needs to dedicate considerable efforts to building its legitimacy to engage policies in sectors other than health care. In addition, the complex and shifting rationalities of public policy-making still largely elude health promotion. Even when competency benchmarks explicitly frame a role for the profession in the policy process (see de Leeuw and Breton, Chapter 2 in this volume), researchers and practitioners alike struggle to make sense of public policies and lack the appropriate tools to engage effectively in this enterprise. Several authors concur in saying that these difficulties stem from a certain 'naivety' about politics and the process of public policy-making on the part of health promoters (Bambra et al., 2005; Egan et al., 2009; Sparks, 2009). Others emphasize the path dependence of policies around health, which tend to focus on individual lifestyle factors despite current discourse insisting on the importance of acting on health determinants at the societal level (Popay et al., 2010). Greater knowledge about the policy process is necessary if health promotion is to overcome this 'lifestyle drift' and take full advantage of its own definition of health as being the product of political, social, and environmental factors. This will also contribute to reinforcing the legitimacy of health promotion within the policy arena.

Conceptualizing health as political and as being produced through political action has several practical implications. First, it takes the responsibility of producing health out of the hands of just medical doctors and other health care professionals. While health as political may seem like a truism within the ranks of health promotion, the proportion of public spending on prevention and public health services versus the total amount of health spending in Organisation for Economic Co-operation and Development (OECD) countries testifies to the limited entrenchment of this idea. Indeed, most countries, including Australia, Denmark, France, Germany, and the United States, allocate only 2–3.5% of their health spending to prevention and public health services, with Canada and New Zealand spending the most, at 6.6% and 7% respectively (OECD, 2012).

A second consequence of the assertion that health is inescapably political is that health is usually seen as beyond the reach of the mere health promotion practitioner. However, these practitioners may, in fact, have considerable control over health education and community empowerment processes thanks to their training and competency in the behavioural sciences. They may be particularly adept at creating supportive environments, reorienting health services, and, above all, creating healthy public policy. Influencing the social determinants of health at the policy level, as called for in the strategies outlined in the Ottawa Charter, requires dealing with organizations and issues from other policy sectors as well as with governments and politics. Such collaboration and reach, to health promotion, remains largely uncharted territory.

This book steps into this breach: it considers that health promoters have a legitimate claim when they seek to influence public policy, and that they need appropriate tools to increase their legitimacy within the policy arena. To this end, we argue that focusing on how public policies work makes it possible for health promoters to move beyond the more behavioural 'health education' and into translating political statements into effective political strategies. This book, therefore, makes a strong case for the use, in health promotion research, practice, and policy, of theories of the policy process that researchers in political science and its related disciplines have been developing and using for many years.

Public policy and the policy process

Looking closely at the relationship between health promotion and public policy, we suggest that the reason public policies are elusive for health promotion is two-fold. On the one hand, the characteristics of public policies make it challenging to identify their contours, to keep track of their changes, and to isolate the different influences that shape them. On the other hand, health promotion is currently ill equipped to fully understand and work with these characteristics of public policy.

An abstract construct

The first defining feature of public policy that makes it hard for health promoters to grasp is that it is largely invisible. Let us be clear: it is not the abstract nature of public policies that makes them difficult for health promotion researchers and practitioners to identify. On the contrary, health promoters are generally quite skilled at dealing with the abstract, as they do when studying attitudes, beliefs, and social norms (e.g. Fishbein and Ajzen, 1975; Godin and Kok, 1996). Rather, health promotion tends to 'materialize' public policy, to conceive of it not as an abstraction but rather as a document that can be held, leafed through, and (ultimately) rewritten. It is not uncommon for health promotion researchers and practitioners to consider a law or plan—namely the visible, concrete portion of public policy—and take it to be the only representation of the policy (Bernier and Clavier, 2011; Breton and de Leeuw, 2011).

But this is limiting. Of course, analysts can read the strategy documents, laws, and programmes that form the basis of a policy like, for example, Quebec's energy policy. But these documents merely state, in this case, the government's intention to rely on hydroelectricity and to give some support to wind energy. They give an incomplete picture of the policy. First, laws, programmes, and policy statements do not explain the historical process that led to the particular framing of the issue embodied in these texts. In this case, energy policy based on hydropower has been a flagship for Quebec's economic nationalism since the 1940s, in contrast to the historical influence of US markets and US capital on the production of energy in the province (Faucher, 1992; Gattinger, 2005). This is an important factor to consider when trying to explain Quebec's attachment to hydroelectricity and to the province-owned company that produces hydropower, a phenomenon that can only be understood with a historical perspective. Second, laws, programmes, and policy statements say nothing about current controversies between different coalitions of actors trying to push for distinct conceptions of an issue. This requires a thorough study of the actors involved, including those who do not have access to governmental policy arenas. In the case of Quebec's energy policy, the three coalitions of actors promoting the development of wind energy do not agree on the economic model underlying the development of alternative, renewable energy sources. One defends a government-owned wind power policy, while the other two favour privately owned wind power plants (Jegen and Audet, 2011). In sum, laws and programmes 'mask' these complexities because they only give a picture of the policy orientations at a given moment in time. How configurations of power have shaped values, actors, and policy ideas in one direction at the expense of another can only be understood in relation to the broader context of the policy and the actors involved.

Indeed, there is more to public policies than documents fixed in time and content. Public policy is 'anything a government chooses to do or not to do' (Dye, 1972: 2). Understanding the options that governments choose not to follow, and why they choose to follow one policy option at the expense of others, requires researchers to observe the controversies and debates surrounding policy decisions. A policy is, therefore, a programme of action (or inaction) that is consciously decided upon and implemented by public authorities. In this sense, while laws and plans have the legal authority of public action and express the interpretation of an issue at a given moment in time, in no way do they represent the full complexity of the issue.

Jenkins provides further insight into the complexity of public policy when he defines it as:

> a set of interrelated decisions taken by a political actor or group of actors concerning the selection of goals and the means of achieving them within a specified situation where those decisions should, in principle, be within the power of those actors to achieve.
>
> (Jenkins, 1978: 15)

This definition emphasizes the ideas and knowledge underlying policy content, the dynamic process leading to government action, and the latter's capacity (alone or with other actors) to carry out the action.

A public policy, therefore, can be defined as the programme of action (or inaction) of a government to achieve specific goals. The study of public policy is thus 'the study of the State in action' (Hassenteufel, 2008: 7; Jobert and Muller, 1987). To make sense of these programmes analysts need to understand their emergence (why?), their contents (how?), and their effects. The study of public policies does not start, or stop, with the study of decision-making. It encompasses the emergence of so-called public problems. It engages, both before and after a decision is taken, a range of actors that are not necessarily mentioned in the law or plan, such as citizens, public administrations, municipalities, and interest groups. Public policy is also composed of objectives, ideas, and values that are sometimes implicit; of resources in the form of credits, workforces, and knowledge; and of instruments such as taxes, information campaigns, and regulations (Howlett et al., 2009). Public policies, therefore, cannot be grasped at a single glance: for the analyst, it is a task in itself to delineate their contours and to determine which of their elements are relevant to a given issue.

Dynamic policy processes

The second reason public policies are elusive is that they are dynamic, iterative processes. In this book, we conceptualize the policy process as 'the manner in which governmental policies get formulated and implemented, as well as the effects of those actions on the world' (Sabatier, 1991: 147). The concept of the policy process follows from what we have just said about public policies—namely, that they are more than a decision set in time and in content. Rather, the policy process encompasses actors, ideas, and institutions that are part of making and implementing policy. Sabatier, one of the leading authors in policy studies, sums up the complexity of the whole policy process in just one sentence:

> Understanding the policy process requires knowledge of the goals and perceptions of hundreds of actors throughout the country involving possibly very technical and legal issues over periods of a decade or more while most of those actors are actively seeking to propagate their specific "spin" on events.
>
> (Sabatier, 2007: 4)

To make sense of these processes, the policy studies literature has defined them as a set of stages: emergence of a public problem (agenda-setting), formulation of a policy, formal decision-making, implementation of the policy, and evaluation of the policy (Jones, 1970; Lasswell, 1956). These stages, however, do not work in a neat and orderly fashion: new events or new actors may change the definition of a problem, thereby forcing a re-evaluation of the policy's formulation; the widespread public perception of a problem may not translate into a policy; or policy evaluation may not inform a renewed, improved public policy (an experience, no doubt, with which many of you are familiar). In fact, the 'stages model' has been much criticized in policy studies, precisely for not taking into account the complex and iterative nature of the policy process. For the policy-making stages to achieve their full heuristic value, they need to be seen as 'milestones' within an iterative process and not as a representation of a rational and linear policy process (deLeon, 1999) (see Figure 1.1).

In the past three decades, policy analysts have also developed a number of theories to make sense of the complex rationalities of the policy process. These theories make

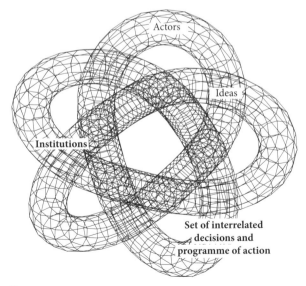

Figure 1.1 The policy process.
Source: Image © Shutterstock 2013.

different assumptions about how public policies are made, how they are changed and why, and what effects they have. While some place greater emphasis on institutions (e.g. institutional rational choice), others focus on ideas and belief systems (the advocacy coalition framework), the interactions between problems, policy solutions and political issues (the multiple streams theory) (Sabatier, 2007), or the complex interrelations between policy decisions and actions across levels of government (Hill and Hupe, 2006). More recently, network analysis, social movement theories, and political sociology have expanded the role of actors in the policy process (politicians, elite civil servants, experts, and intermediary actors) (Hassenteufel et al., 2010; Marsh and Rhodes, 1992; Tantivess and Walt, 2008).

Policy change

Attempts to understand public policy are further complicated by the issue of policy change. This is what governments claim to achieve with each new 'reform', and also what health promoters aim to accomplish through actions of influence on public policies. But what, precisely, is policy change, and what causes it?

First, policy change may occur at different moments in the policy process, for instance following elections and the rise to power of a new government, or following a crisis like an epidemic or economic turmoil. It occurs under the influence of new knowledge or in response to a shifting balance of power among the different actors involved in a policy.

Second, the scope of public policy change varies greatly. Some changes are the product of sweeping paradigm shifts, as when the British economic policy changed radically from Keynesian-inspired State involvement to neo-liberalism (with talk of deregulation and the free market) in the 1980s (Hall, 1993). Public policies also change through small steps (Lindblom, 1959), a process concomitant with public policy development and implementation (Sabatier, 2007). The various actors involved in the implementation of a policy interpret and adapt the original decision, making a series of smaller-scale decisions to fine-tune roles and responsibilities, budgetary issues, and so on. In fact, incremental policy change is most often invoked as the reason for continuity and inertia in public policies. Nevertheless, the accumulation of small-scale changes may progressively lead to more radical policy change.

Studies of the policy process have highlighted different types of policy change. For instance, Hall distinguishes between three orders of policy change (Hall, 1993). Changes of the first order occur when a policy instrument is used in a different way. This could happen, for example, when taxes are used to promote changes in smoking behaviour or to encourage industry to reduce polluting emissions. Changes of the second order occur when new instruments are introduced into a policy, as when the government of Quebec or the European Union added health impact assessments to their repertoire in public health policy. First and second order changes correspond to incremental changes; they do not affect the overall objectives of the policy. By contrast, third order changes are paradigm changes that occur when the very ideas that form the basis of a policy are replaced with a new set of values and ideas. Building healthy public policy and replacing the biomedical approach to health would be such a major policy change.

Other authors have pointed out that different dimensions of public policy can change. Expanding on Hall's typology, Hassenteufel proposes four dimensions of policy change: the use and creation of policy instruments; policy actors, who may be created/disappear or strengthened/weakened; the institutional rules of the game; and the values and ideas embedded in and driving the policy (Hassenteufel, 2008). Contrary to Hall's three orders of change, these four dimensions are not hierarchical but rather strongly intertwined. Changes in institutional rules, such as creating a new administrative body, may strengthen some actors at the expense of others, while a new set of policy ideas may lead to the reformulation of policy instruments and institutional rules, and a shift in power relations among policy actors.

This perspective also helps us understand resistance to policy change. For instance, in all probability, the introduction of new policy instruments such as health impact assessments will be met with some opposition from advocates of the biomedical approach to health or from economic policy actors, whose rationale for action is based on a different set of values and policy ideas.

The third characteristic of public policies is that they are socially and historically embedded: in large part, they are the product of past choices and institutional arrangements. As several other choices or institutions depend on, or are based on, the original choice, the cost of change is very high. Labelled 'path dependence' (Pierson, 2000), this phenomenon has been shown to explain the adoption of technological innovations, even when there are more efficient competing technologies on the market. For instance, the adoption of the QWERTY keyboard was largely due to the development of touch typing (typing with all your fingers) using the QWERTY keyboard, thus making it more 'unlikely' that typists and businesses would choose a different technological solution (David, 1985).

The phenomenon of path dependence has two major implications. First, along with incrementalism, it explains policy continuity or inertia. It explains why, for example, pension systems based on solidarity between generations of workers cannot be radically reformed to become systems based on individual savings. For one thing, current workers would have to pay for retired workers as well as for themselves, thus paying twice. For another, coalitions defending the solidarity-based systems still wield strong influence on political decision-making. This does not mean that pension systems are not being reformed; instead, these changes are occurring gradually and are being adapted to the particular institutions of individual countries (Palier, 2007; Pierson, 2000).

The other implication of this phenomenon is that policy students need to redefine the frontiers of their study in order to better observe and understand policy change. The existence of a historical legacy means that the time frame selected for the study of a policy will influence the perception of policy change. To fully understand whether, and to what extent, public policies change, policy analysts need to look at them across relatively long periods of time. For example, a newcomer to the field of public health studying health policy since the mid-1980s would certainly pinpoint 1986 and the promulgation of the Ottawa Charter as a landmark. And rightly so: the Ottawa Charter crystallized change towards a more collective-oriented health policy, focusing not only on care to individuals, but also on the social, environmental, and political determinants of health. However, to get a fuller picture, the new analyst would need to look back to other landmarks, such as the Lalonde Report on the health of Canadians, which first put some of these social determinants in a policy document a decade before the Ottawa Charter; to the emancipatory social movements of the 1960s and 1970s, which put community engagement on the map; and, much earlier, to the hygienists' understanding of the role of environmental factors, such as sewage systems and insalubrious housing in the propagation of epidemics (de Leeuw and Clavier, 2011; Porter, 1994; Porter, 1997). With a historical perspective, policy changes garner new depth and meaning. What seemed so radically innovative now appears less so, and a variety of new questions arise: what circumstances explain why the Ottawa Charter has had such staying power, not only with health professionals but also with policy-makers? Why then: would the Charter have had the same impact ten years earlier?

In sum, the policy process is far from linear: it evolves in response to changes that can occur at any time, and it is embedded in existing societal and policy constraints. To make sense of, and to be able to effectively influence, the policy process, analysts need to consider the broader picture: both the social and institutional constraints under which an issue is being debated and the positions of the different actors with an interest in the issue in question.

The politics of policy-making

Finally, public policies are elusive and difficult to describe because of their relationship with political power. In their work, Klein and Marmor bring together the actions of governments (*policies*) and the ideologies and conflicts of interest characteristic of the struggle for political power (*politics*). They add to Dye's definition that public policy 'is about politics, resolving (or at least attenuating) conflicts about resources, rights, and morals' (Klein and Marmor, 2008: 892). In their view, what analysts need in order to make sense of public policy is to understand the paradigms underlying policy-makers' choices, the institutions within which governments operate, and the interests of the different political actors involved. Political ideologies and institutions, the rules of electoral competition, the power of interest groups, media coverage of an issue, public opinion, the economy, and diplomatic ties all contribute to the definition and evolution of public policies.

The politics of the welfare state provide rich illustrations of the ambiguous influence of party ideologies on public policy. Some studies have shown that countries run by social democratic governments over long periods of time tend to fare better than countries run by liberal governments because of their commitment to redistributive policies (Navarro and Shi, 2001). Attaining equity in societies, however, is not a prerogative of social democracy (Wilkinson and Pickett, 2011). The ongoing philosophical debate on the nature of social justice and its contribution to redistributive politics, and therefore health, has amply demonstrated the complexity of the issue (e.g. Nussbaum, 2006; Rawls, 1971; Sen, 1992). Without delving too deeply into this debate, let us simply note the complexity and ambivalence of short-term party politics on health policy.

For instance, and contrary to what would be expected, Danish social democrats, who were once the founders and strong defenders of the Danish universal welfare state, have also been responsible for its liberalization in recent years. In the early 1990s they introduced more flexibility into the labour market and imposed means-related criteria on what had previously been universal social benefits. Social democrats had a great advantage over their centre-right predecessors in trying to implement such changes because no one believed they would introduce changes that could jeopardize the integrity of the welfare state. Paradoxically, this situation enabled them to introduce very significant reforms (Clasen, 2002; Green-Pedersen, 2002). Even though party rhetoric may be strong, policy choices can be mitigated by other constraints, such as an economic crisis, unstable government coalitions, or any other conjunction of events.

Public policies, therefore, are abstract constructs—albeit with very tangible effects—that result from complex, iterative, and socially embedded processes. Studying the policy process necessitates looking beyond policy contents and outcomes to the whole set of conditions under which policies are developed (Sabatier, 2007).

Implications for health promotion

On one level, this conception of public policy and the policy process is in tune with recent developments in health promotion. The past decade has seen considerable and notable steps towards broadening the intellectual apparatus of health promotion in order to take into account the complexity of health and its social dimensions. McQueen, Kickbusch, and their colleagues have argued that modernity calls for a full theoretical understanding of health within its social context (McQueen and Kickbusch, 2007). Specifically, they point out that sociobehavioural theories alone, because they are too deeply rooted in causal reasoning, cannot provide this understanding; we need social theory. They have explored, among other theories, the potential of sociology, social capital studies, actor–network theory, and cultural theory.

Hawe and Potvin (2009) seek to reinvigorate thinking about health intervention around the concept of population-level health intervention research. Set in the Canadian tradition of population health research, their approach advocates the study of all policies and programmes that aim to change the distribution of a given social risk and that could have consequences for the distribution of health risk across populations. This approach is also firmly entrenched in complexity and systems thinking.

Other, more 'classic' models for health promotion planning have also incorporated complexity and systems thinking by encouraging the identification and use of all kinds of theories that may explain a phenomenon, including those used in social sciences. The latest version of the PRECEDE–PROCEED framework and, to a greater extent, the intervention mapping approach, encourage theory-based planning and intervention in a less linear way (Bartholomew et al., 2001; Green and Kreuter, 2005). Interestingly, Lawrence Green and Marshall Kreuter's title for their book on the well-known PRECEDE (and in later editions, the PRECEDE–PROCEED) framework went through a number of incarnations: *Health Education Planning: A Diagnostic Approach* in the 1980s, then *Health Promotion Planning: An Educational and Environmental Approach* in the 1990s, and, finally, *Health Program Planning: An Educational and Ecological Approach* in the new millennium. These changes are not merely rhetorical: they reflect a change in perspective from a more behaviourist to a systems view.

However, significant discrepancies remain between the conception of the policy process developed in policy studies and that permeating current health promotion research and practice. Existing planning and intervention models in health promotion favour, even if only implicitly, a linear understanding of the policy process that is reminiscent of the causal reasoning that reigns supreme in biomedical health sciences. In such models, concerned primarily with explaining the health of populations, public policy is considered to be simply a contextual factor that influences behaviour that, in turn, influences health. The planning and intervention process is assumed to be a rational process whereby, upon the identification of a problem, data (preferably evidence-based) are gathered, a decision is made, a law is enacted, a programme is implemented and, finally, the programme is evaluated. Such planning models place too little emphasis on the complexity and essential political nature of the policy process. In fact, these models do not consider the influence of political institutions and ideologies, competing interests, and the implementation stage at all. In other words, classic (i.e. behavioural) planning models in health promotion limit the lines of investigation about public policy in that they see critical elements of the policy process as 'black boxes', and try to explain or change policy processes through inappropriate (often psychological health) approaches.

Current strategies to engage public policy—namely evidence building and knowledge transfer—reflect the ambiguity of the knowledge base of health promotion. While these strategies are rooted in a linear understanding of planning and intervention processes, their practice signals a move towards a more comprehensive, complex understanding of public policy-making. For instance, recent advances in evidence-based policy-making encourage the co-production of research agendas by both academics and knowledge users (de Leeuw and Skovgaard, 2005; Hunter, 2009; Whitehead et al., 2004). The underlying argument is that evidence building will not only produce a better fit between knowledge and practice but also raise awareness about health issues within governments and their administrations (Gagnon et al., 2007). Recently, current practices of knowledge transfer have also been called into question on the grounds that they are overly linear (de Leeuw et al., 2008; Macintyre, 2012).

We concur with this assertion. Like these authors, we do not deny the importance of evidence building and knowledge transfer for shaping the causal pathways between public policy and health. However, we argue that the real issue is how health promotion can effectively engage public policy, knowing that the policy process is far from linear.

Generally speaking, the political science literature is rife with cases where it is not the accumulation of evidence that triggers public intervention but rather some other factor. For instance, although the risks associated with the use of contaminated blood had been well established scientifically, it took considerable media coverage of public scares and scandals for public authorities to finally take action and regulate the conditions of blood donation (Farrell, 2006; Marchetti and Champagne, 2004). Although most policy cases are not quite so dramatic, this example highlights the fact that public policy-making answers to a set of rules, values, and norms that are radically different from those prevailing in the fields of academic research and health promotion.

Consequently, we assert that engaging in the policy game with the rules by which health promotion currently plays is ineffective. The health promotion realm has been very good at talking the talk of the policy world, with lofty statements on healthy public policy, the social determinants of health, and the like, but it has failed to walk the walk of the complex, iterative, and quintessentially power-driven policy process. This process engages and thrives through a set of rules, values, and norms—sometimes explicit, often implicit—in which the ideal of health does not always predominate. While the welfare state is not alone in efforts at health promotion (in fact, the Nairobi Call to Action and the Yanuca Healthy Island Declaration both link the health promotion perspective with a human and economic development agenda outside high-income nation states), a critical look at such efforts within welfare states provides a point in case. The rules, values, and norms driving welfare state development and sustainability are a result of raw politics, normative positions, and blunt differences in political philosophies, and these forces drive radically different approaches to a goal that all welfare states seem to share but which never seems to materialize: equal health for all (Bambra, 2011).

Health promoters need to become more knowledgeable about aspects of the policy process like 'raw politics'. This would help with knowledge transfer strategies. More importantly, in our view, theories on the policy process could then be effectively applied earlier in the research process. Such theories would allow us to formulate new research questions and guide practice in health promotion, thereby expanding the scope of health promotion research to, as yet, under-explored areas of knowledge on health policy (Breton and de Leeuw, 2011).

Other authors have taken a position similar to ours. Among them, most notably, are O'Neill et al. (2011), whose book presents a method for the political analysis of health initiatives, and Gilson (2012), who has published a reader on health policy analysis (see Boxes 1.1 and 1.2). Lee also has brilliantly argued for increased knowledge about the processes of governance and policy-making (Lee, 2010). While this particular research does not explicitly address the theories behind arguments for global governance, it aptly illustrates their importance in understanding and acting upon pressing health issues. Health promotion, Lee argues, needs to understand the rules of issue competition and agenda-setting in order to compete for space on the policy agenda, alongside issues of economic globalization and security. In these processes, lack of knowledge about health issues among policy-makers is often pointed out as an obstacle, but it turns out that

Box 1.1 A manual for political analysis of health interventions

O'Neill et al. (2011) propose a powerful method for analysing the political dimension of interventions designed to improve health and its social determinants. Whether they take place at the policy level, such as adopting an anti-tobacco bylaw in a municipality, or at the organization level, such as implementing a caring philosophy of clinical intervention within a hospital, health interventions are fraught with power relationships between the different parties involved. Not taking these into account may thwart even the most evidence-based intervention efforts. This is where their method comes in. Carefully crafted over the past 15 years, it has been used to assess the feasibility of such interventions and to identify strategies for their implementation. The first step of the method is to clarify what the intervention is going to be: the problem to address, the historical precedents, and the objectives of the intervention. The second step draws on theories of the policy process to characterize the network of actors involved in the proposed intervention: what actors will potentially be concerned; what their arguments and position will be regarding the problem to address; what their potential influence will be, given their respective positions in the political space; what alliances could be made; and whether the intervention is feasible. The third and final step of the method is devising strategies to advocate the proposed solution: consensus building, preparing a political platform, cooperation, campaign, and protest.

A hands-on manual designed for practitioners, decision-makers, managers, and citizens, this book provides practical tools like tables, guidelines and an interactive website to help practitioners draw insights from political studies and apply them to real-life situations. In this sense, readers will find it of great practical value. Nevertheless, although clearly rooted in political science works, the manual provides little explanation of the theories behind the method's three steps. Readers will find that the underlying theory is reminiscent of both network analysis and the multiple streams theory in that it assesses solutions in their search for a political opportunity (see de Leeuw et al., Chapter 8). However, the approach could also be complemented with knowledge of the advocacy coalition framework (see Breton et al., Chapter 3) or actor–network theory (see Potvin and Clavier, Chapter 5).

values and ideas (about the economy, for instance) are far more of an obstacle to political attention to health issues than is lack of knowledge. This is an important consideration for health promoters when devising knowledge transfer and advocacy strategies. Lee also raises the question of how formal governance structures affect health policy: in a world where non-state actors like philanthropic organizations and the pharmaceutical industry exercise increasing power, and where issues and interests cut across state boundaries, how relevant and effective are state-based institutions in global health governance?

Box 1.2 A reader on health policy and systems research

Lucy Gilson (2012) has created a comprehensive reader for analysts, teachers, and students engaged in health policy and systems research, with a strong focus on low- and middle-income countries. The studies included focus on health care systems, clinical practitioners, hospital management, family planning, community-based care, and so on. After an introduction to the boundaries of health policy and systems research and to the research process, there are ten theoretical papers, each of which proposes a different conceptual framework for making sense of health policy and health systems. These include systems thinking, theories of decision-making, and studies of governance, decentralization, and financing issues. The reader also collates a broad selection of empirical papers pertaining to different methodological perspectives: cross-sectional studies, case studies, ethnographic studies, impact evaluations, studies of policy and system change, cross-national analyses, and action research. The studies draw on multiple disciplines: political science, health economics, sociology, organizational studies, anthropology, and epidemiology. This reader is of great practical value because it covers the range of theoretical and methodological approaches to health systems and policy research, showing how this diversity is needed to make sense of, and support, contemporary transformations of health care systems and policies. It does not, however, propose any systematic pedagogical approach to any of the conceptual frameworks featured.

Bringing theory back in

So how can we take public policy processes into account in health promotion research and practice? Two possible, not necessarily contradictory, solutions emerge. The first is to bring into the field people with a background and interest in public policy studies. Of course, social scientists have been invited to collaborate in public health research before, notably when a public health professor encouraged sociologists to investigate the emergence of chronic diseases in the 1960s (Rogers, 1968). Similarly, Green (2006) called on systems specialists to help unravel the intricacies of networks, partnerships, and knowledge transfer. However, for all its appeal, this strategy has some limitations, especially in the short term. A study in Canada asked how health scientists on committees examining grant applications related to health and social issues would define 'legitimate science' in health (Albert et al., 2008). The answer given by clinicians and biomedical researchers was that legitimate science is experimental and quantitative biomedical research. Cultural boundaries between the health and social sciences, as well as their deep entrenchment within institutions governing health research, certainly make it more challenging to fund social science research on the health policy process. The Australian Public Health Research Advisory Committee (2008) in its 'Nutbeam Review' (named after its chair) substantiates this position.

No less challenging, but nevertheless promising, is the second solution: encouraging health promotion researchers to familiarize themselves with policy studies and to integrate theories on the policy process into their own theoretical frames of reference. Mirroring the first solution, this may require involving specialists in policy studies. There is a difference in degree, however, as the second solution advocates more than cursory collaboration. Rather, it aims to expand the existing foundations of health promotion theories. It is this solution that is the focus of this book. We argue for a theory-based way of making sense of public policies and their impact on health. We assert that health promotion would benefit from bringing theories on the policy process into its growing corpus, and that theory-based thinking is practical.

As Kurt Lewin famously said, and as many like-minded researchers have since reiterated, there is nothing as practical as a good theory (Lewin, 1945). At first, this seems like quite a paradox, since the essence of a theory is its abstract nature. Theories do not refer to any particular empirical phenomena; rather, they synthesize myriads of observations about similar empirical phenomena into 'a clear and logically interrelated set of propositions, some of them empirically falsifiable' (Breton and de Leeuw, 2011: 83). But theories are practical precisely because of this abstract and aggregate character. They establish relationships between the different elements in society, a policy process, or a programme. These relationships can be causal (how A influences B), systemic (interdependencies between A and B within the system they form), structural (how A is positioned in relation to B, as in network theories for instance), comprehensive (exploring the meaning of social and human actions), or agency-based (uncovering the strategies behind actors' actions). In this sense, theory is practical because it allows for an in-depth, critical understanding of social processes, including policy processes. Theory is also practical because the patterns it establishes can help in problem-solving (Bartholomew et al., 2001). Following the principles of theory-based evaluation, theory used in the analysis of programmes or policies helps produce knowledge of whether these programmes and policies work and, most importantly, of how and in what circumstances they work (Birckmayer and Weiss, 2000; Pawson, 2003; Weiss, 1995).

Chapter 2 by de Leeuw and Breton builds on this premise. Having established the importance of public policy in health promotion, the authors explain how theories of the policy process help make sense of governments' actions. Such theories, they argue, could become powerful tools for the health promotion profession in its efforts to develop healthy public policy. To determine whether theories are already part of the repertoire of health promotion research, they review the current use of theories of the policy process in peer-reviewed publications on health promotion. Their findings suggest that they are not yet widely in use, although the situation is improving. They identify five conditions for achieving more robust, theory-based health promotion research and practice on healthy public policy.

The 'Understanding Policy' section contains four chapters that take a critical look at public policies for health and their underlying values and principles. Each draws on a specific theory to analyse the policy process.

Chapter 3 by Breton, Richard, Gagnon, Jacques, and Bergeron proposes a detailed analysis of the process that led to the adoption of the anti-tobacco law in the Province of Quebec in the late 1990s. Using Sabatier's advocacy coalition framework and Lemieux's theory of coalition building, the authors explain how different coalitions of actors, including regional public health officers, the tobacco industry, and the media interacted to influence the government's policy. The authors' analysis highlights both the complexities of the interactions between the different coalitions—each structured around their own values and interests—and the impact of contextual factors, such as the tobacco contraband crisis.

In Chapter 4, Bryant adopts a political economy approach, conceptualizing public policy choices as the result of several forces, including the State, the market, political ideology, and power relationships. This work draws on Esping-Andersen's classification of the welfare state, which is based on the extent and type of social stratification and the role of the State in service provision. Applying these frameworks to Canada, Bryant identifies the ideology of neo-liberalism as a primary obstacle to the development of a comprehensive policy addressing the social determinants of health.

Potvin and Clavier, in Chapter 5, explore a recurring theme in health promotion research and practice: actors from different policy sectors, professions, and organizations must collaborate in order to carry out health promotion programmes. They use actor–network theory, a conceptual framework originating from the social studies of technology, to describe the networks of actors that constitute health promotion programmes and to analyse the characteristics of their interactions in building shared understandings of situations and joint action. They provide a practice-oriented understanding of what the theory calls 'translation'. Their argument is based on a critical analysis of several health promotion programmes and initiatives in Canada.

In Chapter 6, de Leeuw, Townsend, Martin, Jones, and Clavier address the forces of globalization in health policy-making. Increased interdependence between countries has affected how we think about health at the global level, forcing us to consider the global social determinants of health and to take global action. Drawing on theories of global health governance, this chapter presents three case studies of how globalization affects health policy-making. The first examines the influence of the Doha Declaration on trade agreements and intellectual property for access to essential medicines in low-income countries. The second analyses the implementation of the Framework Convention on Tobacco Control in remote Pacific islands. The final case study proposes a different approach: it shifts the research focus from global governance mechanisms to national policies concerned with global health.

The 'Making Policy' section includes four chapters that take a hands-on, theory-based approach to health promotion policy-making. They provide accounts of real-life experiences and tools, such as questionnaires, software, and practice guides that are theory-based and of practical use to health promoters. The authors used insights from theories on the policy process to guide their work and build the tools presented.

In Chapter 7, Hunter is concerned with the complexity of putting knowledge into practice. His chapter recounts the experience of FUSE, a UK-based collaborative research centre that studies how stakeholders use knowledge on health promotion in their own practice. He also analyses his own contribution, as an academic, to a WHO Regional Office for Europe policy-making process. Using three theoretical frameworks—the concept of wicked issue, systems thinking, and theories on knowledge transfer and exchange—he advocates the co-production of knowledge by academic researchers and practitioners. He argues that knowledge production should incorporate a deeper understanding of how decisions are made and of the political context of policy-making.

In Chapter 8, de Leeuw, Keizer, and Hoeijmakers focus on policy-making for health at the local level, with a view to how these processes can be supported. Some of their earlier studies were based on a now classic theory of the policy process, Kingdon's multiple streams theory. For all its relevance in showing the intricacies of politics and policy, the theory has fallen short in highlighting the networked relationships of local actors. In this chapter, the authors present an interactive software they have developed based on both Kingdon's model and network analysis. This highly practical tool allows local actors to visualize, and eventually strengthen, their own position within the network.

Rütten, Gelius, and Abu-Omar's approach, in Chapter 9, also seeks to support policy-making processes at several levels, but it is rooted in a different theoretical tradition. Using action theory as their foundation, the authors have studied the determinants of individual action (goals, resources, constraints, and opportunities) along with their impact, and adapted the theory to policy-making processes. Relying on this theoretical framework, they have developed and empirically tested their own ADEPT model, a quantitative questionnaire designed to evaluate processes, outputs, and outcomes in policy development and policy implementation.

In Chapter 10, Baum, Lawless, and Williams recount the development of the Health in All Policies by the government of South Australia. Their analysis is rooted in three main theoretical approaches: Kingdon's multiple streams theory, theories on organizational change, and systems theory. Combining these theories allows them to identify the strategies used to gain, and retain, the attention of policy-makers. The authors study the process of how the Health in All Policies approach was put on the government agenda, as well as the implementation stages of the approach (awareness, adoption, implementation, and institutionalization). Their chapter highlights issues, opportunities and obstacles in the actual formulation and implementation of a government policy that brings together all governmental sectors and ministries.

Finally, in Chapter 11, de Leeuw and Clavier conclude with a discussion of the contributions of theories on the policy process to health promotion research and practice. Theories, they argue, are valuable because they enable us to analyse and understand the processes and factors underlying health policy-making in different contexts. Theories are also practical in a more pragmatic sense: they can be used to build tools that can be used by both practitioners and policy-makers in their quest to participate in the policy-making process.

References

Albert, M., Laberge, S., Hodges, B. D., Regehr, G., and Lingard, L. (2008). Biomedical scientists' perception of the social sciences in health research. *Social Science & Medicine*, **66** (12), 2520–31.

Bacigalupe, A., Esnaola, S., Martin, U., and Zuazagoitia, J. (2010). Learning lessons from past mistakes: how can Health in All Policies fulfil its promises? *Journal of Epidemiology and Community Health*, **64** (6), 504–5.

Bambra, C. (2011). Health inequalities and welfare state regimes: theoretical insights on a public health 'puzzle'. *Journal of Epidemiology and Community Health*, **65** (9), 740–5.

Bambra, C., Fox, D., and Scott-Samuel, A. (2005). Towards a politics of health. *Health Promotion International*, **20** (2), 187–93.

Bartholomew, L. K., Parcel, G. S., Kok, G., and Gottlieb, N. H. (2001). *Intervention Mapping*. Mountain View, CA: Mayfield Publishing Company.

Bernier, N. F. and Clavier, C. (2011). Public health policy research: making the case for a political science approach. *Health Promotion International*, **26** (1), 109–16.

Birckmayer, J. D. and Weiss, C. H. (2000). Theory-based evaluation in practice: what do we learn? *Evaluation Review*, **24** (4), 407–31.

Breton, E. and de Leeuw, E. (2011). Theories of the policy process in health promotion research: a review. *Health Promotion International*, **26** (1), 82–90.

Clasen, J. (2002). Modern social democracy and European welfare state reform. *Social Policy & Society*, **1** (1), 67–76.

Colgrove, J. (2002). The McKeown Thesis: a historical controversy and its enduring influence. *American Journal of Public Health*, **95** (2), 725–9.

CSDH (2008). *Closing the Gap in a Generation. Health Equity through Action on the Social Determinants of Health. Final Report of the Commission on Social Determinants of Health*. Geneva: World Health Organization.

David, P. (1985). Clio and the economics of QWERTY. *American Economics Review*, **75** (2), 332–7.

de Leeuw, E. and Clavier, C. (2011). Healthy public in all policies. *Health Promotion International*, **26** (Suppl. 2), ii237–ii244.

de Leeuw, E. and Skovgaard, T. (2005). Utility-driven evidence for Healthy Cities: problems with evidence generation and application. *Social Science & Medicine*, **61** (6), 1331–41.

de Leeuw, E., McNess, A., Crisp, B. and Stagnitti, K. (2008). Theoretical reflections on the nexus between research, policy and practice. *Critical Public Health*, **18** (1), 5–20.

deLeon, P. (1999). The stages approach to the policy process: what has it done? Where is it going?, in P. A. Sabatier (ed.) *Theories of the Policy Process (1st edn.)*, pp. 19–34, Boulder, CO: Westview.

Dye, T. R. (1972). *Understanding Public Policy* Englewood Cliffs, NJ: Prentice Hall.

Egan, M., Bambra, C., Petticrew, M., and Whitehead, M. (2009). Reviewing evidence on complex social interventions: appraising implementation in systematic reviews of the health effects of organisational-level workplace interventions. *Journal of Epidemiology and Community Health*, **63** (1), 4–11.

Farrell, A.-M. (2006). Is the gift still good? Examining the politics and regulation of blood safety in the European Union. *Medical Law Review*, **14** (2), 155–79.

Faucher, A. (1992). La question de l'électricité au Québec dans les années trente. *L'Actualité Économique—Revue d'Analyse Économique*, **68** (3), 415–32.

Fishbein, M. and Ajzen, I. (1975). *Belief, Attitude, Intention and Behavior: An Introduction to Theory and Research*. Reading, MA: Addison-Wesley.

Gagnon, F., Turgeon, J., and Dallaire, C. (2007). Healthy public policy. A conceptual cognitive framework. *Health Policy*, **81** (1), 42–55.

Gagnon, F., Turgeon, J., and Dallaire, C. (2008). L'évaluation d'impact sur la santé au Québec: lorsque la loi devient levier d'action. *Téléscope*, **14** (2), 79–94.

Gattinger, M. (2005). From government to governance in the energy sector: the states of the Canada–U.S. energy relationship. *American Review of Canadian Studies*, **35** (2), 321–52.

Gilson, L. (ed.) (2012). *Health Policy and Systems Research: A Methodology Reader*. Geneva: World Health Organization.

Godin, G. and Kok, G. (1996). The theory of planned behavior: a review of its applications to health-related behaviors. *American Journal of Health Promotion*, **11** (2), 87–98.

Green, L. W. (2006). Public health asks of system science: to advance our evidence-based practice, can you help us get more practice-based evidence? *American Journal of Public Health*, **96** (3), 406–9.

Green, L. W. and Kreuter, M. W. (2005). *Health Program Planning: An Educational and Ecological Approach*. Boston, MA: McGraw-Hill.

Green-Pedersen, C. (2002). New public management reforms of the Danish and Swedish Welfare states: the role of different social democratic responses. *Governance*, **15** (2), 271–94.

Hall, P. A. (1993). Policy paradigm, social learning and the state. *Comparative Politics*, **25** (3), 275–96.

Hancock, T. (1985). Beyond health care: from public health policy to healthy public policy. *Canadian Journal of Public Health*, **76** (Suppl. 1), 9–11.

Hassenteufel, P. (2008). *Sociologie Politique: l'Action Publique*. Paris: Armand Colin.

Hassenteufel, P., Smyrl, M., Genieys, W., and Moreno-Fuentes, F. J. (2010). Programmatic actors and the transformation of European health care states. *Journal of Health Politics, Policy and Law*, **35** (4), 517–38.

Hawe, P. and Potvin, L. (2009). What is population health intervention research? *Canadian Journal of Public Health*, **100** (1), I8-I14.

Hill, M. and Hupe, P. (2006). Analysing policy processes as multiple governance: accountability in social policy. *Policy & Politics*, **34** (3), 557–73.

Howlett, M., Ramesh, M., and Perl, A. (2009). *Studying Public Policy. Policy Cycles & Policy Subsystems*. Don Mills, ON: Oxford University Press.

Hunter, D. J. (2009). Relationship between evidence and policy: a case of evidence-based policy or policy-based evidence? *Public Health*, **123** (9), 583–6.

Illich, I. (1976). *Medical Nemesis: The Expropriation of Health*. New York: Pantheon.

Jegen, M. and Audet, G. (2011). Advocacy coalitions and wind power development: insights from Quebec. *Energy Policy*, **39** (11), 7439–47.

Jenkins, W. (1978). *Policy Analysis: A Political and Organizational Perspective*. London: Martin Robertson.

Jobert, B. and Muller, P. (1987). *L'Etat en Action. Politiques Publiques et Corporatismes*. Paris: PUF.

Joffe, M. and Mindell, J. (2004). A tentative step towards healthy public policy. *Journal of Epidemiology and Community Health*, **58** (**12**), 966–8.

Jones, C. (1970). *An Introduction to the Study of Public Policy*. Belmont, CA: Wadsworth.

Kemm, J. (2001). Health impact assessment: a tool for healthy public policy. *Health Promotion International*, **16** (1), 79–85.

Kickbusch, I. and Buckett, K. (2010). *Implementing Health in All Policies: Adelaide 2010*. Adelaide: Department of Health, Government of South Australia.

Kickbusch, I., McCann, W., and Sherbon, T. (2008). Adelaide revisited: from healthy public policy to Health in All Policies. *Health Promotion International*, **23** (1), 1–4.

Klein, R. and Marmor, T. R. (2008). Reflections on policy analysis: putting it together again, in M. Moran, M. Reid and R. E. Goodin (eds.) *The Oxford Handbook of Public Policy*, pp. 892–911, Toronto: Oxford University Press.

Koivusalo, M. (2010). The state of Health in All Policies (HiAP) in the European Union: potential and pitfalls. *Journal of Epidemiology and Community Health*, **64** (6), 500–3.

Lasswell, H. D. (1956). *The Decision Process: Seven Categories of Functional Analysis*. College Park, MD: University of Maryland Press.

Lee, K. (2010). How do we move forward on the social determinants of health: the global governance challenges? *Critical Public Health*, **20** (1), 5–14.

Lewin, K. (1945) The Research Center for Group Dynamics at Massachusetts Institute of Technology. *Sociometry*, **8 (2)**, 126–36.

Lindblom, C. E. (1959). The science of 'muddling through'. *Public Administration Review*, **19** (2), 79–88.

Link, B. G. and Phelan, J. C. (2002). McKeown and the idea that social conditions are fundamental causes of disease. *American Journal of Public Health*, **92** (5), 730–2.

Lock, K. (2000). Health impact assessment. *British Medical Journal*, **320**, 1395–8.

Lock, K. and McKee, M. (2005). Health impact assessment: assessing opportunities and barriers to intersectoral health improvement in an expanded European Union. *Journal of Epidemiology and Community Health*, **59** (5), 356–60.

Macintyre, S. (2012). Evidence in the development of health policy. *Public Health*, **126** (3), 217–19.

McKeown, T. and Record, R. G. (1962). Reasons for the decline of mortality in England and Wales during the nineteenth century. *Population Studies*, **16**, 94–122.

McQueen, D. V. and Kickbusch, I. (eds.) (2007). *Health & Modernity. The Role of Theory in Health Promotion*. New York: Springer.

Marchetti, D. and Champagne, P. (2004). The contaminated blood scandal. Reframing medical news, in R. Benson and É. Neveu (eds.) *Bourdieu and the Journalistic Field*, pp. 113–34, Cambridge: Polity (publié dans Actes de la recherche en sciences sociales, n°101–102, 1994).

Marsh, D. and Rhodes, R. A. W. (1992). *Policy Networks in British Government*. Oxford: Clarendon Press.

Milio, N. (1981). *Promoting Health through Public Policy*. Philadelphia, PA: F. A. Davis Co.

Navarro, V. (ed.) (2002). *The Political Economy of Social Inequalities: Consequences for Health and Quality of Life*. Amityville, NY: Baywood.

Navarro, V. and Shi, L. (2001). The political context of social inequalities and health. *Social Science & Medicine*, **52** (3), 481–91.

Nussbaum, M. C. (2006). *Frontiers of Justice: Disability, Nationality, Species Membership. Cambridge, MA*: Harvard University Press.

O'Neill, M., Roch, G., and Boyer, M. (2011). *Petit Manuel d'Analyse des Politiques de Santé*. Sainte-Foye: Presses de l'Université Laval.

OECD (2012). *OECD Health Data 2012*. Paris: OECD Publishing.

Palier, B. (2007). Tracking the evolution of a single instrument can reveal profound changes: the case of funded pensions in France. *Governance*, **20** (1), 85–107.

Pawson, R. (2003). Nothing as practical as a good theory. *Evaluation*, **9** (4), 471–90.

Pierson, P. (2000). Path dependence, increasing returns, and the study of politics. *American Political Science Review*, **94** (2), 251–67.

Popay, J., Whitehead, M., and Hunter, D. J. (2010). Injustice is killing people on a large scale—but what is to be done about it? *Journal of Public Health*, **32** (2), 148–9.

Porter, D. (ed.) (1994). *The History of Public Health and the Modern State*. Amsterdam: Rodopi.

Porter, R. (1997). *The Greatest Benefit to Mankind. A Medical History of Humanity from Antiquity to the Present*. London: Fontana Press.

Public Health Research Advisory Committee (2008). *Report of the Review of Public Health Research Funding in Australia. Prepared by the Public Health Research Advisory Committee chaired by Professor Don Nutbeam (The 'Nutbeam Review')*. Canberra: National Health and Medical Research Council.

Rawls, J. (1971). *A Theory of Justice*. Cambridge, MA: Harvard University Press.

Ritsatakis, A. and Järvisalo, J. (2006). Opportunities and challenges for including health components in the policy-making process, in T. Ståhl, M. Wismar, E. Ollila, E. Lahtinen and K. Leppo (eds.) *Health in All Policies: Prospects and Potentials*, pp. 145–67, Helsinki: Ministry of Social Affairs and Health; Brussels: European Observatory on Health Systems and Policies.

Rogers, E. S. (1968). Public health asks of sociology...: can the health sciences resolve society's problems in the absence of a science of human values and goals? *Science*, **159** (3814), 506–8.

Sabatier, P. A. (1991). Towards better theories of the policy process. *PS: Political Science and Politics*, **24** (2), 147–56.

Sabatier, P. A. (ed.) (2007). *Theories of the Policy Process* (2nd edn.). Boulder, CO: Westview.

Sen, A. (1992). *Inequality Re-Examined*. Cambridge, MA: Harvard University Press.

Simos, J. (2006). Introducing health impact assessment (HIA) in Switzerland. *Sozial- und Präventivmedizin/Social and Preventive Medicine*, **51** (3), 130–2.

Smith, K. E., Fooks, G., Colin, J., Weishaar, H., and Gilmore, A. B. (2010). Is the increasing policy use of impact assessment in Europe likely to undermine efforts to achieve healthy public policy? *Journal of Epidemiology and Community Health*, **64** (6), 478–87.

Sparks, M. (2009). Acting on the social determinants of health: health promotion needs to get more political. *Health Promotion International*, **24** (3), 199–202.

Ståhl, T., Wismar, M., Ollila, E., Lahtinen, E., and Leppo, K. (2006). *Health in All Policies: Prospects and Potentials*. Helsinki: Ministry of Social Affairs and Health; Brussels: European Observatory on Health Systems and Policies.

Tantivess, S. and Walt, G. (2008). The role of state and non-state actors in the policy process: the contribution of policy networks to the scale-up of antiretroviral therapy in Thailand. *Health Policy and Planning*, **23** (5), 328–38.

Veerman, J. L., Bekker, M. P. M., and Mackenbach, J. P. (2006). Health impact assessment and advocacy: a challenging combination. *Sozial- und Präventivmedizin/Social and Preventive Medicine*, **51** (3), 151–2.

Weiss, C. H. (1995). Nothing as practical as good theory: exploring theory-based evaluation for comprehensive community initiatives for children and families, in J. L. Connell, A. C. Kubisch, L. B. Schorr and C. H. Weiss (eds.) *New Approaches to Evaluating Community Initiatives. Concepts, Methods, and Contexts*, pp. 65–92, Washington, DC: The Aspen Institute.

Whitehead, M., Petticrew, M., Graham, H., Macintyre, S. J., Bambra, C., and Egan, M. (2004). Evidence for public health policy on inequalities: 2. Assembling the evidence jigsaw. *Journal of Epidemiology and Community Health*, **58** (10), 817–21.

WHO (1986). *First International Conference on Health Promotion. The Ottawa Charter for Health Promotion*. Geneva: World Health Organization.

WHO (1988). *Conference Statement of the 2nd International Conference on Health Promotion: The Adelaide Recommendations—Healthy Public Policy*. Geneva: World Health Organization.

WHO and Government of South Australia (2010). *Adelaide Statement on Health in All Policies: Moving Towards a Shared Governance for Health and Well-being*. Adelaide: World Health Organization and Government of South Australia.

Wilkinson, R. G. (1996). *Unhealthy Societies: The Afflictions of Inequality*. London: Routledge.

Wilkinson, R. G. and Pickett, K. (2011). *The Spirit Level: Why Greater Equality makes Societies Stronger*. New York: Bloomsbury Press.

Chapter 2

Policy change theories in health promotion research: a review

Evelyne de Leeuw and Éric Breton

Introduction

Health is made outside the health care sector. This obvious idea started to get empirical and theoretical traction with the work, in the late 1960s and early 1970s, of authors such as Laframboise (1973), Blum (1974), Waitzkin (1974), Mechanic (1986), and Navarro (1986). Ivan Illich (1976) even demonstrated that the health care sector was sometimes detrimental to health. Although their arguments have been potent drivers of change, the impact of the ideas has been limited by their commitment to the pathogenic epistemology.

Pathogenic epistemology is possibly the most powerful, and yet also the most evasive, idea that drives health policy towards biomedical rather than social solutions for population health challenges. When in the course of the 19th century the germ theory replaced other notions of the causalities between health and the environment, the search for—and identification of—micro-biological pathogens shaped entire disciplines and industries, including the strict professionalization of medical training and practice. This 'biomedical model of health' was challenged in the years after the Second World War by a 'social model of health'. The rise of the complementarity of both models seems to have culminated, at least rhetorically, in the publication in the early 21st century of influential works on health equity and the social determinants of health. Yet, as Antonovsky (1984) and Kelly and Charlton (1995) have shown, the core epistemology of the discourse has not challenged the pathogenic paradigm that governs it: mechanistically and rationally it remains critical to identify cause and effect, whether in terms of virus activity or toxins affecting cell integrity, or of poverty and climate change affecting disease patterns. Many might believe that in the 'social model of health' it is important to distinguish between so-called upstream (systems), mid-stream (population) or downstream (behavioural) determinants of health, but Nancy Krieger (2008) has convincingly argued that such 'stream' rhetoric only confirms and reinforces the epic search for causalities of disease, and, in attempting to mimic the biomedical model of the pathogenic paradigm, fails to address the politics of health (rather than disease).

Further, the role of the medical establishment and its intimate symbiosis with politics is an issue that merits further scrutiny. Didier Fassin (1996) has shown that when the collective management of health and disease was first introduced into the realm of governments, physicians and scientists sought to guarantee the autonomy of public health from both medicine and politics. The constitution of a specific corpus and dedicated profession were considered instrumental in this process. However, the extent of this autonomy is more than questionable even today. Rudolf Virchow (1848)—one of the fathers of the germ theory—is often heralded by social science scholars of health as having argued that medicine and politics do go hand in hand ('Die Politik ist weiter nichts, als Medicin im Grossen'). Two slightly more cynical alternative interpretations of Virchow's statement are also possible. First, it might reflect a simplistic and naive notion of politics being medicine on a grander scale, deciding 'who gets what' (cf. Lasswell, 1936), as in the triage process. But second, and even more insidiously, it would suggest that medical doctors in fact perceive that they have a legitimate and determining veto (beyond a mere stake) in public policy deliberations. Rarely has this close and hungry connection to power been visible as blatantly as in Chile in 1973, when the country's Colegio Medico was instrumental in the coup d'état success of the right-wing Pinochet junta (Goldman, 1985). At the other end of the political spectrum, Salvador Allende himself was an eminent pathologist, and the archetypical revolutionary of the left, Che Guevara, trained to be a dermatologist. More widespread still, mayors or heads of government often grant medical doctors a de facto competency to make health policy decisions because of their professional skills (Clavier, 2009). Thus, ministers of health are often medical doctors, and so are the councillors in charge of health policy in city councils, even though caring for individual patients has little in common with making policy decisions for the public's health. Particularly prominent in the health sector, this tendency to appoint ministers or councillors based on a reputation of competency has worked against the entrenchment of 'healthy public policy' ideas by making health the business of medical doctors at the policy level.

Another development towards recognition of the intricate interface between medicine and politics came from the emancipatory movements that started in the 1960s. While the fathers of the public health movement were frequently based within the medical establishment, its 'mothers' grounded themselves in more activist and community-based experiences and perspectives, which were often driven largely by women (Ehrenreich and English, 1973; Marieskind and Ehrenreich, 1975; Boston Women's Health Book Collective, in Zola, 1991). Although the strong community base of these developments has had its merits, it may also have hindered access to the political system, even when feminists were actively recruited into government bureaucracies. These 'femocrats' (cf. Williamson, 1999; Sawer, 2007) have been criticized as being co-opted by the status quo, rather than continuing to exercise the ability to challenge it.

Towards healthy public policy

The work of these health scientists and social movements paved the way for a more grounded perspective on political intervention for health. But the idea that health was influenced from outside the health sector still had to be brought into the realm of public policy. The first national policy to formally recognize the contribution of factors beyond the health care sector was the Canadian Lalonde Report (1974). Along the lines of the traditional biomedical determinants of health—human biology, lifestyle, health care services—this report acknowledged the influence of the social and physical environments, emphasizing that these would bring the biggest changes to the health of the population. It nevertheless put much of the responsibility for health on the individuals who should make the right choices for their own good. Then, in the 1980s, the works of two scholars/activists were instrumental in shaping the idea of healthy public policy—that is, how other sector policy does and should contribute to the health of populations.

Nancy Milio, a scholar with a solid foundation in community nursing, was the first to integrate activism and astute academic analysis in *Promoting Health through Public Policy* (1981, reprinted 1985 in Canada). With a massive intellectual effort she compiled the evidence on how, and to what extent, sectors such as agriculture, social services, and defence influence human health, and how the inclusion of health considerations in other sector policies would contribute significantly to the health of populations. She observed that governments had failed to integrate health as an overarching social policy ambition in public decision-making. Her argument was that, regardless of other health efforts (in either the clinical environment or in lifestyle change), public policy across sectors could be seen as having the most profound impact on population health. If there was any truth in the often-heard rhetoric that governments were to take care of their constituencies, she maintained, they should build health through public policy. Milio continued to explore such intersectoral policy linkages, using the farm–food–nutrition triad as a compelling case study that demonstrated the feasibility of integrated policy perspectives in food-rich countries such as Norway (Milio, 1990) and in community health (1988; 1992).

Around the time that Milio started to transcend her community activism a young British doctor moved to Canada, where he found exciting opportunities to engage in novel, and often futuristic, notions based at the interface of ecological considerations, sustainability, the inability of bureaucracies to respond to (community health) crises, and health. Trevor Hancock co-founded the Canadian Green Party in 1983 and contributed significantly to health innovations in the City of Toronto in 1984. His influential and visionary work is possibly best characterized by his piece (with Clem Bezold) 'Possible futures, preferable futures'. In it, the authors write: 'Futures thinking is a tool for wiser action that stimulates the imagination, encourages creativity, identifies threats and opportunities, and allows us to relate possible future choices and consequences to our values' (Hancock and Bezold, 1994: 29). Choosing between possible, plausible, probable, and preferable futures, it appears that Hancock has consistently followed the last path, dreaming large and presenting his arguments in a compelling fashion. In an act of serendipity he presented healthy public policy ideas at the City of Toronto 'Beyond Health Care' conference (Hancock, 1985), which celebrated the tenth anniversary of the publication of the Lalonde Report. The conference culminated in the formulation of the birth of the 'healthy city' concept.

Whether through the ideas of Rudolf Virchow, Louis-René Villermé (1840/1971) (linking 'L'argent, la vie, la mort' in the first systematic epidemiological review) or Edwin Chadwick (1842), health and society are inseparably connected. Further connecting the brief definition of politics by one of the fathers of political science, Harold Lasswell (1936) ('who gets what, when, how'), with the ambitions of health promotion suggests that the inclusion of a call to build healthy public policy in the Ottawa Charter for Health Promotion (WHO, 1986) was inevitable. The process of enabling individuals and communities to control the determinants of health, in these terms, is a political act in itself. The healthy public policy perspective gained further prominence through the second conference on health promotion in Adelaide, where the Adelaide Recommendations (WHO, 1988) viewed it as policy enacted by the various levels of government, 'characterized by explicit concern for health and equity in all areas of policy and by accountability for health impact'.

Today, virtually every health promotion textbook or government statement pronounces the importance of policy considerations for health promotion. In celebration of the silver jubilee of healthy public policy we investigated whether research practice has followed this enthusiastic rhetorical embrace of 'policy'. To that end, we carried out a systematic review of the health promotion literature with a view to identifying the host of material that empirically applies theoretical insights from political science to health promotion.

Policy, politics, political science, and health promotion

Political science harbours hundreds of theories, and Paul Sabatier, a key figure in contemporary political science, has taken it upon himself to identify a set of theories that 'are clear enough to be proven wrong' (2007: 5). A theory is a clear and logically interrelated set of propositions, some of them empirically falsifiable, to explain fairly general sets of phenomena (de Leeuw, 1989a). Applying this presupposition to the field of political science, Sabatier finds a distinction between conceptual frameworks, theories, and models, which operate on a continuum from broadly applicable to any situation to (preferably mathematical) modelling for highly specific situations. A 'good' theory of the political process should explain goals and perceptions, actions and events, among potentially hundreds of stakeholders in the process, leading to specific sets of policy deliverables and outcomes.

It should be noted that in our view there is a useful difference between 'policy theories' and 'theories of the policy process'. 'Policy theories' describe the set of assumptions and values (for instance, between cause and effect, about the efficacy of policy actions, or the—normative—acceptability of such actions) espoused by policy-makers (Hoogerwerf, 1984; de Leeuw, 1989b). Policy analyses usually examine the consistency and effectiveness of such policy theories. The father of Dutch policy studies, Hoogerwerf, unequivocally states that the better validated the policy theories through scholarly insights, the more easily the policy will be implemented, and the more profound its impact (1984). On the other hand, theories of the policy process—which are the focus of this chapter—rather formulate propositions on the conditions under which certain policy phenomena (e.g. preferences for certain types of interventions, decisions on implementation issues, allocation of resources, inclusion or exclusion of certain stakeholders, etc.) are observed and have an impact on policy outcomes (e.g. Breton et al., 2008; de Leeuw, 2007). Theories of the policy process look at parameters that determine policy theories. It should be recognized that these parameters are intimately connected to issues of power.

The body of knowledge developed in the political sciences around the concept or definition of 'policy' is extensive, and generally not used unequivocally in health science writings. Although we prefer to define policy as the 'explicit formal decision by an executive agency to solve a certain problem through the deployment of specific resources, and the establishment of specific sets of goals and objectives to be met within a specific time frame' (de Leeuw, 2007: 51), there are numerous examples in the health literature where the concept is either not defined at all, or is merely seen as 'the law' or 'a plan'.

The traditional perspective of the policy process is that of the 'stages heuristic': the notion that the policy process follows clearly distinguishable steps from problem definition, through alternative specification, to resource allocation and implementation. Although this conceptual framework seems to have served a purpose since Lasswell (1956) originally proposed it (e.g. Cobb and Elder, 1983; de Leeuw and Polman, 1995), it has since become the subject of devastating criticism, predominantly focusing on the fact that the stages heuristic fails to address the dynamics of multiple, interacting, iterative, and incremental cycles of action at many different levels of mutual and reciprocal action at the same time (deLeon, 1999). Anyone active at the policy development coalface realizes that although thinking in neatly compartmentalized stages serves an analytical purpose, the muddling-through character of policy development makes for often messy decision-making. There are so many a priori contextual factors that 'problem definition', for instance, cannot and should not be separated from pre-existing implementation challenges. Thus, where policy development work along the stages heuristic might be beneficial for the sanity of bureaucrats and practitioners, it is an inappropriate approximation of the ever-changing, fluctuating, and pulsating policy game. Often the rules of the game seem counterintuitive, as John Maynard Keynes famously stated: 'There is nothing a Government hates more than to be well-informed; for it makes the process of arriving at decisions much more complicated and difficult' (Keynes and Moggridge, 1982: 409). Theories of the policy process have therefore increasingly divorced themselves from stages and levels, and have attempted to incorporate the feedback loops, a priori contexts, first and second order changes, and most of all the dynamics between stakeholders, institutions, and agencies.

A good theory enables validated explanation, sometimes with conditional predictions, of the phenomena studied. Sabatier established the following parameters to assess appropriate theoretical frameworks of the policy process.

> 1. Each framework must do a reasonably good job of meeting the criteria of a scientific theory; that is, its concepts and propositions must be relatively clear and internally consistent, it must identify clear causal drivers, it must give rise to falsifiable hypotheses, and it must be fairly broad in scope (i.e., apply to most of the policy process in a variety of political systems).

2. Each framework must be the subject of a fair amount of recent conceptual development and/or empirical testing. A number of currently active policy scholars must view it as a viable way of understanding the policy process.

3. Each framework must be a positive theory seeking to explain much of the policy process. The theoretical framework may also contain some explicitly normative elements, but these are not required.

4. Each framework must address the broad sets of factors that political scientists looking at different aspects of public policymaking have traditionally deemed important: conflicting values and interests, information flows, institutional arrangements, and variation in the socioeconomic environment.

(Sabatier, 2007: 8)

Four such frameworks, also pertinent to health policy development, were identified by Sabatier as meeting these parameters. These are the event-driven multiple streams theory empirically developed by John Kingdon (2002); the punctuated equilibrium framework by Baumgartner and Jones (1993), in which long periods of policy stability are alternated with general shifts in policy perspectives and ambitions; the advocacy coalition framework (Sabatier, 1988; Sabatier and Jenkins-Smith, 1993), which emphasizes the importance of coalition formation of camps of proponents and opponents to new policy directions; and the policy domains approach, which derives from different perspectives on network governance (e.g. Laumann and Knoke, 1987; Börzel, 1998). Other theoretical frameworks that seem applicable, but are not extensively empirically validated, are the social movement theory (e.g. McCarthy and Zald, 1977), which argues that disenchanted people will join social movements to mobilize resources and political opportunity so that policy is changed to serve their interests; neo-corporatism (e.g. Olson, 1986), which advocates that (semi-)political organizations in the social environment mimic business models rather than social morality to maximize competitiveness; and a host of hybrid approaches that mix these perspectives or address specific processes such as coalition structuring (Breton et al., 2008).

Kurt Lewin said that 'Nothing is as practical as a good theory' (1945: 129). We certainly believe that good theories can be very practical in describing, analysing, and assessing healthy public policy processes, and would thus allow for improved policy-making capacity and engagement. Following the principles of the theory-based evaluation framework by Birckmayer and Weiss (2000), the rigorous application of theory to the analysis of development and outcomes of policy processes would not just highlight *whether* policy has achieved its intended objectives, but also *how* this has happened. In answering how change has come about we will add an important layer of evidence to the health promotion cake.

A good theory is especially important for the further refinement of evidence-based policy research: it would identify processes, issues, events, and actors that have facilitated or compromised the effectiveness of policy. Or, again in the words of Lewin (1951): 'If you want truly to understand something, try to change it'.

Theories of the policy process and the health promotion profession

The stated purpose of health promotion is 'to enable individuals, groups, and communities to increase their control over the determinants of health, and thereby improve their health' (WHO, 1986). Action on policy, or the building of healthy public policy, is a key strategy that would assist in achieving this purpose. In fact, many health promotion practitioners around the world are actively engaged in developing policy strategies, focusing on the reorientation of health services, creating supportive environments for health, or supporting community development and personal skills for health.

The capacity to develop and assess policy processes for health promotion has been appreciated and formalized by a number of regional and global statements. For Europe, the *CompHP Core Competencies Framework for Health Promotion Handbook* states that: 'A competent workforce that has the necessary knowledge, skills and abilities in translating policy, theory and research into effective action is recognised as being critical to the future growth and development of global health promotion' (Dempsey et al., 2011: 1). Paragraph 5.7 of the Australian Health Promotion Association's *Core Competencies for Health Promotion Practitioners* (2009) states that 'an entry level health promotion practitioner is able to demonstrate knowledge of: health promotion strategies to promote health—health education, advocacy, lobbying, media campaigns, community development processes, policy development, legislation'. Interestingly, the most detailed listing of policy competencies is provided by the US National Commission for Health Education Credentialing under section '7.5 Influence Policy to Promote Health':

> 7.5.1 Use evaluation and research findings in policy analysis;
> 7.5.2 Identify the significance and implications of health policy for individuals, groups, and communities;
> 7.5.3 Advocate for health-related policies, regulations, laws, or rules;
> 7.5.4 Use evidence-based research to develop policies to promote health;
> 7.5.5 Employ policy and media advocacy techniques to influence decision-makers.
>
> (Doyle, 2010)

It will be obvious that health promotion practitioners and their representative bodies have embraced the need to engage in the policy process. The responsibilities and competencies listed from around the world range from merely understanding policies and policy development to actively participating in policy development with the appropriate skills and world views. It should be recognized, however, that most health promotion practitioners do not have a remit to spend substantial parts of their time on scholarly efforts in policy process research; the research most of them partake in, as reflected in the above competencies, relates to policy analysis (that is, considering the question of whether a policy achieves its intended objectives), and to acting at the interface between research, policy and practice (de Leeuw et al., 2008). It seems that in the latter realm the opportunities within government health promotion agencies to devote substantial time to knowledge co-generation, brokerage, or commissioning high-quality rigorous research are very limited (Jansen et al., 2010; Harting et al., 2010). In this volume, the chapters by Potvin and Clavier, and Hunter take a closer theoretical look at these issues.

We are not arguing here that health promotion practitioners should apply more theories on the policy process to their work. What we do argue, however, is that the rigorous application of theory to health promotion issues is critical if we want to achieve sustainable and equitable health development (cf. the intervention mapping approach as developed by Bartholomew et al., 2011). This seems even more important in the policy arena, because we suggest that there are very few solid health promotion policy inquiries. A more profound and reciprocal understanding between health promotion researchers and practitioners, the communities they serve, and the policy world would grow out of such a process.

Methods

We have shown the interface between health promotion and policy development and demonstrated that healthy public policy (or rather 'health policy'; cf. the chapter by de Leeuw, Keizer and Hoeijmakers in this volume) is an integral part of the health promotion mission. We have also established that health promotion practitioners support and incorporate these views. Based on the argument so far we were curious to know how much rigorous research had been carried out on the policy process in health promotion. Should there be an abundance of such research, we could formulate recommendations on how that work could become part of the practice repertoire of health promoters. But if there were a research deficit it would be necessary to ask completely different questions as a consequence.

To report on the state of policy research in the health promotion field, we first needed to assemble a corpus of peer-reviewed journals that could confidently be said to contribute to the scholarly development of the field. These journals were identified by applying a set of rigorous criteria (see Table 2.1) and search terms using the MedLine and CINALH databases. The core assumption on which we based the identification of the journals was that their editorials would be reflective of their interest for the health promotion movement. The first search yielded 141 articles from 61 journals. We then collected information on these journals to appraise their mission statements, relevance, and targeted readership, and to ascertain that they regularly publish papers in English and/or French. This exercise reduced the number of journals to 17. The final set was established by retaining only those in which at least 10% of all their titles or abstracts contained 'health promotion', 'promotion de la santé' or derivatives of these terms. This threshold was set to reduce the number of articles to a manageable level. The final list of 11 journals was validated by colleagues and experts well acquainted with the health promotion field (see Table 2.2).

We developed a second set of criteria to identify the articles eligible for analysis (see Table 2.1). As was the case for the journals, the search was conducted through MedLine and CINALH, but this time with a validation search through Academic Search Premier,

Table 2.1 Inclusion criteria for the identification of the journals and articles

Criteria for the identification of the journals pursuing the scholarly development of health promotion	Criteria for the identification of the journal articles reporting on policy research
The journal:	The article:
	◆ was published in one of the eligible journals;
◆ is indexed in Medline or CINALH databases;	◆ is indexed in Medline or CINALH databases;
◆ features papers either in English or French;	◆ is in English or French;
◆ covers a diversity of health issues, age and population subgroups;	◆ was published between January 1986 (the year of the 'birth' of health promotion in the Ottawa Charter) and June 2006;
◆ targets a broad readership representing a diverse set of disciplines and professions;	◆ features either in its abstract, title or subject headings the search terms: 'politi*', 'polic*', 'advoca*' or 'coalition';
◆ had, between January 2000 and January 2006, at least: ◆ one editorial title featuring: 'health promotion', 'promot* health' or 'promotion * santé'; ◆ 10% of its titles or abstracts featuring the aforementioned search terms.	◆ either reports on issues at the local, regional, state, national or supra-national level related to: ◆ the content or nature of a policy, i.e. (foreseen) components; effectiveness; impact; evolution; ◆ the policy change process, i.e., advocacy intervention or strategy, capacity building for advocacy, evidence and knowledge shaping policy-making, theoretical and methodological issues in policy analysis.
	◆ addresses a policy or policy process that goes beyond the walls of a specific workplace, school or other organizational settings.

which yielded one additional article (from *Critical Public Health*). These searches returned 591 articles by applying the search terms defined above. These were then manually assessed against the inclusion criteria. We considered that papers addressing organizational policy issues associated with a specific workplace or school were not eligible, since other theories have already been specifically developed for organizational settings (e.g. innovation theory, diffusion theory, etc). The application of these criteria resulted in a total of 119 eligible articles.

Having identified the corpus of articles to analyse, we set out to assess whether insights from political science had guided the research projects or the theoretical reflections they reported. To do this, we examined how the cited works from the political science literature contributed to the writing either on a specific policy or on the policy process. When an article was reporting on the result of a research project, we appraised whether the

Table 2.2 Peer-reviewed academic journals pursuing the scholarly development of health promotion selected for inclusion in the review

Journal	Indexed in/since	No. of articles retrieved from the databases	No. of articles retained for analysis
American Journal of Health Promotion	CINAHL & Medline 1986 vol 1(1)	95	27
Health Promotion International	CINAHL 1994 vol 9(1)	101	24
Health Education & Behavior	CINAHL 1997 vol 24(1)	91	16
Health Education Research	CINAHL 1986 vol 1(1)	106	12
Promotion & Education	CINAHL & Medline 1993 Special first issue	43	12
Health Education Journal	CINAHL & Medline 1986, vol 45(2)	50	9
Critical Public Health	CINAHL & Medline 1998, vol 8(2)	17	6
Health Promotion Journal of Australia	CINAHL 2000, vol 10(1)	25	6
Sozial- und Präventivmedizin	CINALH & Medline 1986 vol 31(1)	49	6
International Journal of Health Promotion & Education	CINAHL 1999 vol 37(1)	11	1
Journal of the Royal Society for the Promotion of Health	CINAHL 2002 vol 122(1)	3	0
Total		**591**	**119**

theory, model or framework had driven data collection and analysis. For the theoretical papers not reporting on a specific research project, we scrutinized the concepts used and examined whether these concepts were integrated into a framework suggested by the theory mentioned. In short, we were not interested in mere rhetoric around theory, but in seeing how theoretical frameworks drove explanatory conceptualizations of the research problem identified.

Findings

As we can see from Figure 2.1, the absolute number of eligible policy-related articles has increased over time. This can be attributed to two factors: first, the growing number of new health promotion journals since 1986; and second, improved indexing of the journal articles by the two databases of the literature we used to conduct this review. A third explanation could be that the interest in policy research has substantively increased in

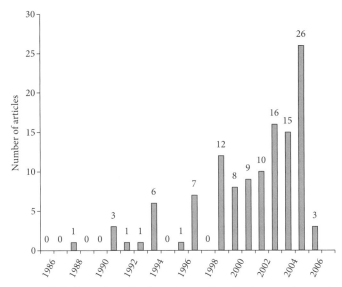

Figure 2.1 Frequency of eligible policy-related articles published in 11 journals pursuing the scholarly development of health promotion (Jan 1986–Jun 2006).

Table 2.3 Number of eligible articles applying a validated theoretical framework of the policy process

The article is about...	Number of eligible articles	Referring to a theoretical framework?	
		Yes	Of these, from political science
The content and nature of a policy	44	6	3
The policy process	70	31	18
Both content and process	5	2	0
TOTAL	119	39	21

Reproduced with permission from Breton, E. and de Leeuw, E., Theories of the policy process in health promotion research: a review, *Health Promotion International*, Volume 26, Issue 1, pp. 82–90, Copyright © 2011 Oxford University Press.

the period. This finding cannot be supported or rejected by our research as 7 of the 11 journals were either not published or not indexed in 1986. Moreover, by 1996 only six journals were indexed by the databases we searched.

Of the 119 articles that were found eligible for our analysis, 39 (or 32.7% of the 119) did apply to some degree a theoretical framework, while 21 (or 17.6% of the 119) referred to a theoretical framework from political science. Table 2.3 gives a breakdown of the categories of articles.

Articles addressing issues related to the policy process

We found scant references to theoretical frameworks of the policy process. Only two articles reported on results guided by the advocacy coalition framework (Bryant, 2002) and by the multiple streams theory (Bryant, 2002; Yeatman, 2003). Three others were based on the social movement theory (Herman et al., 1993; Nathanson, 2005; Zakocs and Earp, 2003), while the remainder borrowed from a broad array of frameworks that guided data collection and analysis. The majority of the remaining articles used theories of the political sciences in a more superficial way and in some cases only as a token of acknowledgement of the existence of a policy process (e.g. Altman et al., 1999; Lavis et al., 2001; Stanton et al., 2002).

A few articles reporting on policy processes applied theories from outside the realm of political science. The models used here included notably Roger's diffusion of innovation theory (Hallfors and Godette, 2002; Pankratz et al., 2002; Simons-Morton et al., 1997), a strategic management learning model (Powis et al., 2002), and some social theories (e.g. Rütten et al., 2003a; 2003b). More puzzling was the recourse to Bandura's social learning theory (Scheepers et al., 2004) and to Fishbein and Ajzen's theory of planned behaviour (Gottlieb et al., 2003), which stand as applications of behavioural micro level theories to systems meso/macro level processes. This might be construed as committing an error of the third kind ('answering the wrong question') (e.g. Mitroff and Featheringham, 1974; Breton and de Leeuw, 2010).

Articles addressing issues related to the content or nature of a policy

Of the eight articles addressing issues in line with the content or nature of a policy, only three (Ståhl et al., 2002; Taylor et al., 2000; Wold et al., 2004) directly referred to the body of literature from the political sciences. The five others put forward different frameworks, drawing from sociology (Rütten et al., 2003a; 2003b), public health (Orleans et al., 1999), psychology (Smith et al., 2000), and management (Pucci and Haglund, 1994).

We also wondered whether certain (public) health issues were represented more than others in our final set of selected papers. We identified the categories of problem addressed by the 119 articles and established the number of articles dealing with each issue (see Table 2.4). Unsurprisingly, most policy work was concerned with behavioural risk factors associated with communicable or non-communicable diseases, injuries, and health care services. Considering the foundations of the health promotion field and profession, it comes as no surprise that the large majority of papers looked at policies to shape or change lifestyles and behaviours. It is noteworthy that tobacco use came out as the most prominent problem targeted (in almost a third of the articles published).

Unfortunately, and in spite of the well-acknowledged problem of inequalities in health, only four policy papers addressed this issue, while only another four touched upon some of the social policies key to good living conditions such as education and housing. Clearly, health promotion policy research is challenged not only in the appropriate

Table 2.4 Public health issues addressed in policy process research in health promotion (some papers counted more than once when they addressed multiple issues)

Issue	Number of papers
Tobacco	39
Health promotion in general	27
Alcohol and drug use	16
Health care services and prevention of specific diseases	11
Diet and nutrition	11
Injuries (road, gun, etc.)	10
Sedentary lifestyle	6
Health promotion in specific settings (e.g. Healthy Cities)	5
Environmental health	4
Health inequities/inequalities	4
Sexual practice	4
Social policies as determinants of health (education, housing)	4
Other topics (urban planning, mental and oral health)	4

application of political theory but also in choosing a range of complementary levels of analysis, ranging between the individual and the systems perspective ('the causes of the causes'; cf. Marmot, 2005: 1102).

Discussion

The body of knowledge developed by political science has still made few inroads in health promotion policy research as assessed through the lens of our review of 11 journals. We consider this a disappointing finding. First of all, (healthy public) policy studies only feature nominally in leading journals in the field (in 591 out of 8337 articles, or 7%). Second, of those articles that met our inclusion criteria (n = 119), only 39 claim to use some sort of theoretical foundation, and among these, only 21 (18%, or 0.2% of the grand total of health promotion articles) rigorously apply a theory that draws on political science.

These results point towards a seriously impeded capacity for the health promotion field to learn from policy research. A common problem is the adherence to a narrow conceptualization of policy as a legislation, regulation, or law—a perspective that runs against a whole array of contemporary theoretical constructs. This conceptualization is no stranger to the long-discredited stages heuristic perspective of the policy process to which we found allusions in a number of papers (e.g. Durrheim et al., 2003; Taylor et al., 2000).

It therefore comes as no surprise that many critical issues for effective policy advocacy practice and research are left unanswered. Let us consider the articles presenting results of content analyses of the media coverage of a specific problem (e.g. Smith and Wakefield, 2005; Wakefield et al., 2005), of interventions to mobilize community members (e.g. Blaine et al., 1997; Conway, 2002; Freudenberg, 2004), and of extensive analyses of public opinion (e.g. Forster et al., 1991; Stanton et al., 2002). Although conducted with the utmost rigour, all these contributions failed to provide answers to critical questions such as: *How* do the media influence the policy process? *What* do actors and their coalitions need to achieve to successfully influence the process? *How* does public opinion feed into and influence the policy process? And *how* is health promotion policy informed by evidence? For the period covered by our review of the literature, these questions are barely addressed; when they are, the answers given unfortunately resort largely to intuition.

Without proper theoretical grounding, successes and failures cannot be satisfactorily explained and remain all but anecdotal accounts. To explain the role an advocacy strategy can play, one needs first and foremost to have a clear concept of what a policy is about, both in order to distinguish between mere policy adjustments and significant policy changes, and to come up with a clear theoretical map of the possible factors associated with a change of policy. Only then can one appraise and weigh the respective contributions of the hypothesized factors and processes to preferred or defined policy developments.

There is little doubt that a sound theoretical repertoire can also offer an invaluable guide to policy advocacy practice. For one thing, it can orient health promotion professionals towards the critical policy analyses required to achieve a clear understanding of the barriers to change. Sabatier and Jenkins-Smith's (1993) advocacy coalition framework hypothesizes some prerequisites of significant policy change that can only (if ever) be achieved over many years—a situation that calls for persistent and well-planned advocacy work.

On a more positive note, our review of the literature may have shown that, although still in its infancy, the volume of policy research articles in the health promotion field has increased and may continue to increase over time. The health promotion and health policy research community should by now be well-poised to transcend its naive and largely atheoretical approach. However, in order to achieve this, five issues need to be considered.

First, health promotion practitioners and researchers will have to abandon the models that served them well for conceptualizing behaviour change at the micro level and embrace the complexity of the policy change process and its new requirements in terms of both theoretical frameworks and levels of change. Research questions should drive the selection of theory, and not—as seems to have been the case for at least the last twenty-odd years—researchers' disciplinary preferences. The need for such a shift was recognized nearly a decade ago by the influential Institute of Medicine (Smedley and Syme, 2001) but still seems to have made little headway.

Second, therefore, training programmes and qualifications in health promotion and public health will need to include more rigorous theory-based policy perspectives. There is a role for accreditation bodies to adopt and adapt such perspectives.

Third, the funding base for appropriate health policy research needs to be addressed. In Australia, for instance, the Nutbeam Review of funding parameters for health research found that 'current arrangements did not offer flexibility in response to opportunities to test and/or evaluate changes to government policy' and identified a need for research that 'supports partnerships between researchers and health agencies, especially in the development of intervention research, and the development and evaluation of health policy' (Public Health Research Advisory Committee, 2008: 27). Clearly, this challenge is not unique to Australia and must be taken up by other research bodies around the world.

Fourth, new theories of the policy process need to be developed to reflect the broad diversity of political systems encountered across the world. Without exception, the most authoritative conceptualizations mentioned here were modelled on Western-style democratic governance systems and may therefore have little relevance for significant sections of the world population. Efforts urgently need to be invested in modelling other democratic systems and, even more challengingly, in understanding policy change under authoritarian regimes.

Fifth, and perhaps most dominantly, there is a role for (political) theoreticians to communicate the value and benefits of their work better to students, scholars, politicians, and bureaucrats. Colloquially, there seems to be an aversion to theory being abstract, difficult, and tedious. In our own communications with students and policy-makers, though, we have seen that there can be much excitement when theory-driven research results yield tangible outcomes for policy change.

Without such changes, health promotion policy research is unlikely to offer much help to practitioners willing to influence the policy process; nor is it likely to contribute to improving current models. As health promotion needs to translate its words into actions—which more often than not implies addressing at a political level the scandalous and widening disparities in health and wealth—it is inconceivable to think that we can do this without a proper theoretical lens.

Acknowledgements

During the data collection phase of this study, Éric Breton was the recipient of a doctoral research award from the Canadian Institute of Health Research (NST-42826).

References

Altman, D., Strunk, B. and Smith, M. (1999). Newspaper and wire service coverage of tobacco farmers. *Health Education Research*, **14**, 131–7.

Antonovsky, A. (1984). The sense of coherence as a determinant of health, in J. D. Matarazzo (ed.) *Behavioral Health. A Handbook of Health Enhancement and Disease Prevention*, pp. 114–29, New York: Wiley.

Australian Health Promotion Association (2009). *Core Competencies for Health Promotion Practitioners*. Maroochydore: AHPA, University of the Sunshine Coast.

Bartholomew, L. K., Parcel, G. S., Kok, G., Gottlieb, N. H., and Fernández, M. E. (2011). *Planning Health Promotion Programs: an Intervention Mapping Approach*. San Francisco, CA: Jossey-Bass.

Baumgartner, F. R. and Jones, B. D. (1993). *Agendas and Instability in American Politics.* Chicago, IL: University of Chicago Press.

Birckmayer, J. D. and Weiss, C. H. (2000). Theory-based evaluation in practice: what do we learn? *Evaluation Review,* **24** (4), 407–31.

Blaine, T. M., Forster, J. L., Hennrikus, D., O'Neil, S., Wolfson, M., and Pham, H. (1997). Creating tobacco control policy at the local level: implementation of a direct action organizing approach. *Health Education and Behavior,* **24** (5), 640–51.

Blum, H. L. (1974). *Planning for Health Development and Application of Social Change Theory.* New York: Human Sciences Press.

Börzel, T. A. (1998) Organizing Babylon: on the different conceptions of policy networks. *Public Administration,* **76** (2), 253–73.

Breton, E. and de Leeuw, E. (2010). Multiple streams theory in Sweden: an error III. *Health Promotion International,* **25** (1), 134–5.

Breton, E. and de Leeuw, E. (2011). Theories of the policy process in health promotion research: a review. *Health Promotion International,* **26** (1), 82–90.

Breton, E., Richard, L., Gagnon, F., Jacques, M., and Bergeron, P. (2008). Health promotion research and practice require sound policy analysis models: the case of Quebec's Tobacco Act. *Social Science & Medicine,* **67** (11), 1679–89.

Bryant, T. (2002). Role of knowledge in public health and health promotion policy change. *Health Promotion International,* **17** (1), 89–98.

Chadwick, E. (1842). *Report on an Inquiry into the Sanitary Condition of the Labouring Population of Great Britain.* Republished by M. W. Flynn, Edinburgh: Edinburgh University Press.

Clavier, C. (2009). Les élus locaux et la santé: des enjeux politiques territoriaux. *Sciences Sociales et Santé,* 27 (2), 47–74.

Cobb, R. W. and Elder, C. D. (1983). *Participation in American Politics: the Dynamics of Agenda-Building.* Baltimore, MD: The Johns Hopkins University Press.

Conway, K. (2002). Booze and beach bans: turning the tide through community action in New Zealand. *Health Promotion International,* **17** (2), 171–7.

de Leeuw, E. (1989a). *Health Policy. An Exploratory Inquiry into the Development of Policy for the New Public Health in The Netherlands.* Maastricht: Maastricht University.

de Leeuw, E. (1989b). Concepts in health promotion: the notion of relativism. *Social Science & Medicine,* **29** (11), 1281–8.

de Leeuw, E. (2007). Policies for health: the effectiveness of their development, adoption, and implementation, in D. McQueen and C. M. Jones (eds.) *Global Perspectives on Health Promotion Effectiveness,* pp. 51–66, New York: Springer.

de Leeuw, E. and Polman, L. (1995). Health policy making: the Dutch experience. *Social Science & Medicine,* **40** (3), 331–8.

de Leeuw, E., McNess, A., Crisp, B., and Stagnitti, K. (2008). Theoretical reflections on the nexus between research, policy and practice. *Critical Public Health,* **18** (1), 5–20.

deLeon, P. (1999). The stages approach to the policy process: what has it done? Where is it going?, in P. A. Sabatier (ed.) *Theories of the Policy Process* (1st edn.), pp. 19–34, Boulder, CO: Westview.

Dempsey, C., Battel-Kirk, B., Barry, M. M., and the CompHP Project Partners (2011). *The CompHP Core Competencies Framework for Health Promotion Handbook.* Paris: IUHPE.

Doyle, E. (ed.) (2010). *A Competency-Based Framework for Health Education Specialists – 2010.* Whitehall, PA: National Commission for Health Education Credentialing (NCHEC), Society for Public Health Education (SOPHE), American Association for Health Education (AAHE).

Durrheim, D. N., Williams, II. A., Barnes, K., Speare, R., and Sharp, B. I.. (2003). Beyond evidence: a retrospective study of factors influencing a malaria treatment policy change in two South African provinces. *Critical Public Health*, **13** (4), 309–30.

Ehrenreich, B. and English, D. (1973). *Witches, Midwives, and Nurses: A History of Women Healers*. Old Westbury, NY: Feminist Press.

Fassin, D. (1996). *L'espace Politique de la Santé. Essai de Généalogie*. Paris: PUF.

Forster, J. L., McBride, C., Jeffery, R., Schmid, T. L., and Pirie, P. L. (1991). Support for restrictive tobacco policies among residents of selected Minnesota communities. *American Journal of Health Promotion*, **6** (2), 99–104.

Freudenberg, N. (2004). Community capacity for environmental health promotion: determinants and implications for practice. *Health Education & Behavior*, **31** (4), 472–90.

Goldman, B. (1985). Chilean medical college battles doctor participating in torture. *Canadian Medical Association Journal*, **132** (12), 1414–16.

Gottlieb, N. H., Goldstein, A. O., Flynn, B. C., Cohen, J. E., Bauman, K. E., Solomon, L. J., Munger, M. C., Dana, G. S., and McMorris, L. E. (2003). State legislators' beliefs about legislation that restricts youth access to tobacco products. *Health Education & Behavior*, **30** (2), 209–24.

Hallfors, D. and Godette, D. (2002). Will the 'Principles of Effectiveness' improve prevention practice? Early findings from a diffusion study. *Health Education Research*, **17** (4), 461–70.

Hancock, T. (1985). Beyond health care: from public health policy to healthy public policy. *Canadian Journal of Public Health*, **76** (Supp1), 9–11.

Hancock, T. and Bezold, C. (1994). Possible futures, preferable futures. *The Healthcare Forum Journal*, **37** (2), 22–9.

Harting, J., Kunst, A. E., Kwan, A., and Stronks, K. (2010). A 'health broker' role as a catalyst of change to promote health: an experiment in deprived Dutch neighbourhoods. *Health Promotion International*, **26** (1), 65–81.

Herman, K. A., Wolfson, M., and Forster, J. L. (1993). The evolution, operation and future of Minnesota SAFPLAN: a coalition for family planning. *Health Education Research*, **8** (3), 331–44.

Hoogerwerf, A. (1984). Het ontwerpen van overheidsbeleid: een handleiding met toelichting [The design of public policy: an annotated manual]. *Bestuurswetenschappen*, **38** (1), 4–23.

Illich, I. (1976). *Medical Nemesis: The Expropriation of Health*. New York: Pantheon.

Jansen, M. W. J., van Oers, H. A. M., Kok, G. and de Vries, N. K. (2010). Public health: disconnections between policy, practice and research. *Health Research Policy and Systems*, **8** (37), 1–13.

Kelly, M. P. and Charlton, B. (1995). The modern and the postmodern in health promotion, in R. Bunton, S. Nettleton and R. Burrows (eds.) *The Sociology of Health Promotion*, pp. 78–90, London: Routledge.

Keynes, J. M. and Moggridge, D. (eds.) (1982). *The Collected Writings of John Maynard Keynes, Vol. 21. Activities 1931–1939; World Crisis and Policies in Britain and America*. London: Macmillan; New York: Cambridge University Press; for the Royal Economic Society.

Kingdon, J. (2002). *Agendas, Alternatives and Public Policies* (2nd edn.). Boston; Toronto: Little Brown & Company.

Krieger, N. (2008). Proximal, distal and the politics of causation: what's level got to do with it? *American Journal of Public Health*, 98 (2), 221–30.

Laframboise, H. L. (1973). Health policy: breaking the problem down into more manageable segments. *Canadian Medical Association Journal*, 108, 388–93.

Lalonde, M. (1974). *Nouvelle Perspective sur la Santé des Canadiens [A New Perspective on the Health of Canadians]*. Ottawa: Gouvernement du Canada.

Lasswell, H. D. (1936). *Politics: Who Gets What, When, How*. New York: McGraw-Hill.

Lasswell, H. D. (1956). *The Decision Process: Seven Categories of Functional Analysis*. College Park, MD: University of Maryland Press.

Laumann, E. O. and Knoke, D. (1987). *The Organizational State: Social Choice in National Policy Domains*. Madison, WI: University of Wisconsin Press.

Lavis, J. N., Farrant, M. S. R., and Stoddart, G. L. (2001). Barriers to employment-related healthy public policy in Canada. *Health Promotion International*, **16** (1), 9–20.

Lewin, K. (1945) The Research Center for Group Dynamics at Massachusetts Institute of Technology. *Sociometry*, **8 (2)**, 126–36.

Lewin, K. (1951). *Field Theory in Social Science: Selected Theoretical Papers*. London: Tavistock.

McCarthy, J. D. and Zald, M. N. (1977). Resource mobilization and social movements: a partial theory. *American Journal of Sociology*, **82** (6), 1212–41.

Marieskind, H. I. and Ehrenreich, B. (1975). Toward socialist medicine: the women's health movement. *Social Policy*, 6, 34–42.

Marmot, M. (2005). Social determinants of health inequalities. *The Lancet*, **365** (9464), 1099–104.

Mechanic, D. (1968). *Medical Sociology: A Selective View*. New York: Free Press.

Milio, N. (1981). *Promoting Health through Public Policy*. Philadelphia, PA: F. A. Davis Co.

Milio, N. (1988). *A Mosaic of Australian Community Health Policy Development*. Canberra: Australian Government Publishing Service.

Milio, N. (1990). *Nutrition Policy for Food-Rich Countries: a Strategic Analysis*. Baltimore, MD: The Johns Hopkins University Press.

Milio, N. (1992). Keeping the promise of community health policy revival under Hawke 1983–85, in F. Baum, D. Fry and I. Lennie (eds.) *Community Health Policy and Practice in Australia*, pp. 28–47, Sydney: Pluto Press.

Mitroff, I. I. and Featheringham, T. R. (1974). On systematic problem solving and the error of the third kind. *Behavioral Science*, **19**, 383–93.

Nathanson, C. A. (2005). Collective actors and corporate targets in tobacco control: a cross-national comparison. *Health Education & Behavior*, **32** (3), 337–54.

Navarro, V. (1986). *Crisis, Health, and Medicine: a Social Critique*. New York: Tavistock.

Olson, M. (1986). A theory of the incentives facing political organizations: neo-corporatism and the hegemonic state. *International Political Science Review*, **7** (2), 165–89.

Orleans, C. T., Gruman, J., Ulmer, C., Emont, S. L., and Hollendonner, J. K. (1999). Rating our progress in population health promotion: report card on six behaviors. *American Journal of Health Promotion*, **14** (2), 75–82.

Pankratz, M., Hallfors, D., and Cho, H. (2002). Measuring perceptions of innovation adoption: the diffusion of a federal drug prevention policy. *Health Education Research*, **17** (3), 315–26.

Powis, B., Nga, N. H., and Ireland, J. (2002). National environmental health planning in Vietnam: flying some kites. *Health Promotion International*, **17** (4), 373–81.

Public Health Research Advisory Committee (2008). *Report of the Review of Public Health Research Funding in Australia. Prepared by the Public Health Research Advisory Committee chaired by Professor Don Nutbeam (The 'Nutbeam Review')*. Canberra: National Health and Medical Research Council.

Pucci, L. G. and Haglund, B. (1994). 'Naturally Smoke Free': a support program for facilitating worksite smoking control policy implementation in Sweden. *Health Promotion International*, **9** (3), 177–87.

Rütten, A., Lüschen, G., von Lengerke, T., Abel, T., Kannas, L., Rodríguez Díaz, J. A., Vinck, J., and van der Zee, J. (2003a). Determinants of health policy impact: a theoretical framework for policy analysis. *Sozial- und Präventivmedizin/Social and Preventive Medicine*, **48** (5), 293–300.

Rütten, A., Lüschen, G., von Lengerke, T., Abel, T., Kannas, L., Rodríguez Díaz, J. A., Vinck, J., and van der Zee, J. (2003b). Determinants of health policy impact: comparative results of a European policymaker study. *Sozial- und Präventivmedizin/Social and Preventive Medicine*, **48** (6), 379–91.

Sabatier, P. A. (1988). An advocacy coalition framework of policy change and the role of policy-oriented learning therein. *Policy Sciences*, **21** (2–3), 129–68.

Sabatier, P. A. (2007). The need for better theories, in **P. A. Sabatier** (ed.) *Theories of the Policy Process* (2nd edn.), pp. 3–17, Boulder, CO: Westview.

Sabatier, P. A. and Jenkins-Smith, H. C. (1993). *Policy Change and Learning: an Advocacy Coalition Approach*. Boulder, CO: Westview.

Sawer, M. (2007). Australia: the fall of the femocrat, in M. Sawer, J. Outshoorn and J. Kantola (eds.) *Changing State Feminism*, pp. 20–40, Basingstoke: Palgrave Macmillan.

Scheepers, E., Christofides, N. J., Goldstein, S., Usdin, S., Patel, D. S., and Japhet, G. (2004). Evaluating health communication: a holistic overview of the impact of Soul City IV. *Health Promotion Journal of Australia*, **15** (2), 121–33.

Simons-Morton, B. G., Donohew, L., and Crump, A. D. (1997). Health communication in the prevention of alcohol, tobacco, and drug use. *Health Education & Behavior*, **24** (5), 544–54.

Smedley, B. D. and Syme, S. L. (eds.) (2001). *Promoting Health: Intervention Strategies from Social and Behavioral Research*. Washington, DC: Institute of Medicine, National Academy Press.

Smith, K. C. and Wakefield, M. (2005). Textual analysis of tobacco editorials: how are key media gatekeepers framing the issues? *American Journal of Health Promotion*, **19** (5), 361–8.

Smith, M. H., Altman, D. G., and Strunk, B. (2000). Readiness to change: newspaper coverage of tobacco farming and diversification. *Health Education & Behavior*, **27** (6), 708–24.

Ståhl, T., Rütten, A., Nutbeam, D., and Kannas, L. (2002). The importance of policy orientation and environment on physical activity participation: a comparative analysis between Eastern Germany, Western Germany and Finland. *Health Promotion International*, **17** (3), 235–46.

Stanton, W. R., Saeck, L., Purdie, J., Balanda, K. P., and Lowe, J. B. (2002). Public support in Australia for restrictions on cigarette smoking. *Health Promotion Journal of Australia*, **13** (1), 32–8.

Taylor, M.-L., Haglund, B. J. A., and Tillgren, P. (2000). Policy content and context for health promotion in Swedish schools: an analysis of municipal school plans. *Health Promotion International*, **15** (3), 185–95.

Villermé, L.-R. (1840/1971). *Tableau de l'état Physique et Moral des Ouvriers Employés dans les Manufactures de Coton, de Laine et de Soie*. Textes choisis et présentés par Yves Tyl. Paris: Union générale d'Éditions.

Virchow, R. (1848). Der Armenarzt. *Die medizinische Reform*, 18, 125.

Wakefield, M., Smith, K. C., and Chapman, S. (2005). Framing the Australian newspaper coverage of a secondhand smoke injury claim: lessons for media advocacy. *Critical Public Health*, **15** (1), 53–63.

Waitzkin, H. and Waterman, B. (1974). *The Exploitation of Illness in Capitalist Society*. Indianapolis, IN: Bobbs-Merrill.

WHO (1986). *First International Conference on Health Promotion. The Ottawa Charter for Health Promotion*. Geneva: World Health Organization.

WHO (1988). *Conference Statement of the 2nd International Conference on Health Promotion: The Adelaide Recommendations—Healthy Public Policy*. Geneva: World Health Organization.

Williamson, C. (1999). Reflections on health care consumerism: insights from feminism. *Health Expectations*, **2** (3), 150–8.

Wold, B., Currie, C., Roberts, C., and Aaroe, L. E. (2004). National legislation on school smoking restrictions in eight European countries. *Health Promotion International*, **19** (4), 482–8.

Yeatman, H. R. (2003). Food and nutrition policy at the local level: key factors that influence the policy development process. *Critical Public Health*, **13** (2), 125–38.

Zakocs, R. C. and Earp, J. A. L. (2003). Explaining variation in gun control policy advocacy tactics among local organizations. *Health Education & Behavior*, **30** (3), 360–74.

Zola, I. K. (1991). Bringing our bodies and ourselves back in: reflections on a past, present, and future "medical sociology". *Journal of Health and Social Behaviour*, **32** (1), 1–16.

Chapter 3

Coalition advocacy action and research for policy development

Éric Breton, Lucie Richard, France Gagnon, Marie Jacques, and Pierre Bergeron

Introduction

Although the power of the State to improve population health through public policies has been acknowledged for hundreds of years—including, more recently, by proponents of the health promotion movement (WHO, 1986; WHO, 1988)—advances in the 'art and science' of policy advocacy interventions have been modest in the health sector. As argued in Chapter 2, and in Breton and de Leeuw (2011), very few researchers have adopted a theoretically grounded approach to the analysis of policy advocacy interventions and strategies. We believe this has impeded advances in advocacy practice. In fact, only a few of the papers we reviewed explicitly refer to the policy change process. But without a valid theoretical lens, it is doubtful that health promoters can draw any valuable lessons from descriptions of what advocates have done for a specific policy.

There is general consensus among health promoters that the building of a strong coalition of organizations and influential policy stakeholders is instrumental to any policy change. In the public health literature, the term 'coalition' has many different meanings and definitions, ranging from a loosely structured group of people with little commitment to a common cause to a fully fledged strategic alliance in which members invest resources and take risks. Peer-reviewed journals are peppered with accounts of programmes aimed at building local coalitions to address a specific public health problem such as AIDS or asthma, and some coalitions aim directly to influence policies and policy decision-making. In many cases, coalitions are groups of individual or organizational actors that work together to some degree. However, accounts of their activities rarely hint at any power struggles, either within or external to the coalition, that could prevent them from reaching their goals.

In this chapter, we are interested in coalitions of actors (individual or organizational) that are striving to bring about policy change or to protect current policies from being modified or repealed. Our aim is to provide an explanatory framework that encompasses both the processes that lead to policy change, or that prevent policy change from taking place; and the building of capacity to influence these processes. We first present two theoretical frameworks for understanding policy advocacy. We then apply these theories to an analysis of a coalition that was successful in its advocacy for the 1998 Tobacco Control Act in the Province of Québec (Canada).

Theories for analysing advocacy coalitions in the policy change arena

In this chapter we draw on two theoretical contributions from political science that are useful tools for understanding the policy change process. The first is the Advocacy Coalition Framework (ACF) of Sabatier and Jenkins-Smith (1993; 1999). The other is Lemieux's (1998) theory of coalition structuring, which identifies the challenges/constraints and strategies of actors who are trying to influence the policy process through pooling their resources.

The Advocacy Coalition Framework

Paul Sabatier and Hank Jenkins-Smith proposed the ACF to explain the emergence of, and changes in, public policy. They maintain that policies are the product of the belief systems of the actors in a given policy subsystem (e.g. tobacco or transport). Actors include not only legislators but also civil servants and representatives of interest groups, and other groups concerned by the issue in question, such as journalists and academics. Together these actors make up the policy elite of the subsystem. In the words of Sabatier and Jenkins-Smith, the subsystem 'consists of those actors from a variety of public and private organizations who are actively concerned with a policy problem or issue, such as air pollution control, and who regularly seek to influence public policy in that domain' (Sabatier and Jenkins-Smith, 1999: 119).

Policies emerge from numerous confrontations and negotiations between different coalitions of actors in the subsystem (see Figure 3.1). Each coalition forms around a belief system that conveys a worldview and its own hierarchy of values. To better grasp these belief systems, Sabatier and Jenkins-Smith divide them into three strata: deep core, policy core, and secondary aspects. These strata are differentiated by their content (beliefs, values, and precepts), their resistance to change, and the scope of their field of application to the overall system, or to the subsystem or part of the subsystem of the policy in question. The deep core stratum of the belief system determines such things as the actors' views on the nature of man and the relative priority attributed to ultimate values (e.g. is health more important than freedom?). These deep core values are inherently extremely resistant to change. The policy core stratum is the expression of this deep core stratum in a specific policy subsystem. It concerns such aspects as the basic causes of the problem and the priority accorded to various policy instruments. Finally, there are the secondary aspects of the belief system, which are the most likely to evolve because they usually only apply to parts of the subsystem. Most decisions concerning administrative rules address the secondary aspects of the belief system (Sabatier and Jenkins-Smith, 1999). As administrative rules are relatively easy to change, so are the secondary aspects of the advocacy coalition's belief system.

In the policy subsystem, one coalition typically predominates over others, imposing its vision of problems and solutions—a vision that is compatible with its belief system. This coalition enjoys important strategic advantages from the standpoint of resources and opportunities. According to the model, the accumulation of new knowledge and the struggle waged by one or more challenger coalitions can achieve only limited policy change—i.e. modifications in the secondary aspects of the policy. Only events outside the subsystem, such as external perturbations or shocks, are likely to significantly upset the predominant coalition's advantages and resources (Sabatier and Weible, 2007). Such events allow a challenger coalition to impose the policy core of its belief system (see Figure. 3.1). It can do so by changing, for instance, the rules, resources, and individuals in charge of institutions, or by adopting legislation that imposes its own vision of the problems and solutions. This being the case, Sabatier and Jenkins-Smith believe that external events are a necessary, albeit insufficient, condition to changing the policy core attributes of a governmental programme or policy, because the challenger coalition still has to mobilize its resources to take advantage of the opportunities stemming from such events.

Lastly, Sabatier and Jenkins-Smith note that the decisions underlying policies are determined, in part, by a series of parameters, including basic attributes of the problem area and fundamental sociocultural values, which are highly stable over time and over which coalitions exercise virtually no control. Such parameters are, in fact, contextual variables that establish the realm of possibilities surrounding the discourse of coalitions

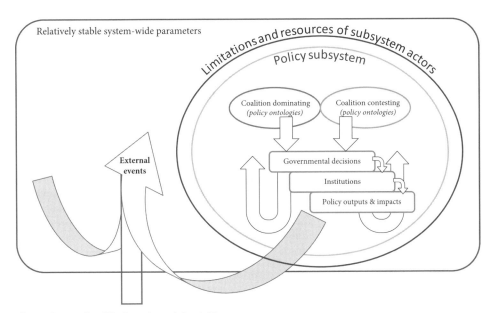

Figure 3.1 A simplified version of the ACF.
Source: Data from Sabatier, P. A. and Jenkins-Smith, H. C., *Policy Change and Learning: an Advocacy Coalition Approach*, Westview Press, Boulder, Colorado, USA, Copyright © 1993.

(for instance, whether discussions on welfare regime can venture away from the conservative view of men as sole breadwinners). They thus have a constraining effect on the nature and outcome of policy debates.

With the ACF, we now have a model of the policy change process that explains why policy advocates find it difficult to induce *significant* change in policies. It explains why policy subsystems are highly stable over time, a characteristic that has been repeatedly observed by a number of political scientists (Baumgartner and Jones, 1993; Hall, 1993; Heclo, 1974). For significant policy changes to take place—that is, change in the policy core of the dominant coalition—the ACF posits that there must first be a change in the subsystem's external environment. Sabatier and Jenkins-Smith's first hypothesis on the policy change process reminds us that such a change in the external environment can either shift the power balance between advocacy coalitions or result in having another jurisdiction impose a new course of action on the dominant coalition.

> Policy Change Hypothesis 1: The policy core attributes of a governmental program in a specific jurisdiction will not be significantly revised as long as the subsystem advocacy coalition that instituted the program remains in power within that jurisdiction except when the change is imposed by a hierarchically superior jurisdiction.
>
> (Sabatier and Jenkins-Smith, 1999: 124)

However, as noted by several authors (Mintrom and Vergari, 1996; Schlager, 1995; Schlager and Blomquist, 1996), the ACF falls short in providing a satisfactory explanation of what conditions lead to effective policy-oriented collective action, and on how disputes between actors are prevented and resolved such that an alliance may form. For such issues, we need to consider the problems and rationales behind collective bargaining for the pursuit of a common policy goal.

The theory of coalition structuring

Political scientists have mostly devoted their energy to studying coalitions that rule governments. The exception is the work of Gamson (1961), subsequently developed into the theory of coalition structuring by Lemieux (1998), which sheds light on the functioning of coalitions that seek to achieve a change in policy or to maintain the status quo. Lemieux conceptualizes coalitions as:

> concerted and temporary sets of individual or organizational actors experiencing cooperative and conflicting rapports in respect to their relationships, transactions and controls, and who strive through a proper structuration of their powers to predominate over their opponents so they can gain greater benefits than what they would have achieved outside the coalition.
>
> (Lemieux, 1998: 35)

An important feature of Lemieux's definition is that coalitions are not meant to last: rather, they disband as soon as they have fulfilled their purpose. Lemieux postulates that actors' decisions and actions reflect their assessment of the coalition's external environment, and that it is this assessment that somehow dictates the power structure and the level of resources needed by the coalition to succeed. Success is understood to be either the safeguarding of the status quo or a change in the external environment that is in line with the expectations and interests of coalition members.

Lemieux claims that in order for a system to control its external environment, it must exhibit a greater degree of diversity than its environment (Lemieux, 1998: 61). This implies that there is a threshold in diversity of resources towards which coalitions must strive—resources like the social/professional network, and access to the media and key decision-makers. This threshold pertains not only to the coalition's diversity of resources, but also to the coalition's control over its internal environment. Resources can only be put to use in a strategic fashion when the coalition is able to exert the necessary level of control over them. It is in reaching this threshold that a coalition succeeds in subordinating its external environment to its choices and preferences. That a coalition has reached this state is shown by its ability to force on its external environment the decisions and options that it favours.

For coalitions formed by political parties in order to rule a government, it is possible to quantify and objectively appraise the contribution of each party involved by using the number of seats secured. While it is pretty straightforward in this case, it becomes murkier when considering the threshold for coalitions that form with the goal of advocating, or blocking, policy change. The respective contributions of coalition members are more difficult to evaluate, as are their motives for entering the coalition and what is needed to overcome opposition in terms of level of resource diversity and control. The difficulty is also exacerbated by the continuously evolving nature of the coalition's external environment and by the fluctuation of the threshold over time, both of which add a great deal of uncertainty for members.

The three core dimensions of a coalition

As mentioned above, coalition members continuously monitor their external environment. Such appraisal has a direct impact on the three core dimensions that frame the social system making up the coalition: transactions, relationships, and controls.

Transactions correspond to the benefits and advantages sought by each individual member of the coalition. The benefits are weighed against the resources that need to be invested (costs). According to Lemieux, the coalition will not see the light of day or survive unless its potential members feel, upon appraising the external environment, that the actual or potential benefits associated with their involvement in the coalition exceed the costs. The same holds true if the members deem they could get comparable results at a lower cost by working outside the coalition. This added value of investing resources in a coalition points to its main advantage.

As the members appraise the resources they invest in the coalition based on the threshold for resource diversity and control, a sudden increase in this threshold may lead them to reconsider their involvement in order to avoid any further resource loss in an enterprise that now seems bound to fail. Another issue related to transactions concerns the distribution of benefits achieved through the coalition's operations. Members who invest heavily in the coalition but benefit little are likely to question the contribution of those who invest little but benefit greatly. Such a situation, if not settled in a satisfactory manner, may generate conflict and cause members to quit the coalition or, in the worst case scenario, lead to the disbanding of the coalition. An illustration of this problem can be found in Traynor and Glantz's (1996) analysis, which studied the efforts of a group of organizations to induce the government to levy a special tax on cigarettes.

The second core dimension of coalitions is relationships (*les liens* in French, which also translates as 'links'). These are what bring the members together and what forms the basis of their cooperation. Obviously, actors that share similar views and ideologies are more likely to collaborate. Bringing together people with a long history of collaboration, as opposed to people with a history of conflict with each other, will also be easier and more conducive to effective coalition work. The quality of the relationships within the coalition will also determine its capacity to resolve disagreements and conflicts that arise during difficult times. Lemieux also notes that cohesion between members can sometimes be strengthened when there is hostility towards them from actors in the external environment.

The last dimension, controls, relates to the coalition's capacity to exert control over its resources (i.e. members) and its opponents in order to shape to its liking the most critical elements of its external environment. To reach the necessary threshold, the coalition must adopt a power structure that will allow it to mobilize and put to use its resources. This is what Lemieux dubs 'controlled diversity'.

As the coalition is a form of alliance into which actors may freely decide to integrate or not, it is natural for a coalition to have a collegial structuring of power, whereby all members have a say in all decisions regarding the allocation of resources being pooled. A coalition naturally takes the form of a network, with each member of the network in direct contact with all other members. However, coalitions structured in this way are not very effective when faced with a threat from their external environment, and they usually struggle to control resource diversity. Members must hold talks and agree on a new course of action in the face of a threat, which takes time and may delay their response to the threat. Faced with an alarming change in their external environment, coalitions either dissolve—the costs are too great compared to the expected benefits— or change their structure in order to achieve better control of their diversity. The coalition's structure is, therefore, likely to evolve from a network to a quasi-network. For members, this transition comes, as one can imagine, at the price of their close oversight on all decisions regarding the coalition's daily business. The coalition will probably select a coordinator, or a team of coordinators, that will be granted some leeway in running the coalition and, more importantly, in deploying coalition strategy and interventions. Electing to have this kind of structure does not mean that coalition members totally relinquish their oversight on the coalition's activities. Having agreed on the extent of its latitude in dealing with common, and not so common, threats from the external environment, the coalition will gain in its capacity to act upon them quickly and to better seize upcoming opportunities, thereby increasing its advantage over opponents.

Thus, the coalition, in Lemieux's definition, is a temporary strategic alliance that is formed for a specific goal. This contrasts with Sabatier and Jenkins-Smith's conception of the advocacy coalition, which has a broader constituency, is composed of actors who share a common set of policy beliefs, and can evolve over a long period of time. This conceptualization suggests that as we analyse the evolution of an advocacy coalition over a number of years, we could witness the rise and fall of different *strategic alliances* that have been forged either to actualize specific goals of the advocacy coalition or to secure its hold on the policy subsystem.

Applying the two theories to tobacco control

To illustrate the insights that can be achieved via these theories, we will apply them to the development of Québec's Tobacco Act (1998). This case was documented through interviews (28 informants), policy documents (>200), and newspaper articles (569) (Breton et al., 2008). According to Sabatier and Jenkins-Smith, to analyse a change in public policy properly we must scrutinize its policy subsystem over a period of at least one decade. We have therefore chosen to examine changes in our unit of analysis, the tobacco policy subsystem, between 1986 when the first provincial statute governing the use of tobacco was adopted and 1998 when the Tobacco Act was adopted.

The relatively stable parameters that framed the policy debates

Figure 3.2 summarizes the results of our analysis of the parameters and their influence on the policy elite that comprises the tobacco policy subsystem. We have characterized these parameters as 'relatively stable' since they had already permeated and become part of mainstream policy discourses as far back as 1986.

Figure 3.2 shows very clearly that as early as 12 years prior to Québec's Tobacco Act the two basic attributes of tobacco use—its lethality for smokers and its addictive properties—were well recognized within the policy elite. In 1986, the harm caused by exposure to environmental tobacco smoke (ETS; also called second-hand smoke) was still being debated. The following quotations are from two elected representatives (or MNAs) addressing the National Assembly (Assemblée nationale, 1986).

> We should keep in mind that a cigarette takes on average 12 minutes to burn through, whereas a smoker only inhales smoke for a minute and a half. In addition, an individual exposing himself to the smoke of others doubles his risk of developing lung cancer. I believe that if one examines the statistics, it appears that every year in Québec many deaths are caused by those who smoke.
>
> I would like to bring to your attention, as the Canadian Tobacco Manufacturers Council solicited me to do, to the fact that the [health risks of ETS] have not been agreed on in a definite manner. It is somewhat like the opinion of an engineer or the opinion of a lawyer. There are always disagreements. We do not always agree.

What is more, the policy actors had yet to agree on a definitive French translation of ETS, and different terms were being used concurrently. But this debate was secondary. MNAs and the media seemed more interested in asserting the fundamental right of non-smokers to enjoy a smoke-free environment than in the health consequences of smoking

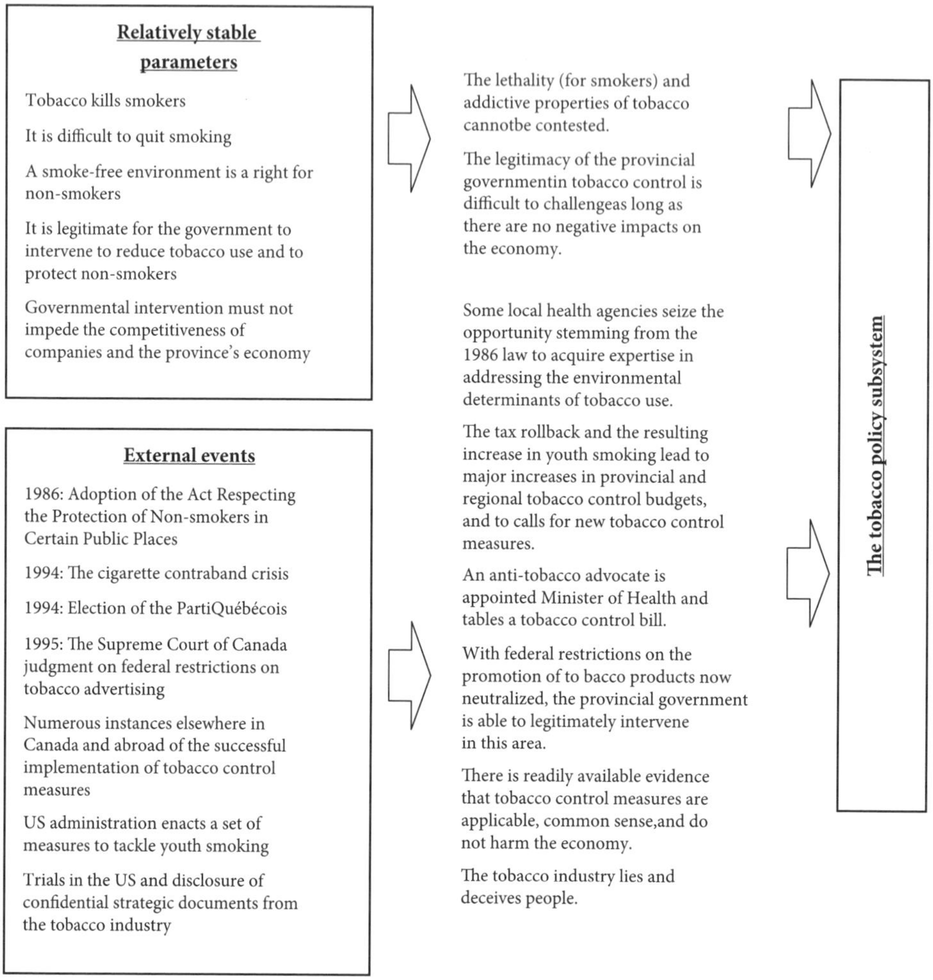

Figure 3.2 Main parameters and events that impacted on the advocacy capacity of the promoters of tobacco control measures (1986–1998).

Reproduced with permission from *Social Science and Medicine*, Volume 67, Issue 11, Breton, E., et al, Health promotion research and practice require sound policy analysis models: The case of Quebec's Tobacco Act, pp. 1679–1689, Copyright © 2008 Elsevier.

for the population. By 1998, the debate around ETS had completely disappeared; only experts mandated by the tobacco manufacturers were still attempting to instil doubt in the policy subsystem.

As for the addictive properties of tobacco, in 1986, despite the fact that interventions on this issue made little mention of nicotine as the dependence-inducing chemical, the media and MNAs repeatedly testified about the danger of addiction. One MNA addressing the National Assembly said: 'I always smoked two or three packs of cigarettes a day, but I quit three weeks ago. I deserve a big round of applause because this is really difficult!' (Assemblée nationale, 1986). In 1998, tobacco use was widely recognized as an addiction, and nicotine as its trigger. Again, only representatives of the tobacco industry kept framing smoking as a matter of personal choice.

> The FTQ [Federation of Québec Workers, the trade union representing tobacco manufacturing workers] does not contest the noxious effects of tobacco on health…nor the need to protect non-smokers. We have always said that it was important. What we say is that tobacco remains a legal product and that smokers have rights, just like they have responsibilities, towards non-smokers.…[the effects of tobacco] on health have forced us to address tobacco use as a choice that must be exercised in a responsible fashion by adults.
>
> (President of the FTQ, in Assemblée nationale, 1998b)

A second observation that emerged from our analysis of the policy discourse from 1986 to 1998 concerns the legitimacy of governmental intervention in tobacco control. Again, in Québec, the policy elite influential in defining tobacco policy generally backed government involvement in tobacco control. This support rested on three arguments: (1) youth smoking is an important public problem, (2) non-smokers make up the majority of the population, and (3) the treatment costs of smoking-related diseases are an undue burden on the universally accessible and publicly funded provincial health care system.

But while recognition of the government's legitimacy in tobacco control was not seriously contested during this 12-year period, the promoters of tobacco control measures still faced a major obstacle in bringing about more stringent tobacco control legislation. Whatever the measure on the table, they had to convince decision-makers that its implementation would not affect the province's economy. This was particularly true in 1998, when, as we will see later, concerns for the economic impacts of the bill on tobacco company-sponsored arts and sports events threatened its adoption.

These observations are important because they provide insights into why the tobacco industry, rather than trying to convince policy actors that smoking is harmless or not very harmful, elected to focus its public relations strategy on the potential economic impacts of tobacco control measures, a dimension of tobacco policy in which it enjoyed much greater leeway and leverage than the health dimension. It is noteworthy that in our analysis of the newspaper coverage and the Hansard of the National Assembly we found only two instances, in 1986 and 1998, of representatives of tobacco manufacturers contesting the lethality of ETS. The CEO of Imperial Tobacco claimed: 'It is bad science.…Science does not prove everything, smoking is not a scientific phenomenon. Smoking is a social and cultural phenomenon' (quoted in Dutrisac, 1998); and when testifying during the parliamentary commission studying the tobacco bill, the spokesperson of the Canadian Tobacco Manufacturers' Council opted not to argue against the health risks to smokers, and left unaddressed the health risks to non-smokers.

> I would say that the industry concedes that there are risks associated with the use of our products and that if you smoke you are at risk of developing a number of diseases. We should not fool ourselves. This is a fact. But is it 10,000, 9,800, 5,000, 2,000 or 13,000 [deaths]? It depends on how it is calculated. I am no accountant, I am no economist.
>
> (Marie-Josée Lapointe, spokesperson, Canadian Tobacco Manufacturers' Council, in Assemblée nationale, 1998a)

The events that influenced the tobacco policy subsystem

The historical narrative suggests that many events may have influenced the course of Québec's tobacco policy, and therefore the adoption of the Tobacco Act, our analysis shows that only a few rank as significant contributors (summarized in Figure 3.2). From the standpoint of the Tobacco Act's adoption, all these external events positively influenced the advocacy capacity of the promoters of tobacco control measures. However, they did not all affect the subsystem in a similar fashion, nor with equal weight.

Looking back at the Act Respecting the Protection of Non-smokers in Certain Public Places, adopted in 1986, we can make a few observations. First, it was tabled by the Ministry of Environment and no reference was made to the health impact of ETS.

> I believe that here again, Québec is showing the way in a manner that is unique because an issue which was supposed to cause so much controversy has been received here in the House with applause when I introduced it. People on both sides, smokers and non-smokers alike, ministers, MNAs and Opposition MNAs alike felt that the time was right and we should do it, that we should go forward. Quietly, we are going forward…in an area which is fundamentally an area of human rights.
>
> (Clifford Lincoln, Minister of the Environment, in Assemblée nationale, 1986)

The second observation is that one of the Act's provisions pre-empted local and regional governments from enforcing more stringent regulations on smoking in public places. Finally, the law was regarded simply as a way of asserting the rights of non-smokers to a smoke-free environment. Certainly, this piece of legislation does not seem to have been a strong forerunner to the Tobacco Act. Nevertheless, the Act of 1986 did give some local public health boards the impetus to start intervening on the environmental determinants of smoking in the province, at a time when most, if not all, tobacco control interventions were exclusively educational in nature and delivered in the school setting. These boards felt that it was part of their mandate to promote the implementation of the Act's provisions in hospitals and clinics. They did this by hiring public health professionals, the majority of whom had no prior experience in tobacco control. A few years later, some of these professionals were to play a key role in advocating, at the provincial and federal level, more stringent measures to fight the tobacco epidemic.

Of all the external events we could identify, the 1994 cigarette contraband crisis is the one that had by far the most significant impact on the tobacco policy subsystem. Pressured by the Opposition, the media, and public opinion, both provincial and federal governments were eager to curb the traffic of cigarettes smuggled in from the US and sold at less than half the price of cigarettes on the legal market.

> Responsibility for contraband tobacco does rest on consumers…it is the government that has overtaxed the product and by doing so generated unfair competition with the American product. When you have a tax of $1 in New York and a tax of $4.60 in Québec then it is the legislators who have caused the problem. And people resisted.. .
>
> (Opposition MNA in the National Assembly, in Assemblée nationale, 1993)

In order to resolve the crisis, both levels of government cut taxes, leading to a halving of the retail price of cigarettes. Acknowledging that its decision could engender a surge in youth smoking, the government of Québec adopted an action plan and a dedicated four-year budget for tobacco control interventions at the provincial and regional levels. For Québec's public health system, this new influx of money was substantial and was said to have brought an estimated 100-fold increase in the total funds available for tobacco control in the province.

> When I was working in tobacco control [before the tobacco tax rollback], we estimated that there was, overall, the equivalent of six full-time professionals in Québec working in this field.... The maximum amount of money available to do little things at the Ministry [of Health] was $50,000 per year. And this was really the maximum we could get.
>
> (Public health professional)

Therefore, when it was shown that the prevalence of youth smoking soared as a result of the tax rollback, public health professionals had not only a solid case when presenting their demands to the elite of the tobacco subsystem but also a significant level of resources to fuel their advocacy interventions. However, following the contraband crisis, suggestions that the cigarette tax be raised again were met with strong criticism in the National Assembly and from the media. Many non-governmental organizations (NGOs) from the health sector that had actively fought the cigarette tax rollback emerged bruised from all the attacks by the media and promoters of the fiscal measures. Hence, they were reluctant to engage in any high-profile promotion of tobacco control measures at the provincial government level.

> [The contraband crisis] generated so many waves, it was such a touchy issue, and we knew that the [tobacco] industry was behind it all. It became almost taboo [to talk about tobacco taxation]. I remember I was delivering a press conference [after the tobacco tax rollback] and in our recommendations we did not ask for a tax increase...we had been briefed beforehand and decided not to address this sensitive issue.
>
> (Volunteer in a health-sector NGO)

A more complete account of the contraband crisis can be found in Breton et al. (2006).

The 1994 elections in Québec brought a new government to power; however, with respect to tobacco policy, it was not very different from the previous one. As the Opposition, this party—the Parti québécois—had strongly supported the cigarette tax rollback and was no more inclined to address the health concerns than was the ruling Liberal Party. The single most notable difference was the appointment of a public health physician as the new Minister of Health, a physician and former executive at the World Health Organization (WHO), who was well acquainted with population-level strategies to reduce smoking. Following the events described below, he proposed a set of legislative measures that was significantly more comprehensive and stringent than those formulated by his predecessor, the goal being to compensate for the cigarette tax rollback.

In 1995, after years of sustained judicial procedures to have the federal Tobacco Products Control Act (1988) scrapped, the tobacco manufacturers finally succeeded in having the Act's provisions prohibiting the promotion of tobacco products overturned by the Supreme Court of Canada. The Act was found to infringe unreasonably on the tobacco manufacturers' freedom of expression as guaranteed under the Canadian

Charter of Rights and Freedoms. Although nothing ever really precluded the provincial government from regulating the promotion of cigarette brands, it appears that the policy elite deemed this area off limits for Québec. The Supreme Court judgment changed the situation drastically, leaving a void that could legitimately be filled by the provincial government. This gave the Minister of Health the impetus to provide the province with a comprehensive tobacco act covering most of the essential measures to reduce smoking.

The Québec tobacco policy subsystem was not impervious to the different legislative initiatives being implemented elsewhere in Canada and abroad, especially in the US. The promoters of tobacco control measures repeatedly quoted the scientific literature, which abounded with evidence that a prohibition on smoking in public places was achievable. They modelled their compensation scheme for the ban on the sponsorship of arts and sports events by tobacco manufacturers on the experience of the State of Victoria in Australia. Studies on the economic impact of various measures implemented in other countries had also shown that the implementation of the proposed Tobacco Act would not be catastrophic (Crémieux et al., 1997).

While the advocacy capacity of the promoters of tobacco control measures increased significantly during the 12-year period analysed, the tobacco industry experienced a constant decline in its public image. The media reported its active involvement in schemes to evade cigarette taxes and duties that led to the 1994 contraband crisis. They also covered the interventions of the US Food and Drug Administration and the various trials in the US that pitted a number of states against tobacco manufacturers. These news stories not only contributed to legitimatizing tobacco control measures but also uncovered manufacturers' strategies to entice new smokers and retain current ones.

As demonstrated by our discussion of the relatively stable parameters and external events, the promoters of tobacco control measures, evolving within a broad anti-tobacco advocacy coalition, were facing both opportunities and constraints in advancing their policy goal. How did they take advantage of these opportunities and convert them into real gains? How did they ensure that the tobacco policy subsystem adopted the core elements of their vision of the tobacco problem and its solutions? This is where Lemieux's theory of coalition structuring proves helpful because it enables us to appraise the advocacy strategy used.

The strategies used to promote the tobacco control bill

The first elements of a strategy to support the tobacco control bill (1994–1996)

As mentioned above, following the 1994 elections, advocates of more stringent tobacco control measures were faced with a significant opportunity: the provincial government's willingness to move on the issue. But as the Minister of Health was disclosing his legislative intentions, it became clear that he would face harsh opposition from tobacco manufacturers, and that action was needed to counter this opposition. In response, a strategy took shape within regional public health directorates, informed mainly by experiences with the cigarette contraband crisis and a thorough diagnosis of the present situation (Anonymous, 1995).

For the heads of the 18 regional public health directorates, the problem in advocating the bill was not whether they would be equipped, for instance, to hold press conferences to stress the impact of tobacco on health, but rather whether they would have the means to participate in debates falling outside the public health realm on topics like the potential economic impacts of the bill. To circumvent this barrier, the directors agreed to pool part of their resources earmarked for tobacco control interventions in order to increase their capacity to advocate the bill outside existing organizational structures. They created a special programme that would fund an NGO to set up an advocacy organization. The NGO acted as a firewall, protecting the strategic coalition of regional public health directorates from any possible backlash to its interventions in public debates.

This advocacy organization was officially launched in April 1996 under the name Québec Coalition for Tobacco Control (CQCT). The group's interventions were based on a policy platform officially endorsed by Québec's most important NGOs in the health sector (e.g. the Québec Division of the Canadian Cancer Society) and by the provincial body of the regional public health directorates. Basically, the platform set forth the legislative measures CQCT could advocate without having to seek authorization from its founding partners. The adoption of this policy platform was crucial to granting CQCT advocates the leeway needed to grasp unexpected opportunities to advance the tobacco bill swiftly and to counter opponents' allegations rapidly. Once adopted by CQCT's core supporters, the platform's content was disseminated to municipalities, health institutions, local and regional organizations, and businesses in an attempt to recruit supporters. By 1997, more than 600 entities had officially endorsed the platform (CQCT, 1997), a situation that no doubt contributed to increasing CQCT's legitimacy in the political sphere.

From the time of its founding until the actual adoption of the Tobacco Act, CQCT, along with the new provincial branch of the Non Smokers' Rights Association, was the most vocal promoter of the tobacco bill. It regularly intervened in the media on different aspects of tobacco control and the tobacco industry, and visited MNAs in their offices. Also, carrying out a core function of its mandate, it fed regional public health directorates updates on the status of the tobacco bill, pinpointed current barriers and loci of resistance within the government, and advised on measures to facilitate the bill's adoption. Tobacco control professionals were also urged at key points in time to present their views to their MNAs.

Facing a new threat to the tobacco bill (1997–1998)

In November 1996, the Minister of Health announced his plan to include in the bill provisions restricting the promotion of tobacco products and the sponsorship of arts and sports events by the tobacco industry. The announcement followed a similar, albeit less restrictive, plan formulated by the federal Minister of Health, which had led to the 1997 bill that replaced the federal act overturned by the Supreme Court.

In the face of public uproar over the federal restrictions on sponsorship in the arts and sports sector, it became clear that if the strategic coalition of 18 regional public health directorates was serious about facilitating the adoption of the bill, adjustments had to be made to its advocacy interventions and to the level of resources devoted to them. The coalition made its own diagnosis of the situation, taking stock of the mobilization of interest groups from the Province of Québec to oppose the federal bill restricting tobacco sponsorship and advertising, and of the favourable response it received in the French-speaking media. It thus anticipated a fierce debate around the projected bill from the Government of Québec. From there, the coalition concluded first that it should strive to reframe the debate in public health terms, and second that it should organize itself to be able to confront the interest groups that were going to oppose Québec's bill (Comité provincial de santé publique sur le tabac et la santé, 1997).

From the tobacco manufacturers' perspective, the provisions on sponsorship were both a clear menace to their profitability and an opportunity to defeat the bill by having the debate drift from the issue of health to the issue of the survival of sponsored events. Opposition to the provisions was spearheaded by a lobby group representing Québec's seven largest arts and sports events: the Ralliement des événements pour la liberté de commandite. This group, which we will refer to as the Sponsorship Freedom Alliance, carried out a number of well-organized public interventions that received intense and mostly favourable media coverage. It even won the support of the Premier of Québec: '[the Premier] acknowledges that tobacco is a threat that needs to be addressed, but jeopardizing international events as is intended by the [federal law] does not make any sense' (government spokesperson, quoted in Delbes, 1997). The promoters of the tobacco bill could not avoid this issue: they had to find ways to neutralize the lobby group's hold on the debate.

Following calls from tobacco control professionals for more effective involvement by government public health agencies (including hospitals) in policy debates, the heads of the 18 regional public health directorates both centralized their strategic planning and increased the level of resources invested in their advocacy strategy. This reaction to a change in the external environment is directly in line with Lemieux's theorizing. The centralized strategic planning body was composed of full-time tobacco control professionals with direct access to the heads of the regional public health directorates. Its operations were funded through a specially allocated budget that was large enough to allow for a string of province-wide media interventions.

The renewed effort of the strategic coalition of regional public health directorates allowed for an additional set of interventions to advocate the tobacco bill. These actions sometimes complemented or enhanced interventions by CQCT. Two main outcomes of the reformulated strategy should be highlighted. First, the central strategic planning body facilitated the intervention of governmental public health agencies by producing a public health-centred rationale to defend the bill's different measures. It also disseminated to tobacco control professionals throughout the province a daily press review of tobacco-related local, national, and international news. One significant result of this facilitative work was that renowned representatives of health care institutions publicly urged the government to table its stalled tobacco bill. A press conference staged by a group of oncologists and other specialists, along with the expressed intention of authorities from another hospital to stage one, helped to convince the Council of Ministers to table the bill. These demonstrations of support from the health care system probably also contributed to fending off the image of the promoters of tobacco control measures as 'tobacco ayatollahs'—a message that opponents had been actively conveying since the early stages of the cigarette contraband crisis.

> As for us, when we did finally speak to the media, to say 'Hey! There will be consequences to a tax rollback!' they threw tomatoes at us. [They would say things like] 'Who do you think you are? What planet do you live on?…you're a bunch of ayatollahs that want us all to stop smoking.' This is how they responded to us, either ignoring us or, if we grabbed people's attention, telling us that it was none of our business and that we were extremists.
>
> (Professional from a governmental public health organization)

The other major outcome was that the central strategic planning body improved coordination between the different interventions conducted by governmental public health agencies like hospitals and local community health centres, and by NGOs. While a certain level of coordination had already been achieved among some NGOs, CQCT had achieved little success in mobilizing governmental public health agencies because it had deliberately been created outside the governmental public health system. Meetings between the strategic planning body and NGOs were held regularly. Among other things, these meetings helped to ensure that the actions of bill promoters would not unnecessarily overlap and that no aspect of the bill would be left unaddressed during advocacy interventions and the parliamentary process. Joint interventions like press conferences were also conducted, and even though these were funded by the central planning committee, they were credited to CQCT, the Non Smokers' Rights Association, or another NGO. These joint interventions proved critical to disseminating the results of opinion polls that demonstrated to journalists and MNAs that the majority of Quebecers supported tobacco control measures. The interventions also contributed to neutralizing support for the Sponsorship Freedom Alliance, which opposed the provisions on tobacco sponsorship.

With regard to event sponsorship, the central strategic planning body, along with its allies, established an organization to lobby the provincial government to use part of its cigarette tax to compensate arts and sports events for the loss of tobacco industry money. The movement advocating the Québec Fund for Culture, Sports and the Arts recruited the support of a wide array of actors from the arts, sports, and health sectors, gathering enough momentum that its representatives gained access to key ministers and MNAs.

> We didn't decide to put our energy into trying to convince people that [tobacco] sponsorship was bad. We thought that people were sufficiently aware of the fact that it would likely be prohibited and this was a problem…instead, we wanted to come up with a solution. Without ever saying sponsorship needs to be banned, we said we need a fund [dedicated to the sponsorship of cultural and sport event]. So we worked on a solution. And 75% of people supported this fund.
>
> (Public health professional)

The official adoption of the tax scheme by the Minister of Finance was a fatal blow to the Sponsorship Freedom Alliance. When the parliamentary commission hearings on the tobacco bill began, this group no longer represented seven arts and sports events. Representatives for these events had opted instead to promote their own organizations and, rather than opposing the bill, to work on amendments to streamline the phasing out of tobacco industry sponsorship.

> We were hoping to get the heads of the events to cross over to our side. They did not, but it shut them up. They were still funded by the tobacco industry. We know that most of them agreed with our idea [of a dedicated fund] but were not in a position to let it be known: 'I receive 2 million per year from the industry, I cannot bite the hand that feeds me.' So [the Québec Fund for Culture, Sports and the Arts] spelled the end of their alliance. We pretty much stopped seeing them hanging out together. When they testified at the parliamentary commission, they were much less assertive. We did not destroy their coalition, but we did make them much less vocal.
>
> (Public health professional)

Explaining the adoption of the Tobacco Act

The theoretical frameworks of the ACF and coalition structuring are crucial to explaining how the Tobacco Act came to be adopted. The previous sections, in which we applied these theories, indicate the key factors underpinning this process. One way to add order to the study of such a complex process is to consider the various effects observed in the short, mid and long term.

In the short term, the Minister of Health's legislative initiative in 1998 was nothing short of *sine qua non* to the Act's adoption, but the Minister would not have succeeded without the support of the strategic coalition of 18 regional public health directorates. The coalition's actions were critical in thwarting an effective public campaign to scrap the bill on the basis of its potential negative economic impacts. Its actions were made even more effective by the bridges it built with NGOs and health care institutions, which led to a broader and more coordinated array of interventions.

> The issue was that we had a minister who wanted the legislation....we had to...contribute in creating an environment supportive to this end. It is quite different from doing lobbying to get the government to act on something...The leader on this dossier, and from the very beginning, has been the Minister of Health and Social Services, who at some point sat down and said, 'We shouldn't have done that, this cigarette tax rollback. We need measures that will tie in with the international trend. We will prepare a bill and have it enacted, and we will make it broad in scope.' And we worked intensively on generating the conditions that would allow the government to succeed.
>
> (Public health professional)

Our analysis of tobacco policy discourses in 1998 is particularly indicative of the success of the promoters of tobacco control measures. The promoters constituted the largest and most diversified group of actors that we have been able to associate with a common general policy discourse and, hence, to an advocacy coalition as defined by Sabatier and Jenkins-Smith. In contrast, most policy actors outside this group advocated the amendment of a single provision of the bill, offered no alternative solution to youth smoking, and did not contest the actual health risks associated with tobacco use.

It is noteworthy that this broad advocacy coalition pressing for tobacco control measures was the only one that offered a satisfactory solution to the problem of youth smoking, a problem that worsened with the cigarette tax rollback in 1994. The tobacco industry's only foray into this area was to suggest renewed efforts via education programmes, something that did little to satisfy MNAs who were sitting on parliamentary commissions studying the issue.

Except for the three main tobacco manufacturers represented by the Canadian Tobacco Manufacturers' Council, the other organizational actors associated with the tobacco economic sector clearly did not share a common vision of the tobacco problem. And when, at the time of the parliamentary commission studying the bill, the Tobacco Council did make a foray into the health impacts of tobacco, MNAs and journalists afforded very little credibility to their views. The MNAs had already been largely won over by the 'diagnosis' formulated by the anti-tobacco coalition.

> And I would particularly like to thank [CQCT] for helping me understand the issue as I now understand it. I do not question the value of the interventions of the other groups, but I greatly appreciated the information they provided during the debate. I think that, thanks to them, we understand the question much better than before.
>
> (MNA from the ruling party addressing the parliamentary commission studying the tobacco bill, in Assemblée nationale, 1998b)

> And, of course, I and everybody else greatly appreciated your [CQCT's] presentation, which demonstrated, I think, one of the things that personally was troubling me...that perhaps I was not giving enough importance to everything related to advertisement and sponsorship. I didn't really see the relationship there, because there is no real scientific evidence on the impact of a given sponsorship program or advertisement. But globally, it is clear that advertisement and sponsorship do have an impact. Otherwise how could we possibly explain this great generosity extended to sports and arts programs?
>
> (Member of the ruling party, in Assemblée nationale, 1998b)

When focused on health issues, public health and health care actors were, by far, the most legitimate interveners in the policy debate.

From a mid-term perspective, it is clear that the Minister and the strategic coalition of 18 regional public health directorates reaped the fruits of the broader anti-tobacco advocacy coalition's efforts throughout the years—the substantial gains that this advocacy coalition had made in advancing its vision of the tobacco problem and its solutions. For instance, when we compare the policy discourses in 1998 to those in 1986, we see not only that smoking had evolved into a public health problem, but also that a clear recognition had taken hold concerning the hazards of exposure to ETS, as well as a recognition of the importance of tobacco sponsorship in strategies to promote tobacco products. Nonetheless, the effect of new knowledge on ETS within the tobacco policy subsystem was not enough to prevent the cigarette tax rollback of 1994. Concerns for the tax regime and criminality eclipsed concerns over the health impact of tobacco use. In the early 1990s, the anti-tobacco advocacy coalition was too disorganized and so unable to turn the tide.

> For tobacco control…we lost a first battle [with the cigarette tax rollback]. [We realized that] we needed to commit money and that we needed other strategies than just saying [tobacco] is harmful to health. We've being saying that for 40 years! This is not the game we need to play. Instead, we had to convince people that we can ban it in restaurants, that we can ban sponsorships and advertisement, that we can reduce sales to minors, and that we have a villain that has millions [of dollars] and a strategy. The classic strategy of the tobacco industry is to kill the messenger; it's the invisible hand. It's [the tobacco industry] that funds retailers, it's [the tobacco industry] that funds cultural events. But it's not them that will defend their interests—it's the heads of the [arts and sports] events who say: 'Come on! How could there be a link between tennis and tobacco?…So they call us ayatollahs, idiots, and lots of other names too. They fund companies, organizations, and events since the product itself cannot be defended.
>
> (Public health professional)

If this broad anti-tobacco advocacy coalition was able to achieve prominence within the tobacco policy subsystem, it is largely due to its success in seizing the opportunities engendered by a series of events external to the subsystem. These events enhanced the advocacy capacity of the promoters of tobacco control by: (1) putting the tobacco problem on the governmental agenda, (2) increasing the level of resources—human and monetary—devoted to it, (3) leading to a tobacco policy entrepreneur being appointed to a key political position as the Minister of Health in the machinery of the State, and (4) providing an opportunity to broaden the scope of the bill by the inclusion of provisions on the promotion of tobacco products.

Lastly, to explain the adoption of the Tobacco Act requires taking into account the long-term effects of some relatively stable parameters that impeded the opponents of tobacco control measures in effectively contesting the health impacts of tobacco use, the addictive properties of tobacco, and the legitimacy of governmental interventions in reducing its consumption—a legitimacy further reinforced by the surge in youth smoking.

Conclusion

Our primary goal in this chapter was to demonstrate the merits of a theoretically grounded approach to policy analysis in health promotion. As coalitions are, more often than not, a necessary condition of successful advocacy for policy change, we need to analyse them through the lens of a theoretical framework that can, at the very least, both place these coalitions within the broader context of the factors and processes that contribute to policy change; and account for the problem of collective bargaining that is likely to take place when individuals or collective actors have to share both the costs and rewards of their efforts.

These theoretical lenses teach us that achieving policy change can be a lengthy enterprise—one that requires a capacity to monitor the discourses of the policy elite and to spot system-wide events that could potentially shift the balance in favour of one actor over another. For health promotion research and practice, there is clear benefit to grounding policy analysis within a theoretically sound framework.

Acknowledgements

The is chapter is adapted with permission from *Social Science and Medicine*, Volume 67, Issue 11, Breton, E., et al, Health promotion research and practice require sound policy analysis models: The case of Quebec's Tobacco Act, pp. 1679–1689, Copyright © 2008 Elsevier.

All translations of interview excerpts were completed by the chapter authors.

References

Anonymous (1995). *Coalition pour la Santé. Projet d'Élaboration d'une Stratégie d'Influence dans le Cadre du Renforcement de la Législation Québécoise contre le Tabagisme.* Montréal: Conseil des directeurs de la santé publique.

Assemblée nationale (1986). *Journal des débats.* Trente-troisième législature, première session, le vendredi 6 juin, **29** (40), 2382–401. Québec: Assemblée nationale.

Assemblée nationale (1993). *Journal des débats.* Trente-quatrième législature, deuxième session, le mardi 26 octobre, 32 (120), 8192–93. Québec: Assemblée nationale.

Assemblée nationale (1998a). *Journal des débats. Commission permanente des affaires sociales.* Trente-cinquième législature, deuxième session, Cahier no. 127, le jeudi 28 mai, 1–60. Québec: Assemblée nationale.

Assemblée nationale (1998b). *Journal des débats. Commission permanente des affaires sociales.* Trente-cinquième législature, deuxième session, Cahier no. 136, le mercredi 10 juin, 1–65. Québec: Assemblée nationale.

Baumgartner, F. R. and Jones, B. D. (1993). *Agendas and Instability in American Politics.* Chicago, IL: University of Chicago Press.

Breton, E. and de Leeuw, E. (2011). Theories of the policy process in health promotion research: a review. *Health Promotion International*, **26** (1), 82–90.

Breton, E., Richard, L., Gagnon, F., Jacques, M., and Bergeron, P. (2006). Fighting a tobacco-tax rollback: a political analysis of the 1994 Cigarette Contraband Crisis in Canada. *Journal of Public Health Policy*, **27** (1), 77–99.

Breton, E., Richard, L., Gagnon, F., Jacques, M., and Bergeron, P. (2008). Health promotion research and practice require sound policy analysis models: the case of Québec's Tobacco Act. *Social Science & Medicine*, **67** (11), 1679–89.

Comité provincial de santé publique sur le tabac et la santé (1997). *Stratégie de Communication. Faciliter l'Adoption d'un Projet de Loi sur le Tabagisme au Québec.* Montréal: Conseil des directeurs de la Santé Publique.

CQCT (1997). *Plate-forme et Liste des Organismes Membres de la Coalition Québécoise sur le Contrôle du Tabac.* Montréal: Coalition québécoise pour le contrôle du tabac.

Crémieux, P.-Y., Fortin, P., Ouellette, P., Lavoie, F., and St-Pierre, Y. (1997). *Projet de Loi sur le Tabac Proposé par le Ministre de la Santé et des Services Sociaux du Québec. Étude d'Impact.* Québec: Ministère de la Santé et des Services Sociaux.

Delbes, M. P. C. (1997). Grand Prix du Canada Lucien Bouchard a eu le plancher à lui tout seul. *Le Droit*, 16-06-1997, 15.

Dutrisac, R. (1998). Produits du tabac: les fabricants dans la ligne de tir. Les groupes antitabac et les gouvernements se liguent pour faire chuter la consommation. *Le Devoir*, 06-05-1998, B1.

Gamson, W. A. (1961). A theory of coalition formation. *American Sociological Review*, **26** (3), 373–82.

Hall, P. (1993). Policy paradigm, social learning and the state. *Comparative Politics*, **25** (3), 275–96.

Heclo, H. (1974). *Modern Social Politics in Britain and Sweden; from Relief to Income Maintenance.* New Haven, CT: Yale University Press.

Lemieux, V. (1998). *Les coalitions: Liens, Transactions et Contrôles.* Paris: Presses universitaires de France.

Mintrom, M. and Vergari, S. (1996). Advocacy coalitions, policy entrepreneurs, and policy change. *Policy Studies Journal,* **24** (3), 420–38.

Sabatier, P. A. and Jenkins-Smith, H. C. (1993). *Policy Change and Learning: an Advocacy Coalition Approach.* Boulder, CO: Westview.

Sabatier, P. A. and Jenkins-Smith, H. C. (1999). The advocacy coalition framework: an assessment, in P. A. Sabatier (ed.) *Theories of the Policy Process* (1st edn.), pp. 117–66, Boulder, CO: Westview.

Sabatier, P. A. and Weible, C. M. (2007). The advocacy coalition framework: innovations and clarifications, in P. A. Sabatier (ed.) *Theories of the Policy Process* (2nd edn.), pp. 189–220, Boulder, CO: Westview.

Schlager, E. (1995). Policy making and collective action: defining coalitions within the advocacy coalition framework. *Policy Sciences,* **28**, 243–70.

Schlager, E. and Blomquist, W. (1996). A comparison of three emerging theories of the policy process. *Political Research Quarterly,* **49** (3), 651–72.

Traynor, M. P. and Glantz, S. A. (1996). California's tobacco tax initiative: the development and passage of Proposition 99. *Journal of Health Politics, Policy and Law,* **21** (3), 543–85.

WHO (1986). *First International Conference on Health Promotion. The Ottawa Charter for Health Promotion,* Geneva: World Health Organization.

WHO (1988). *Conference Statement of the 2nd International Conference on Health Promotion: The Adelaide Recommendations—Healthy Public Policy.* Geneva: World Health Organization.

Chapter 4

Policy change and the social determinants of health

Toba Bryant

Introduction

Two important concepts relevant to understanding health are the social determinants of health and the process of health promotion. The social determinants of health refer to how living and working conditions structure access to a range of resources needed to ensure health and social well-being such as income, employment security and housing security (Raphael, 2008b; 2008c). Health promotion is the related process concerned with enabling people to gain control over and improve their health. Converging evidence shows that the social determinants of health and the health inequalities that result from their unequal distribution are a direct result of how governments develop and implement public policy (Graham, 2004; 2007). International consensus following the Second World War led to the creation of the welfare state in rich, developed countries, and the implementation of public policies that improved the welfare of the population by strengthening the social determinants of health (Cohen and Pulkingham, 2009; Teeple, 2000). The development of social and health programmes such as public health care, unemployment insurance, and public pensions was considered to improve the standard of living and the health of populations by ensuring a more equitable distribution of income and other resources within populations (CSDH, 2008).

Public policies that redistribute income through the provision of pensions, unemployment insurance, child care and conditions of early childhood, and access to food and housing, among others, shape the social determinants of health (Raphael, 2013a; 2013b). Canadian governments have published a number of reports on health promotion and the social determinants of health that are consistent with this view. Evidence indicates, however, that Canadian governments have been resistant to implementing these concepts in public policies (Bryant et al., 2011). Federal government action on health promotion and the social determinants of health has lagged far behind its publication prowess on these issues. There has been a shift away from health promotion and social determinants to the individualization of health and illness (Lupton, 1999). In regard to the most egregious manifestation of health-threatening social determinants of health, the federal and provincial governments have had little to say about poverty and how it leads to poor health outcomes.

Using Canada as a case study, this chapter will identify and discuss some of the supports and barriers to developing public policy that addresses the social determinants of health. It will also discuss what is required to implement a comprehensive health promotion agenda. The aim is to provide a critical perspective on the agenda-setting process in order to identify the barriers to having health promotion and the social determinants of health on the public policy agenda. Agenda-setting is concerned with the recognition of an issue as a social problem requiring government attention and intervention (Baumgartner and Jones, 1993). There is no assurance, however, that once identified as a problem, that government will act to address it. A critical perspective can help to identify the barriers to implementing health-promoting policies in Canada.

This chapter applies a political economy perspective to examine public policy on health promotion and the social determinants of health in Canada, and to identify the barriers to implementing a health promotion and social determinants of health agenda. Political economy and related frameworks such as welfare state analysis are structural and materialist approaches to understanding the development and implementation of public policy (Coburn, 2010). Welfare state analysis helps to illustrate the impact of political ideology on the public policy process and its outcomes, and can identify opportunities to influence the public policy process. The chapter will conclude by identifying and discussing what changes are needed to move forward a health promotion agenda concerned with the social determinants of health, and how health promotion practitioners and citizens can contribute to this process.

Public policy theory and analysis

The purpose of public policy theory is to examine different aspects and stages of the public policy-making process; these explain the workings of the process and its outcomes. It can also identify opportunities to influence the public policy process—in particular health policy, the focus of this chapter. Political economy provides a critical perspective on the public policy process—particularly health policy, and how health and health promotion practitioners and others can influence health policy.

Political economy is a materialist and structural perspective concerned with the roles of the State, the market, political ideology, power, and civil society in the public policy process (Armstrong et al., 2001). It considers how these help or impede the recognition of social and health issues by governments and government efforts to address these issues. Political economy is materialist because it considers ideas and institutions to emerge from the way in which a society distributes social and economic resources such as income and employment, among others, to citizens (Coburn, 2010). It treats economics and politics as fundamentally related, as structuring politics and public policy outcomes, and determining whether and how the needs of citizens will be met (Armstrong et al., 2001). It considers the structural causes of social and health inequalities and explains how economic interests, such as the business and corporate sector, influence the agenda-setting and public policy-making processes. It attempts to illuminate how policy outcomes privilege some issues and societal interests over others (Armstrong et al., 2001; Coburn, 2006; Raphael, 2001). The dimensions of political ideology, political power, and class interests in the public policy process are therefore key components of a political economy approach. Political economy considers the impact of the capitalist economic system on health and recognizes that it thrives on inequalities between groups. The business and corporate sector exerts considerable influence on the public policy process. When applied to health issues, the approach considers how the capitalist economic and political systems shape health outcomes and inequalities in health among people of differing groups (i.e. social class, gender, and race), geographic areas and even different societies.

The role of political ideology in enabling and justifying the extent of State intervention in the market to ensure provision of such public goods as health care and employment to citizens is a critical element of a political economy focus. Political ideology is a set of ideas identifying societal problems and how these should be addressed. It is therefore critical in shaping government decisions on whether to recognize issues, and whether to intervene to address an issue or set of issues. In terms of the present analysis, these decisions would determine whether a government should develop public policies to strengthen the social determinants of health and make their distribution more equitable. In other words, the ideological commitments of governments strongly influence the timing and content of health promotion-related public policy initiatives, as well as the nature of the public policy process itself in terms of preliminary discussion through to the decision on whether to act and what form government action will take.

In short, political ideology shapes the receptivity of governmental authorities to the social determinants of health concept, and to evidence on the impact of the social determinants on the health of populations. In the case of Canada, resistance to government involvement in addressing the living and working conditions that shape health has been buttressed by increasing adherence to neo-liberal ideology. This political ideology and its adherents may work to prevent some issues such as health promotion (WHO, 2009), the social determinants of health (CSDH, 2008), and health inequalities from getting on the public policy agenda (Hofrichter, 2006). A political economy approach and related frameworks do not consider the presence of social and health inequalities as inevitable. Rather, social and health inequalities are considered to be a socially created phenomenon—arising from a capitalist economic system—that can be reduced through public policy. One of these related frameworks—welfare state analysis—captures these concerns and can explain differences in State social provision and action on the social determinants of health and health promotion among wealthy nations.

Welfare state analysis

From a political economy perspective, Esping-Andersen devised a theory of welfare state development in wealthy industrialized nations (Esping-Andersen, 1990). His research identified three clusters of welfare state regimes based on the extent and type of societal stratification and State involvement in social provision: social democratic, conservative, and liberal. These clusters are differentiated on the degree to which citizens are stratified by class and status and can be independent of engagement in paid employment yet still receive public goods and services (decommodification). If the market is the dominant institution, then societal goods and services are largely commodified such that they need to be purchased (commodification). In such conditions, the State is less involved in social provision. The regimes form a continuum, the two extremes being a comprehensive welfare state (social democratic) and a residual welfare state (liberal).

The Nordic countries (Denmark, Finland, Norway, and Sweden) are social democratic welfare regimes that provide cradle-to-grave support to citizens and have the lowest extent of stratification and the highest degree of decommodification among welfare state clusters (Esping-Andersen, 1990). This is because the State is the primary institution responsible for providing a full range of public goods and supports that include numerous universally available social and health programmes such as child care, home care for seniors, unemployment insurance, and pensions. Conservative regimes (Belgium, France, Germany, Luxembourg, Netherlands, and Switzerland)—also termed corporatist or familist regimes—are midway between liberal and social democratic welfare state regimes in their provision of public goods and social supports. While not as generous in their provision of these public goods and services as social democratic regimes, conservative regimes provide more security to citizens than liberal regimes. They have class- and occupation-related social insurance schemes that manage risks such as unemployment, illness, and disability. The family is seen as the primary institution supporting citizens.

Liberal regimes (Australia, Canada, the United Kingdom, and the United States) have as their primary institution the economic marketplace (Esping-Andersen, 1990). As such, the State provides modest support to citizens and most of these support programmes have strict eligibility requirements. The aim of these programmes is to meet the immediate needs of the most disadvantaged citizens and to discourage dependency. There is little attempt to reduce stratification or poverty. The extent of decommodification in liberal regimes is the lowest among the three types of welfare regimes and state supports are usually seen as providing for the most basic needs of those without economic resources. In other words, such programmes tend to be targeted at those most in need.

As suggested by the classification of the regimes, these different orientations to social provision among the social democratic, conservative, and liberal welfare regimes are driven by political and ideological commitments of governments. They have their origins in governance by political parties identified respectively as Social Democratic, Conservative, and Liberal. A number of studies have been carried out applying Esping-Andersen's welfare typology. For example, Navarro and Shi examined the impact of political parties on the degree of inequality in a country, the size and coverage of the welfare state, the employment/unemployment rate, and the health status of the population (Navarro and Shi, 2001). Political party was used as a proxy for political ideology, by which they considered the impact of the dominant political traditions in Organisation for Economic Co-operation and Development (OECD) countries during the immediate post-Second World War period (1945–1980) on health indicators of life expectancy and infant mortality, among others. As noted by Clavier and de Leeuw in Chapter 1 of this volume, social democratic parties emerged as most committed to redistributive policies, and as most successful in reducing health inequalities. In particular, they experienced the highest reductions in infant mortality over the last 50 years. Indeed, social democratic countries had the highest redistributive effect of the State and highest union density (workers belonging to unions or job associations). Subsequent studies have shown a similar pattern (see Muntaner et al., 2006). Although the social democratic (Scandinavian) countries have experienced increases in inequality since 2008, these are modest compared to the degree of inequality in liberal countries such as Canada.

Figure 4.1 shows the Gini coefficients for representative social democratic, conservative, and liberal welfare states. The Gini coefficient is a measure of inequality (OECD, 2011a), showing the degree to which income is distributed equally across the population. As such, it is an excellent indicator of gaps between the rich and poor in a country. The Gini coefficient ranges from 0 (which means no inequality) to 1 (which means one person owns all the wealth in a country).

The social democratic welfare states had lower inequality in 2000 compared to the conservative and liberal nations, but some experienced increased inequality during the first half of the 2000s. By 2009, inequality had increased in three of the four Nordic countries, with the most notable increases occurring in Denmark and Sweden. Inequality rose in Norway from 0.252 in 2000 to 0.275 in 2005, and fell to 0.247 by 2009. In Sweden, the coefficient of inequality fell from 0.244 in 2000 to 0.241 in 2005, only to rise to 0.261 by 2009.

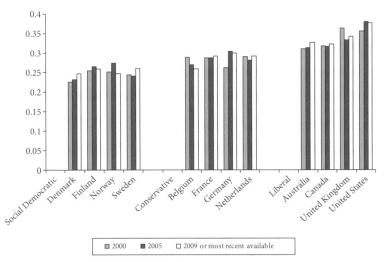

Figure 4.1 Gini coefficients for selected OECD countries, 2000 to 2009 or most recent available
Source: Data from Organization for Economic Cooperation and Development (OECD), *Divided We Stand: Why Inequality Keeps Rising*, OECD Publishing, Copyright © 2011.

Increased income inequality in the Nordic countries may be attributable to political shifts in the national governments in these countries. For example, Sweden, which experienced a notable increase in inequality between 2000 and 2009, has seen a shift in the governmental majority from the left Social Democratic Party to a centre-right party known as the Moderate Party, currently the largest party in the centre-right government. This ideological shift has led to the implementation of some market mechanisms such as an augmented role for private providers in health care. Some see this debate about increasing the role of the private sector in health care as an opportunity to restore health equity to the public agenda (Backhans and Burstromg, 2012).

In spite of these changes, there continues to be broad public support for the Swedish welfare state, which is considered to be one of the most generous. Some see the shift to a centre-right party as temporary; even then the effects of these political shifts are attenuated by the presence of proportional representation, whereby even defeated political parties such as the Social Democratic Party maintain influence on public policy-making. This electoral system allows more political parties—especially left-leaning and small ones—to influence public policy development even when they are not the dominant political party. It is no coincidence that liberal welfare states such as Canada, the US, and the UK do not have this type of electoral system.

Similarly, Norway has a social democratic regime described as committed to solidarity and universalism and to the redistribution of resources among different groups in society (Fosse, 2012). The Norwegian welfare state gives direct transfers to children and provides the conditions to enable women with children to participate in paid employment. Norway has also scored the highest rank on the UN Health Development Index for a number of years. The commitment to universalism and State social and health provision reflects the influence of social democracy in both Norway and Sweden. Nevertheless, some social democratic regimes such as Sweden and Denmark have succumbed to the pressures discussed in the following sections (OECD, 2011b).

In contrast, the Canadian welfare state, in addition to historically providing relatively fewer public goods and social support programmes typical of liberal welfare states, has seen the ratcheting back of even these State provisions since the late 1970s (see Box 4.1). This reduction in federal government transfers for social provision has occurred in tandem with a reluctance to adopt health promotion and the social determinants of health concepts by Canadian governments of all political stripes.

Health promotion and social determinants of health in Canada

Health promotion is a broad term that refers to improving the health of communities and populations (WHO, 1986). Health is defined broadly as a resource for living. Among its many aims, health promotion is about enabling people to act on the social determinants of health to improve health. A key development in health promotion has been the recognition of how social structures and public policy influence the health of populations as

Box 4.1 The rise and fall of the Canadian welfare state

Following the Second World War, the Canadian federal government sought to establish the administrative and financial frameworks for State provision of a broad range of social and health services and programmes in order to improve the welfare of Canadian citizens (Cohen and Pulkingham, 2009). As in other rich, developed countries, Canada initiated a number of social reforms, including the creation of the Canada Pension Plan, unemployment insurance, and Medicare, Canada's public health care programme.

A cornerstone of the welfare state was the Canada Assistance Plan (CAP). Established in 1966, the CAP provided the foundation for cost-sharing between the federal and provincial governments to support a broad range of services and programmes associated with the Canadian welfare state. These included health care, children's services, social assistance, disability allowances, old age security, services for seniors, and institutional care. The 1950s and 1960s marked the period of expanded State intervention in the Canadian economy to ensure the welfare and security of the population. By the end of the 1970s, the Canadian welfare state was beginning to unravel as the federal and provincial governments reconsidered their financial commitments, and focused on reducing deficits.

In 1996, the Liberal Finance Minister Paul Martin replaced the CAP with the Canada Health and Social Transfer (CHST) (Cohen and Pulkingham, 2009). The CHST signified a shift to block funding for health and social programmes. It was funded by a transfer of tax points from the federal government to the provinces and a cash transfer (Pulkingham and Ternowetsky, 1996).

In 2004, the federal government and provincial and territorial governments agreed to create two new transfers—the Canada Health Transfer (CHT) and the Canada Social Transfer (CST) (Department of Finance Canada, 2012). The aim was to ensure transparency and accountability of federal contributions to the provinces and territories. In 2011, the federal government announced its intention to allow the CHT to increase at 6% per year until fiscal year 2016–2017. The CHT will rise consistent with a three-year moving average of nominal gross domestic product (GDP) growth, with funding to increase by a minimum 3% per year, and will increase at its current rate of 3% annually in fiscal year 2014–2015, and beyond. These changes to federal transfers will contribute to further privatization of health care (Walkom, 2012).

The CHT and CST were followed by the Social Union Framework Agreement (SUFA). The SUFA changed the level of funding and the capacity to have national standards to govern the quality of social programmes in each of the provinces. Specifically, it reduced funding and the ability to enforce national standards; this ensured that all Canadians received similar access and treatment, regardless of where they live. In international comparisons, Canada has among the lowest expenditures

(Continued)

Box 4.1 (Continued)

on health and social programmes, and among the fastest growing rates of social and health inequalities among rich countries (OECD, 2011d).

All these changes occurred in conjunction with increasing globalization of the world's economies since the mid-1970s. National governments in Canada and elsewhere have reduced social and health spending to ensure their competitiveness in the new global economy (Bakker, 1996). This has contributed to the decline of the Canadian welfare state. Indeed, the changes in social welfare and health are being shifted away from collective responsibility and redistribution of income and other resources towards making individualized citizens take control of their own affairs.

a whole and of particular vulnerable populations such as women and people of colour, among others (Raphael, 2008a). Intrinsic to this concept is the importance of providing individuals with the prerequisites of health (e.g. shelter, education, food, and income) as the welfare state was intended to do. Tied to this is the idea that individuals and communities can change their environment by initiating activities that enhance their control over the determinants of health (Nutbeam, 1998). More recently, the term 'social determinants of health' replaced the term 'prerequisites of health' in public health discourse. The focus is now on societal conditions that shape health. Consistent with the development of the prerequisites of health concept, the social determinants of health concept also calls for the development of healthy public policy to address the health-promoting needs of citizens.

From the early 1970s through to the early 1990s, Canada contributed to emergent understandings of the social determinants and health promotion concepts. The Canadian government's Lalonde Report, *A New Perspective on the Health of Canadians*, identified social environments as having a significant influence on health (Lalonde, 1974). Although governments and public health practitioners in Canada generally focused on the health behaviours discussed in the report, it was seen by some as launching a new era in public health in which health was conceived as broader than biomedical and epidemiological definitions and categories (Restrepo, 2000). The report seemed to embrace societal factors as having a role in shaping health, but still emphasized lifestyle and behavioural factors such as diet and exercise as fundamentally shaping the health of populations (Labonte, 1997). Public health agencies and federal and provincial government ministries of health seized upon lifestyle and behavioural factors to address health as these were seen as factors over which people had control and could change to improve their health (Legowski and McKay, 2000).

Another Canadian government report, the Epp Report, *Achieving Health for All: A Framework for Health Promotion*, asserted that reducing health inequalities could be achieved by strengthening income security, employment, education, and housing, among others (Epp, 1986). This report was released at the same time as the Ottawa

Charter for Health Promotion (WHO, 1986). Both the Lalonde and Epp reports made important statements about health promotion and how it can improve the health of populations.

The Epp and—to some degree—Lalonde reports identified broad policy themes that were consistent with emerging health promotion concepts (Bryant et al., 2011; Raphael, 2008a). These themes helped to lay the groundwork for further government action to promote the health of the Canadian population at a national level, and at provincial and city levels of government. The take-up and implementation of these concepts occurred primarily at the municipal government level. Indeed, city governments and communities worked in earnest through the 1980s and 1990s to implement healthy communities approaches to improve the health of populations and promote public engagement on these issues in the political realm. Guided by the work of Trevor Hancock and Ronald Labonte, among others (Hancock and Duhl, 1986; Labonte, 1993), communities mobilized around issues such as environmental health (e.g. removing environmental toxins, closing incinerators to improve air quality), or social issues such as poverty, and worked to influence city governments to bring about positive change.

Much work was accomplished in Toronto, Canada, under the leadership of Jack Layton as chair of the Toronto Board of Public Health during the 1980s and early 1990s. During this period, Toronto City Council established a Healthy City Office. This helped to bring together diverse neighbourhood organizations and sectors to build healthy neighbourhoods in Toronto through projects and other activities. In fact, Toronto is often identified as the 'birthplace' of the Healthy Cities movement (Hancock and Duhl, 1986; Raphael, 2008a). Toronto became an exemplar of healthy communities' activities for other jurisdictions wishing to build healthier communities. These represented significant developments in furthering a health promotion agenda at the local municipal level. The federal and provincial governments introduced limited initiatives but remained focused on health care. The Toronto Healthy City Office later closed, the victim of funding cuts during the mid-1990s.

Canada established a public health care insurance programme in 1971 (Campbell and Marchildon, 2007). This popular social programme led to some reductions in income-related health inequalities, particularly for health conditions that are amenable to medical intervention. This may have contributed to the improved life expectancy of Canadians compared to Americans since the 1970s (James et al., 2007). Nevertheless, many health care-related equity issues remain. Canadians with low incomes face barriers to accessing specialist medical care when they need it, compared to high-income Canadians (McGibbon, 2008). In addition, Canadian Medicare does not cover some prescription medications or drugs, or some rehabilitation services. As a result, coverage of health care expenses and services provided under Canada's public health care system ranks among the lowest (70% of total costs) among member nations of the OECD (OECD, 2011b).

Movement away from health promotion

During the 1990s, there was a shift among governmental authorities from a 'health promotion' to a 'population health' perspective (Labonte, 1997; Raphael, 2008a; Robertson,

1998). Population health is seen as a competing and regressive health policy discourse, which is described as 'displacing' health promotion with respect to government departments, health policy discourse and rhetoric, and in the distribution of research funding (Raphael and Bryant, 2002; Robertson, 1998). Population health is seen as strongly epidemiologically focused and as depoliticizing health issues. It favours positivist approaches to knowledge to the exclusion of other knowledge approaches, and is rather silent on community involvement or participation in health issues (Raphael and Bryant, 2002). This in turn has contributed to an even greater focus on lifestyle and behavioural approaches to health by public health agencies and departments and among federal and provincial governments in Canada. It has also contributed to an individualization of responsibility for health (Orsini, 2007; Raphael, 2008a).

These shifts have coincided with the concern about controlling deficits among Canadian governments. Hancock equates the attention to population health as consistent with neo-liberal political discourse and governance and the attendant welfare state retrenchment in Canada (Hancock, 2011). Others have documented how these developments have resulted in Canada having one of the weakest national profiles in regard to provision of public goods and services, and being among the worst in terms of poverty rates and income inequality among wealthy developed nations (Bryant et al., 2011; Raphael, 2013b).

It should not be surprising that there is little evidence that health promotion and the social determinants of health discourse has influenced Canadian health policy (Collins and Hayes, 2007; Lavis, 1998; Lavis et al., 2003). The impact of population health has been to shift whatever enthusiasm existed for health promotion principles in universities and community organizations to applying epidemiological approaches to understanding health determinants. There is also less advocacy for public policy that promotes health and increased focus on research activities (Raphael, 2008a; Raphael and Bryant, 2002; Robertson, 1998). This shift is particularly evident in the changes to financing programmes associated with the welfare state, as illustrated in Box 4.1.

This trend has been reinforced by Canada's governing authorities' receptivity to neo-liberal ideology over the past few decades. As a result, health debates tend to be narrowly focused on health care as opposed to concern about income-driven health inequalities and implementing a health promotion agenda to address inequalities. The institutional arrangements that support such conditions are becoming increasingly entrenched, making it even more difficult to change course. Herein lie some of the philosophical or ideological inclinations that lead to resisting the social determinants and related issues to promote health equity.

Making sense of shifts: the impact of neo-liberalism

As welfare state analysis and Box 4.1 show, governments and their public policies result from the election of political parties that campaign on a public policy agenda reflecting their ideological commitments. These commitments can include focus on any number of issues, but in terms of the present analysis the question is whether their campaign agendas include issues related to the strengthening of the social determinants of health and making their distribution more equitable.

Political economists concerned with health outcomes and the factors that drive these kinds of outcome have increasingly focused on the role political ideology plays in these issues. Most recently, the focus has been on the impact of the political ideology of neo-liberalism on both health inequalities and the social inequalities that create them.

Neo-liberalism is a political ideology that promotes the market as the most efficient allocator of resources and supports reduced government intervention in the economy (Coburn, 2001). At one level, neo-liberalism provides the rationale for economic globalization. At a national level, its acceptance has contributed to trade deregulation and restructuring of labour markets, which have contributed to growing inequalities in income and wealth. These changes are justified as inevitable (Bakker, 1996). State regulation of the economy is therefore seen as an artificial impediment to the effective functioning of the market. It has also been associated with growing commodification of public goods and services. This is particularly the case in Canada, which has seen government provision of goods and services reduced and displaced to the market. Neo-liberalism justifies governments ratcheting back social and health programmes and adopting austerity measures as necessary to ensure competitiveness in the global economy.

Adoption of neo-liberalism as a governing imperative has been linked to higher rates of social and health inequalities including poverty rates, as seen in Canada and the other liberal welfare states (OECD, 2008; 2011a). Countries in which the market is already the primary institution—as in the liberal welfare states of Canada, the UK, and the US—are more receptive to neo-liberal ideas and have increased market/private sector roles in numerous areas including health care provision and public transit. In other areas such as employment security and unemployment benefits—and this is certainly the case in Canada—governments have reduced benefits and made eligibility for such benefits more restrictive (see Box 4.1). The impact of neo-liberalism is especially evident in the health policy field (see Box 4.2). The federal and provincial governments have adjusted housing policy, thereby making it difficult for low-income households to access affordable rental accommodation in major Canadian cities such as Vancouver and Toronto.

In liberal nations such as Canada, the sources of these shifts are seen as reflecting resurgent business and corporate sectors that see little need to balance their interests with those of other societal sectors such as the labour movement and groups associated with civil society (Langille, 2009). In addition, union density in Canada has remained at less than 30% since the late 1990s (OECD, 2011c). Declining union density reflects the diminished power of the labour movement and the resurgence of business and corporate interests. Corporate class interests have exercised considerable influence in shifting governments towards neo-liberal ideas and public policies. For example, the Canadian Council of Chief Executive Officers was instrumental in getting free trade on the national public policy agenda (Langille, 2009). The negotiation of the Free Trade

Box 4.2 Case study of housing as a social determinant of health in Canada

The Ottawa Charter identifies housing as a prerequisite of health (WHO, 1986). Access to quality and affordable housing is a key determinant of the health of populations. A housing crisis has brewed in Canada since the mid-1980s when homelessness began to grow exponentially in urban and rural areas across Canada. Recent federal and provincial housing policy changes since the 1990s have contributed to growing housing insecurity for many Canadian households.

Many critics attribute an increasing homeless population and insecurely housed Canadians to reduced State intervention in the housing sector (Shapcott, 2009). During the 1990s, the federal, provincial, and territorial governments reduced funding and programmes to build new social housing. As a result, there is increased reliance on private rental housing and ownership markets to provide housing for Canadians. The 2009 federal stimulus budget set Canada on a path of declining transfers for social housing. In addition, the province of Ontario was the site of radical housing policy changes. In 1995, the provincial government reversed 25 years of Ontario governments' commitment to ensuring an affordable private rental market for modest- and low-income households.

These policy changes led to modest- and low-income households spending significant proportions of their incomes on housing (Bryant, 2008). Indeed, the Canada Mortgage and Housing Corporation (CMHC) identifies housing affordability as a critical issue, especially for renter households (Engeland et al., 2005). Many Canadian households spend more than 30% of their incomes on housing. Research shows that such insecurity has damaging effects on the health of children and adults, with many developing chronic health conditions (CMHC, 2003; Marsh et al., 1999; Shaw, 2001; Shaw et al., 1999).

Agreement between Canada and the US, and later the North American Free Trade Agreement signed by Canada, the US, and Mexico, reflect the influence of the Council in steering the national public policy agenda (Grieshaber-Otto and Sinclair, 2004). These agreements led to trade deregulation and labour market restructuring in Canada, such as the proliferation of precarious employment. These changes have occurred at the same time as the shift from health promotion to population health.

The federal government promised to negotiate provisions to protect Canadian Medicare, but many trade authorities consider these provisions to be inadequate (Grieshaber-Otto and Sinclair, 2004). More disturbingly, the free trade agreements led to increasingly precarious employment for many Canadians, particularly women and populations of colour, and growing income-related health inequality (Block, 2010; Curry-Stevens, 2008; Galabuzi, 2005). The greater concern among the progressive community in Canada about preserving Canadian Medicare has directed attention away from growing income inequalities and the concomitant health inequalities, and from the need to focus on health-promoting public policies to address the social determinants of health.

Implications for health promotion and social determinants of health

These developments cannot be attributed to a lack of awareness or understanding of the social determinants and health promotion by Canadian governments. Rather, they can be located in the political economy of Canada and understood within the context of how governments decide whether to provide citizens with public goods and services, and of the political will to act on these issues. The actions of Canadian governments must be understood as deliberate decisions to privilege some interests over others, driven by ideological commitments.

When considering the differences among wealthy developed nations, a distinction has been made between liberal market economies and social market economies (Pontusson, 2005). Esping-Andersen's welfare state typology shows the continuum of coverage provided by social democratic, conservative, and liberal welfare regimes. Pontusson's distinction between liberal market economies and social market economies accentuates the differences especially between social democratic and conservative states and liberal welfare states.

In this taxonomy, the social democratic Nordic nations and the conservative regimes are combined in a single cluster, with the liberal regimes as a separate cluster. These clusters differentiate between those countries that attempt to manage the operation of the economy (social market economies) and those that do not (liberal). The primary difference between conservative and social democratic regimes is in their approach to gender equity issues and tax-supported (social democratic) as opposed to contributory, social insurance-based (conservative) provision of public goods and services (Pontusson, 2005). This is a useful distinction when considering how Canada's political economy shapes its public policy approaches towards the social determinants of health.

The liberal market economies are characterized by lower levels of intervention in the economy, which is associated with lower levels of attention to the provision of public goods and services to citizens (Esping-Andersen, 1990; 2002; Teeple, 2000). Lower levels of such provision are associated with higher levels of commodification of resources, which are associated with lower-quality social determinants of health (Menahem, 2010). Since commodification refers to the state in which citizens are reliant on their incomes and the market to obtain basic goods and services, the social market economies tend towards decommodifying (higher State intervention in social provision) the resources associated with the social determinants of health. The State provides them as entitlements of citizenship. This distinction helps to explicate recent public policy trends in Canada that have resulted in retrenchment of the welfare state and growing income-driven health inequalities.

There has been debate about the validity of these kinds of welfare state typology. Nevertheless, while Bambra identified 12 welfare state typologies, in six of the seven typologies in which Canada is included, it is identified with a liberal welfare state-type cluster variously named as minimal or basic security, liberal, or Anglo-Saxon (Bambra, 2005). The only dimension in which Canada appears in the conservative cluster is in health care provision.

Indeed, health care is one of the few social policy programmes that has remained relatively intact over the past few decades, although the federal government has reduced its transfers or contributions to the provincial and territorial governments over the years. The reduced federal contributions have been a point of contention between the federal and provincial governments. Reduced federal transfers have placed more financial burden for health care on provincial governments. This has in turn contributed to provincial governments choosing market mechanisms such as an expanded private sector role for delivering health care. These mechanisms include using public–private partnerships (P3s) to build hospitals, highways, and other public resources, and expanding private sector involvement in health care delivery (Canadian Health Coalition, 2009).

More recently, however, the federal government pledged to increase its health care transfers to the provinces by 6% until fiscal year 2016–2017 (Walkom, 2012). Thereafter, any increases will be tied to economic growth, including inflation, by about 4% and will not fall below 3%. Such choices are consistent with a liberal welfare state because this initiative will limit future federal contributions to provincial health care programmes. This may well undermine Canadian Medicare, as provincial governments may increasingly turn to privatization schemes to finance health care. This will reduce access to health care, particularly for low-income populations. It is also likely to mean no action on the social determinants of health, since the federal and provincial governments are focused on health care.

Welfare state analyses show a strong relationship between the public policy choices of government and action/inaction on the social determinants of health (Raphael, 2013a; 2013b). These choices are strongly influenced by the ideological commitments of governments. Neo-liberalism is the dominant ideology in Canada: Canadian federal and provincial governments support its claims to promote economic growth and better manage the economy. It emphasizes freedom from government (Ham and Hill, 1984), or less government intervention, and thus provides the rationale for reduced social and health spending. The ideological commitments of governments strongly influence their will to take action on the social determinants of health and health inequalities. For example, Canada's social spending is 17% of GDP compared to 27% in Sweden and 28% in France (OECD, 2011d). Its health spending is 8% of GDP, which falls below the OECD average of 9%. Countries with higher social spending tend to have more equal income distribution.

Next steps for health promotion practitioners

A political economy analysis suggests that there is value in bringing public health and social and other citizen movements together to mobilize the Canadian public around a health promotion agenda. An engaged citizenry is considered essential to helping to bring about policy change to realize a health promotion agenda to reduce social and health inequalities.

Health promotion practitioners, many of whom work in public health departments, need to work closely with social and health movements to help communities in their efforts to address issues that impact their health. This will involve engaging local communities—as was accomplished with some success during the 1980s and 1990s with the commitment of Toronto City Council and the Board of Health—to implement healthy communities initiatives. This will create opportunities to recognize how health behaviours interact with and are shaped by the broader social, economic, and political context in which people live (Orsini, 2007).

Health promotion practitioners need to be mindful of these interactions and to concentrate their efforts on working with and focusing on communities, rather than on changing individual health behaviours. This will require public health departments to recognize the role of social determinants and to identify ways that they can intervene to improve the health of populations. Fundamentally, this focus will need to draw on a broader range of evidence beyond epidemiological studies to include qualitative studies and social science research on income-related health inequalities and health, for example, to help to guide action. These should include collaborative activities with communities. It will also need to bring receptive ministries and departments of federal and provincial governments into the discussion and press for shifting investments to strengthen social determinants of health.

Conclusion

This chapter has applied a political economy perspective to explain the barriers to implementing health-promoting public policies to strengthen the social determinants of health. A particular focus was how the political ideology of governments strongly influences their receptivity to health promotion and the social determinants of health, and their willingness to implement health-promoting policies to improve the social determinants of health.

Since the 1970s, Canadian governments have published numerous reports on emergent health promotion and social determinants of health concepts, but their actions have lagged far behind their publications on these issues. Current health and social spending reflects little commitment to addressing the social determinants of health. In Canada, government resistance to health promotion concepts such as the social determinants of health is related to calls to weaken the Canadian welfare state and minimize government intervention in the market. Policy change to strengthen the social determinants requires a shift in government ideology to greater redistribution. This will require a mobilized and politically engaged citizenry to call for government action on the social determinants of health. As the welfare state analyses show, this will be a particular problem in liberal welfare states such as Canada. Yet such commitment in social democratic governments will also require ongoing citizen action to safeguard the advances already made.

A political economy analysis of these issues highlights the role of political ideology in shaping the public policy choices of government, or the State. Political ideological commitments determine whether governments will apply health promotion and social determinants of health concepts in the service of supporting health and reducing social and health inequalities.

In Canada, the marginalizing of a health promotion agenda since the 1990s reflects the neo-liberal commitments of Canadian governments and the lack of political will to improve the health of the Canadian population. These same forces are present elsewhere but have been more actively resisted than is the case in Canada. In all countries, public health practitioners must recognize these developments. They must forge and nurture partnerships with communities to resist these health-threatening forces. By working with communities on issues that communities identify as affecting their health, the factors can be identified and means of resisting them in the service of health implemented (Bryant et al., 2007).

References

Armstrong, P., Armstrong, H., and Coburn, D. (eds.) (2001). *Unhealthy Times: The Political Economy of Health and Care in Canada*. Toronto: Oxford University Press.

Backhans, M. C. and Burstromg, B. (2012). Swedish experiences, in D. Raphael (ed.) *Tackling Health Inequalities: Lessons from International Experiences*, pp. 209–228, Toronto: Canadian Scholars' Press.

Bakker, I. (1996). Introduction: the gendered foundations of restructuring in Canada, in I. Bakker (ed.) *Rethinking Restructuring: Gender and Change in Canada*, pp. 3–25, Toronto: University of Toronto Press.

Bambra, C. (2005). Worlds of welfare and the health care discrepancy. *Social Policy and Society*, **4**, 31–41.

Baumgartner, F. R. and Jones, B. D. (1993). *Agendas and Instability in American Politics*. Chicago, IL: University of Chicago Press.

Block, S. (2010). *Ontario's growing gap: the role of race and gender*. Ottawa: Canadian Centre for Policy Alternatives.

Bryant, T. (2008). Housing and health: more than bricks and mortar, in D. Raphael (ed.) *Social Determinants of Health: Canadian Perspectives*, pp. 235–249, Toronto: Canadian Scholars' Press.

Bryant, T., Raphael, D., and Travers, R. (2007). Identifying and strengthening the structural roots of urban health: participatory policy research and the urban health agenda. *Promotion and Education*, **14** (1), 6–11.

Bryant, T., Raphael, D., Schrecker, T., and Labonte, R. (2011). Canada: A land of missed opportunity for addressing the social determinants of health. *Health Policy*, **101** (1), 44–58.

Campbell, B. and Marchildon, G. P. (eds.) (2007). *Medicare: Facts, Myths, Problems and Promise*. Toronto: James Lorimer.

Canadian Health Coalition (2009). P3s=Private profits, public pays, *Medicare Privatization*, March 2009, Ottawa: Canadian Health Coalition.

CMHC (2003). *Housing Quality and Children's Socio-emotional Health*. Ottawa: Canada Mortgage and Housing Corporation.

Coburn, D. (2001). Health, health care, and neo-liberalism, in **P. Armstrong**, **H. Armstrong** and **D. Coburn** (eds.) *Unhealthy Times: The Political Economy of Health and Care in Canada*, pp. 45–65, Toronto: Oxford University Press.

Coburn, D. (2006). Health and health care: a political economy perspective, in **D. Raphael**, **T. Bryant** and **M. Rioux** (eds.), *Staying Alive: Critical Perspectives on Health, Illness, and Health Care*, (1st edn.), pp. 59–84, Toronto: Canadian Scholars' Press.

Coburn, D. (2010). Health and health care: a political economy perspective, in **T. Bryant**, **D. Raphael** and **M. Rioux** (eds.) *Staying Alive: Critical Perspectives on Health, Illness, and Health Care*, (2nd edn.), pp. 65–92, Toronto: Canadian Scholars' Press.

Cohen, M. G. and Pulkingham, J. (2009). Introduction: going too far? Feminist public policy in Canada, in **M. G. Cohen** and **J. Pulkingham** (eds.) *Public Policy for Women: The State, Income Security, and Labour Market Issues*, pp. 3–48, Toronto: University of Toronto.

Collins, P. and Hayes, M. (2007). Twenty years since Ottawa and Epp: Researchers' reflections on challenges, gains, and future prospects for reducing health inequities in Canada. *Health Promotion International*, **22** (4), 337–45.

CSDH (2008). *Closing the Gap in a Generation. Health Equity through Action on the Social Determinants of Health. Final Report of the Commission on Social Determinants of Health*. Geneva: World Health Organization.

Curry-Stevens, A. (2008). When economic growth doesn't trickle down: the wage dimensions of income polarization, in **D. Raphael** (ed.) *Social Determinants of Health*, pp. 41–60, Toronto: Canadian Scholars' Press.

Department of Finance Canada (2012). *A History of the Health and Social Transfers*. Ottawa: Department of Finance Canada.

Engeland, J., Lewis, R., Ehrlich, S., and Che, J. (2005). *Evolving Housing Conditions in Canada's Census Metropolitan Areas, 1991–2001*. Ottawa: Statistics Canada and Canada Morgage and Housing Corporation.

Epp, J. (1986). *Achieving Health for All: A Framework for Health Promotion*. Ottawa: Health and Welfare Canada.

Esping-Andersen, G. (1990). *The Three Worlds of Welfare Capitalism*. Princeton, NJ: Princeton University Press.

Esping-Andersen, G. (ed.) (2002). *Why we Need a New Welfare State*. Oxford: Oxford University Press.

Fosse, E. (2012). Norwegian experiences, in **D. Raphael** (ed.) *Tackling Health Inequalities: Lessons from International Experiences*, pp. 185–208, Toronto: Canadian Scholars' Press.

Galabuzi, G. E. (2005). *Canada's Economic Apartheid: The Social Exclusion of Racialized Groups in the New Century*. Toronto: Canadian Scholars' Press.

Graham, H. (2004). Social determinants and their unequal distribution: clarifying policy understandings. *Milbank Quarterly*, **82** (1), 101–24.

Graham, H. (2007). *Unequal Lives: Health and Socioeconomic Inequalities*. New York: Open University Press.

Grieshaber-Otto, J. and Sinclair, S. (2004). *Bad Medicine: Trade Treaties, Privatization and Health Care Reform in Canada*. Ottawa: Canadian Centre for Policy Alternatives.

Ham, C. and Hill, M. (1984). *The Policy Process in the Modern Capitalist State*. Brighton: Wheatsheaf Books Ltd.

Hancock, T. (2011). Health promotion in Canada: 25 years of unfulfilled promise. *Health Promotion International*, **26** (Suppl. 2), ii263–ii267.

Hancock, T. and Duhl, L. (1986). *Healthy Cities: Promoting Health in the Urban Context.* Copenhagen: WHO Regional Office for Europe.

Hofrichter, R. (ed.) (2006). *Tackling Health Inequalities Through Public Health Practice.* The National Association of County and City Health Officials and the Ingham County Health Department: Washington DC and Lansing MI.

James, P. D., Wilkins, R., Detsky, A. S., Tugwell, P., and Manuel, D. G. (2007). Avoidable mortality by neighbourhood income in Canada: 25 years after the establishment of universal health insurance. *Journal of Epidemiology and Community Health*, **61**, 287–296.

Labonte, R. (1993). *Health Promotion and Empowerment: Practice Frameworks.* Toronto: Centre for Health Promotion and ParicipAction.

Labonte, R. (1997). The population health/health promotion debate in Canada: the politics of explanation, economics and action. *Critical Public Health*, **7** (1 & 2), 7–27.

Lalonde, M. (1974). *A New Perspective on the Health of Canadians: A Working Document.* Ottawa: Health and Welfare Canada.

Langille, D. (2009). Follow the money: how business and politics shape our health, in **D. Raphael** (ed.) *Social Determinants of Health: Canadian Perspectives*, pp. 305–17, Toronto: Canadian Scholars' Press.

Lavis, J. (1998). *Ideas, Policy Learning and Policy Change: The Determinants-of-Health Synthesis in Canada and the United Kingdom.* Hamilton, ON: MacMaster University, Centre for Health Economics and Policy Analysis (CHEPA).

Lavis, J., Ross, S., Stoddard, G., Hohenadel, J., McLeod, C., and Evans, R. (2003). Do Canadian civil servants care about the health of populations? *American Journal of Public Health*, **93** (4), 658–63.

Legowski, B. and McKay, L. (2000). *Health beyond Health Care: Twenty-five Years of Federal Health Policy Development.* Ottawa: Canadian Policy Research Networks (CPRN).

Lupton, D. (1999). *Risk.* London: Routledge.

McGibbon, E. (2008). Health and health care: a human rights perspective, in **D. Raphael** (ed.) *Social Determinants of Health: Canadian Perspectives*, pp. 318–35, Toronto: Canadian Scholars' Press.

Marsh, A., Gordon, D., Pantazis, C., and Heslop, P. (1999). *Home Sweet Home? The Impact of Poor Housing on Health.* Bristol: Policy Press.

Menahem, G. (2010). *How Can The Decommodified Security Ratio Assess Social Protection Systems?* LIS Working Paper No. 529. Syracuse, NY: Luxembourg Income Study.

Muntaner, C., Borrell, C., Kunst, A., Chung, H., Benach, J., and Ibrahim, S. (2006). Social class inequalities in health: does welfare state regime matter?, in **D. Raphael**, **T. Bryant** and **M. Rioux** (eds.) *Staying Alive: Critical Perspectives on Health, Illness, and Health Care* (1st edn.), pp. 139–58, Toronto: Canadian Scholars' Press: Toronto.

Navarro, V. and Shi, L. (2001). The political context of social inequalities and health. *Social Science & Medicine*, **52** (3), 481–91.

Nutbeam, D. (1998). Evaluating health promotion—progress, problems, and solutions. *Health Promotion International*, **13**, 27–44.

OECD (2008). *Growing Unequal: Income Distribution and Poverty in OECD Nations.* Paris: OECD Publishing.

OECD (2011a). *Divided we Stand: Why Inequality Keeps Rising.* Paris: OECD Publishing.

OECD (2011b). *Health at a Glance: OECD Indicators 2011 Edition.* Paris: OECD Publishing.

OECD (2011c). Labour force statistics: population and labour force, OECD employment and labour market statistics (database). Paris: OECD Publishing.

OECD (2011d). *Society at a Glance, 2011.* Paris: OECD Publishing.

Orsini, M. (2007). Discourses in distress: from 'health promotion' to 'population health' to 'you are responsible for your own health', in **M. Orsini** and **M. Smith** (eds.) *Critical Policy Studies*, pp. 347–63, Vancouver: UBC Press.

Pontusson, J. (2005). *Inequality and Prosperity: Social Europe versus Liberal America*. Ithaca, NY: Cornell University Press.

Pulkingham, J. and Ternowetsky, G. (1996). The changing landscape of social policy and the Canadian State, in **J. Pulkingham** and **G. Ternowetsky** (eds.) *Remaking Canadian Social Policy: Social Security in the Late 1990s*, pp. 2–29, Halifax: Fernwood Publishing.

Raphael, D. (2001). From increasing poverty to societal disintegration: how economic inequality affects the health of individuals and communities, in **H. Armstrong**, **P. Armstrong** and **D. Coburn** (eds.) *Unhealthy Times: The Political Economy of Health and Care in Canada*, pp. 224–46, Toronto: Oxford University Press.

Raphael, D. (2008a). Grasping at straws: a recent history of health promotion in Canada. *Critical Public Health*, **18** (4), 483–95.

Raphael, D. (2008b). Introduction to the social determinants of health, in **D. Raphael** (ed.) *Social Determinants of Health: Canadian Perspectives*, pp. 2–19, Toronto: Canadian Scholars' Press.

Raphael, D. (2008c). Public policy and population health in the USA: Why is the public health community missing in action? *International Journal of Health Services*, **38**, 63–94.

Raphael, D. (2013a). The political economy of health promotion: part 1, national commitments to provision of the prerequisites of health. *Health Promotion International*, **28** (1), 95–111.

Raphael, D. (2013b). The political economy of health promotion: part 2, national provision of the prerequisites of health. *Health Promotion International*, **28** (1), 112–32.

Raphael, D. and Bryant, T. (2002). The limitations of population health as a model for a new public health. *Health Promotion International*, **17**, 189–99.

Restrepo, H. E. (2000). Introduction, in **H. E. Restrepo** (ed.) *Health Promotion: An Anthology*, pp. ix–xi, Washington, DC: Pan American Health Organization.

Robertson, A. (1998). Shifting discourses on health in Canada: from health promotion to population health. *Health Promotion International*, **13**, 155–66.

Shapcott, M. (2009). Housing, in **D. Raphael** (ed.) *Social Determinants of Health: Canadian Perspectives*, pp. 221–34, Toronto: Canadian Scholars' Press.

Shaw, M. (2001). Health and housing: a lasting relationship. *Journal of Epidemiology and Community Health*, **55**, 291–6.

Shaw, M., Dorling, D., Gordon, D., and Smith, G. D. (1999). *The Widening Gap: Health Inequalities and Policy in Britain*. Bristol: Policy Press.

Teeple, G. (2000). *Globalization and the Decline of Social Reform: into the Twenty-First Century*. Aurora, ON: Garamond Press.

Walkom, T. (2012). Will any government stand up for medicare? *Toronto Star*, 18-01-12.

WHO (1986). *First International Conference on Health Promotion. The Ottawa Charter for Health Promotion*. Geneva: World Health Organization.

WHO (2009). *Milestones in Health Promotion: Statements from Global Conferences*, Geneva: World Health Organization.

Chapter 5

Actor–network theory: the governance of intersectoral initiatives

Louise Potvin and Carole Clavier

Introduction

Awareness of the widening gap in health status and well-being between the poor and better-off in society has become a central feature of health promotion discourse in the past two decades. Public authorities at all levels of government are gradually developing strategies and policies aimed at reducing social inequalities in health. However, such interventions are now confronted with a host of challenges. Some of these are more political in nature and require strategic choices to be made, based on epidemiological data, theory, and political values. For instance, some authors argue that to have the greatest and most enduring impact, policies must focus on the determinants of the inequalities, like income or place of residence, rather than on just the health disparities themselves (Frohlich et al., 2006). Other challenges pertain to implementation issues, including the functioning and governance of systems of action involved in these interventions. Of particular importance are the challenges of reaching a shared understanding of a given problem across policy sectors and social perspectives, of building a shared plan for addressing the problem, and of coordinating the strategies and resources of all actors and institutions involved.

Interventions to reduce social inequalities in health powerfully echo what other authors argue in this volume—namely, that health does not belong to any one actor or sector (Baum et al., Chapter 10; Clavier and de Leeuw, Chapter 1; de Leeuw and Breton, Chapter 2). Inequalities in health are the product of inequitable access to the resources and opportunities that constitute the major social determinants of health (Frohlich et al., 2006): income, education, and social support. Interventions to reduce these inequalities and provide equitable opportunities require the bringing together of actors from a variety of different policy sectors. However, such collaboration inevitably raises issues of influence, networking, and governance. Other chapters in this volume address the contribution of intersectoral networks (de Leeuw et al., Chapter 8) and the difficulties associated with the presence of actors from multiple sectors in the process leading to policy formulation (Baum et al., Chapter 10). This chapter takes a different stance: it examines the governance of such intersectoral programmes. The term governance, in this context, refers to the processes of coordinating multiple actors in order to work towards a shared goal (Rhodes, 1996). This examination focuses on the daily operations of partnerships and networks required to formulate or implement intersectoral programmes aimed at reducing social inequalities in health.

In the general area of public health, and more specifically in health promotion, the issue of partnership has been discussed mainly with regard to intersectoral action and participatory research. Advocates of intersectoral action frequently call on the health sector to establish operating partnerships with actors from other sectors. Apart from the recurrent use of the term 'network' to describe the flexibility and, more importantly, the horizontality of this style of coordinated action (Aubry and Bernier, 2012; Berghmans and Potvin, 2005; Bilodeau et al., 2011), the literature on intersectoral action provides few concepts to help us to understand how these partnerships operate and evolve. Moreover, although many studies on participatory research have conducted in-depth investigations of the arrangements and practices behind the co-production of knowledge, the literature skirts the issue of *how* these arrangements work to achieve their objectives, or *how* they can be efficiently coordinated (Cargo and Mercer, 2008).

Consider the case of a local public health organization that is attempting to partner with other local organizations to develop a set of objectives and a work plan for addressing locally relevant social determinants of health. Very early in the process, even before the issues to be addressed are identified, a host of questions arises. What organizations should be invited to join the partnership, and why? How many organizations should be invited? What should be the role of each organization, and what resources should each contribute to the partnership? What type of governance structure should be created to ensure the partnership's success?

In most cases, the answers to such questions are derived empirically through trial and error as the organizations start working together in intersectoral initiatives. It is our experience that because each partner comes from a different perspective with regard to the problem to be solved, and because each has its own specific interest in the situation, coordinating actions to achieve a shared goal invariably leads to controversies. While dealing with this challenge may lead to innovation, it may also lead to the dissolution of the partnership if partners decide the investment is too great given the expected outcomes. When is it time to disengage from a partnership? What are the conditions that support innovative solutions to disagreement?

We believe that such questions are an inherent part of intersectoral collaborative initiatives. Such initiatives do not operate like hierarchical organizations, that is, with a clear line of authority and a clearly articulated mission. Each partner's role, as well as the partnership's *raison d'être*, has to be negotiated among partners, often at the same time as the action is being planned and implemented. The term 'network' has often been used to describe the nature of these partnerships (Berghmans and Potvin, 2005). We believe that among the many theories for conceptualizing networks, actor–network theory (ANT), with its central concept of translation, provides a particularly promising framework for elucidating many of these issues. ANT provides a number of concepts and theoretical propositions, which we have explored and used to study interventions aimed at reducing social inequalities in health. In this chapter, we present the main concepts of ANT and show how we used them to develop a conceptualization of public health interventions as part of the research programme of the Chair on Community Approaches and Health Inequality (CACIS) (Aubry and Potvin, 2012). We show how we translated this conceptualization into research practices, giving examples of the research methods and tools that we designed for actors involved in partnership (or networked) situations. We then consider the utility and limitations of ANT for promoting reflection on such interventions.

ANT

ANT, or the sociology of translation, was developed over the past three decades, chiefly in social studies of technology. It has its origins in a landmark paper by Michel Callon (1986). In this study, Callon examined interactions between engineers, fishermen, and scallops in the Bay of Saint-Brieuc (France) in order to understand how engineers gained the support of both the fishermen and scallops in efforts to develop an innovative solution for shellfish farming in the region. The sociology of translation, as Callon labelled it, rests upon two central assumptions: first, innovation is the product of interactions and connections between previously unrelated entities, and of the alignment of interests between those entities; and second, non-human entities (including animals) are integral to, and influence, these interactions. Translation comprises four operations that are not necessarily sequential: problematization, interestment, enrolment, and displacement. These four operations will be described in detail later, under proposition 2.

The sociology of translation was subsequently clarified, named, and redefined several times over by its creators (Latour, 1987; 1999a; 2005). Bruno Latour was among the first to conduct systematic studies in the anthropology of science (Latour, 1987). Observing researchers at work in the laboratory, he argued that science is a social construction: scientific facts, such as the DNA triple helix, are not just data that are 'revealed' to an astute and passive observer. Rather, they are the outcome of work done by researchers using various devices that are themselves the product of scientific work. The work and practices of a researcher essentially consist in interrelating observations, as well as relating them to established knowledge. Scientific knowledge is built from these various observations and their networks of connections. The facts 'harden' over time as the connections within the networks that support them stabilize. What Latour (1987) calls 'translation' is the process of expanding and strengthening connections in the network, of aligning interests that were formerly disparate. In stabilized networks, translation tends to become less important and is therefore less used.

Although it is not a theory about public policy per se, ANT has been used in policy studies to make sense of the changing ideas underlying public policies. Researchers have used the concept of translation to follow the circulation of policy ideas from one social sphere to another, and to make sense of the adaptations and reinterpretations of these ideas as they circulate (Lascoumes, 1996; 2004). Policy studies—especially in France, where two of ANT's founders come from—have primarily borrowed the concept of translation from the early works of Callon (1986). For instance, the sociology of translation has been used to study actors who serve as mediators between institutions or between actors from different social spheres in public policy. Such actors have been defined as having the 'skills, resources and legitimacy to "translate" (following Callon) knowledge, skills and norms of legitimacy between social or organizational spheres that have to (or wish to) work together but have different frames of reference' (Nay and Smith, 2002: 14—our translation). The sociology of translation has also been used to analyse transnational policy dynamics and the transfer (and adaptation) of public policies from one country to another (Lendvai and Stubbs, 2007).

Other research fields besides social studies of technology and policy studies have also used ANT. The sociology of organizations and management has used it to open up the 'black box' of organizations and analyse how the organization functions as a set of organizational processes and practices (as opposed to an homogenous unit) (Alcadipani and Hassard, 2010). While ANT has been adapted to a variety of different research objects, its underlying purpose has remained the same: to follow the connections between all actors (human and non-human) involved in a given situation and to trace the circulation of the ideas and interests of these actors and the transformations of the network (Lascoumes, 2004). Therefore, ANT is particularly relevant to the study of intersectoral dynamics, whether the object of study is the interactions between actors or the ideas being formed. Applied to health promotion issues and interventions, ANT proves a very practical theory for understanding how interactions between actors from different sectors come to produce (or not) interventions to reduce social inequalities in health.

Case study

In this chapter, we describe how researchers and their partners have used ANT to make sense of intersectoral initiatives to reduce social health inequalities. The propositions presented here are derived from, and tested through, a decade-long research programme of CACIS. This was one of 12 initial Chairs funded by the Canadian Foundation for Health Services Research to foster partnerships between academic researchers and health organization decision-makers, and thereby increase the quality, relevance and use of health research (Aubry and Potvin, 2012).

Since its inception, CACIS has been designed as a partnership between university researchers and the Montreal Public Health Directorate (Potvin et al., 2002). The Chair's mission was to develop and implement a research programme to generate knowledge about the practices and programmes implemented by the Montreal Public Health Directorate to reduce social health inequalities. Once the research programme was underway, we quickly realized that the partnership should bring in other collaborators and partners of the Montreal Public Health Directorate. Regionally, the main partners were programme funders and policy-makers like the City of Montreal and its social development branches, the United Way of Greater Montreal and other charitable organizations, the regional offices of various ministries, elected representatives, and community organizations.

The Chair's main thrust was to develop research projects to accompany, and produce knowledge about, interventions and initiatives planned and implemented by this broad partnership. Very early in this ten-year research programme, the researchers felt the need to develop a framework that would support an understanding of the processes taking place in, and shaping, these partnerships. ANT emerged as the theory best suited to provide such a framework.

From the many concepts and principles developed by Callon, Latour and their colleagues over three decades of work, we formulated four specific propositions that helped us to understand and theorize the interventions we were studying. The first two are direct applications of ANT to intersectoral collaborations, whereas the other two were developed based on ANT to address issues specific to the governance and regulation of intersectoral initiatives.

1. Intersectoral interventions designed to reduce social inequalities in health are sociotechnical networks.

2. Actions in sociotechnical networks take place mainly through a translation process.

3. The governance of intersectoral initiatives requires that actors participate in a multidirectional translation process.

4. The regulation of these complex translation spaces requires specialized practices and tools.

Intersectoral initiatives as sociotechnical networks

In this section, we apply two propositions from ANT to illuminate the nature of intersectoral partnerships and how they work. We end with a presentation of two methodological innovations derived from these propositions.

Proposition 1. Intersectoral interventions designed to reduce social inequalities in health are sociotechnical networks.

Latour (2005) conceptualizes the sociotechnical network as a set of human and non-human entities connected within a network. ANT addresses the nature of the connected entities and the identity they derive from being connected through the network.

With respect to the entities composing the network, the term 'sociotechnical network' reflects an absence of distinction between human and non-human entities. Latour (1987) calls all these entities 'actants' In a sociotechnical network, human and non-human entities participate in symmetrical and reciprocal relationships, and all entities have the capacity to orient action in the network. Whereas the capacity of human beings to orient the action of non-human entities is usually obvious, the symmetrical proposition that non-human entities shape human actions is not self-evident. The notion of the sociotechnical network, however, emphasizes the mediating role of technology that is present in, and shapes, all human practices. In sociotechnical networks, human beings are intrinsically linked with non-human objects.

For Latour (2005), being connected to a sociotechnical network that possesses some degree of stability gives the actants their identity; conversely, an emerging network acquires its identity through the identities of the actants who are linked within the network. Indeed, the actants (human and non-human) that are connected within a network have disparate identities and pursue diverse interests: this is true, for example, of the school teachers, school regulations, nurses, dieticians, and community organizations involved in a health-promoting school programme. But these identities tend to become increasingly aligned as the network stabilizes. For instance, school regulations are changed to accommodate health promotion activities, or dieticians collaborate with teachers to develop joint activities, thus changing their respective positions towards education and health. Actants' identities are derived from all the various roles and functions they perform within the network, but also from those external to the network. An emerging network is made up of actants with heterogeneous identities, and the more heterogeneous these identities, the more unstable the network (Callon, 1999). In essence, more translation is needed to stabilize these connections. Thus, the capacity and purposes of an actor–network are related to the associated actants within it.

There are three reasons why the notions of the sociotechnical network and translation are useful when conceptualizing intersectoral action. First, intersectoral action requires the establishment of connections between disparate entities that originate in a variety of different public service agencies and sectors, and/or community groups that do not share the same mandate, accounting system, or purpose (Moore, 2000). It takes more than good will to make these arrangements work, and any framework that attempts to make sense of what happens in such arrangements needs to account for the work that is required to make them functional. When a public health organization attempts to partner with a school, as is the case in healthy school projects, it needs to align its own interest and identity (which is related to health) with those of the school, which are related to educating youth.

Hawe et al. (2009) use the notion of the network to better understand health promotion programmes. They conceptualize programmes as networks of events that connect people. They define programme implementation as the densification of connections between events and people. We believe that the notion of the sociotechnical network expands on this idea of a network of events and people; it is simply more specific about what entities are connected. Developing and implementing intersectoral actions require the assembling of a great variety of entities, in addition to individuals from the various organizations involved that are physically present and interact during events. Examples of such entities are the economic and material resources needed to create these events, the knowledge bases that inform the planning of events and that differ greatly between sectors, the values and worldviews of the various actors, and the memoranda of agreement that have been negotiated between the partners.

The second reason why the notions of the programme network and translation are useful is that the usual distinction between the context in which an intervention takes place and the intervention itself is often difficult to define, and to observe, when the distinction is posed as a dichotomy between what is attributable to the context and what is attributable to the intervention (Poland et al., 2008). Although the adaptability of an intervention to a particular context is being increasingly recognized as an important issue (Bisset et al., 2009), it is rarely addressed sufficiently, such that workers on the ground can solve the intervention–context problem and optimize the intervention. A sound theoretical framework should enable an in-depth analysis of the interactions between actors, their actions, and the situations in which the actions take place. A socio-technical network is a flexible and dynamic system that is distinguished from its context mainly by the stability and density of its connections. The connections within a system are denser and more stable than the connections that link the system with its context. The actants within a network are stably interconnected by strong links, but because they also belong to other networks, they connect the intervention to its context. The notion of the sociotechnical network also provides a theoretical framework for conceptualizing implementation as the progressive expansion and strengthening of connections, both within the intervention and between the intervention and its context.

Finally, the notion of the sociotechnical network accounts for how interventions and programmes evolve and change as some connections grow stronger and others weaken. Our research has shown that when certain partners are mobilized to resolve a crisis, often related to a lack of resources, parts of the intervention may be reoriented by having new partners joining the programme (Bisset and Potvin, 2007). With respect to inter-sectoral programmes, which bring together highly disparate entities at the outset, ANT points to the need for a major investment in order to help partners to align their interests and identities and thereby stabilize the network. ANT also suggests that entities change their identity as the network becomes more stable. This may explain why Lipp et al. (2012), in their survey of European Healthy City projects, found that the most extensive partnerships developed by participating municipalities were with health sector organi-zations (as opposed to organizations from other sectors), with whom the health identity of Healthy City projects was probably easier to align. One of the main advantages of ANT in the analysis of intersectoral initiatives is that it provides a mechanism to explain the dynamics of intervention implementation. Translation is the dynamic principle of complex programmes.

Proposition 2. Actions in sociotechnical networks take place mainly through a translation process.

According to ANT, translation enables a network to expand by forming new links with other entities, or to stabilize by strengthening established links (Callon and Latour, 1986). Translation is required when situations create uncertainty and ready solutions are not available. Translation takes place through four iterative operations that are not necessarily successive: problematization, interestment, enrolment, and displacement. Initiators of the translation process may vary. Because the rhetoric of intersectoral col-laboration has been heavily promoted by the health sector, public health organizations often play the role of both initiator and translator. This, however, might change in the wake of the Health in All Policies movement. This movement pleads for the health sector to engage in the pursuit of other sectors' agendas in the name of health (WHO and Government of South Australia, 2010). Such a strategy can be interpreted as an openness on the part of the health sector to join partnerships led by other sectors.

In problematization, the groups or entities relevant to a given situation are identified. To problematize is to approach a situation with an open mind, to explore different meanings and areas of uncertainty. It involves establishing a virtual link between a situation and relevant actants (human and non-human) so that the meaning can be appropriately translated for the situation. It also means opening up the meaning to further interpretations that speak to the identity and interests of those interested. It recognizes that actants may not be ready to understand the totality of the situation, and that other viewpoints must be brought to bear. Groups of actants are perceived as relevant insofar as they control the resources and knowledge required to take action, or insofar as they provide access to other actants. Essentially, problematization means situating the programme's social space by anticipating all the connections that need to be established among all the relevant actants in order to reduce uncertainties associated with the intervention. For example, Montreal's Director of Public Health identified poverty as a public health priority for Montreal (Direction de santé publique de Montréal, 1998). He further established that to fight poverty the Public Health Directorate must collaborate closely with municipal authorities (Agence de la santé et des services sociaux de Montréal, 2011). This appeal to the municipal authorities may be interpreted as a problematization of population health as being influenced by local living conditions rather than by the overall structural and economic environment. But it could also mean that, from the point of view of Montreal's Director of Public Health, municipal authorities are more accessible and easier to mobilize than provincial elected representatives, to whom he would have to appeal in order to effect broader structural change.

In ANT, interestment reinforces and confirms the validity of the problematization by defining and stabilizing the roles (and identities) of the relevant actors. Here, the idea is to get the relevant actants to associate their roles and interests with the issue the network is addressing by giving them a good reason to align their own interests with those of the network and to engage in the intervention. Whereas the problematization situates relevant actants in relation to each other within the problematized space, interestment shapes the content of their interactions with each other and with the problem of interest. Through concrete devices and either implicit or explicit negotiations, the actants align their interests within the network and are dissociated from other interests and identities. Our studies have shown how, in a school nutrition programme, the nutritionists who held cooking and nutrition workshops in classrooms were actually using a form of micro-interestment with the teachers, students, parents, and school administration to link the various components of the programme with the school's normal operating procedures (Bisset et al., 2009). Hawe and Stickney (1997) have also shown how interestment devices, in the form of flyers presenting preliminary evaluation results, were created based on the preliminary results of an evaluation of an intersectoral food coalition.

The purpose was to 'raise Committee members' interest in attending the following meeting for the full presentation and discussion of findings' (Hawe and Stickney, 1997: 221).

The operation of enrolment may be understood as a successful interestment: the actants have aligned their interests and accepted their assigned roles and identities. Because translation is an iterative process and interestment may involve negotiations, the initial problematization may be transformed through these negotiations. Interestment devices, which become entities in the sociotechnical network, may also require substantial investment to ensure that they succeed in stabilizing the network and enrolling key actants. In our relationships with various partners of the Chair, we repeatedly observed that the partnership framework we negotiated at the start of our collaborative initiative served as an interestment device for enrolling community partners in our participatory research projects (Aubry and Bernier, 2012). Because the partnership framework problematized the relationships between community groups, government agencies, and—to some extent—research programmes, it facilitated the discussion of certain action-related issues that acquired new meanings in the context of specific partnership agreements (Mantoura et al., 2007).

The operation of displacement, as Callon (1986) calls it, is the actual engagement of the network in coordinated actions. It entails a re-examination, in situation and in action, of the roles and identities of the actants in the network. It means testing, through coordinated action, the actants' enrolment and the stability of the network's connections. With respect to mobilization, ANT proposes the notion of the spokesperson. Insofar as the roles and identities within the network are stable and accepted, the spokesperson, if legitimate, can *displace* (i.e. speak for and direct) the network so that it acts intelligibly and predictably, with some inevitable minor adjustments. The presence of controversy indicates that the network or significant parts of it cannot be appropriately displaced, leading to a renegotiation of roles and identities. Thus, network stabilization is not a linear process; rather, it requires some give-and-take, which occurs through the problematization, interestment, enrolment, and displacement operations. Solutions to the controversies that arise during these processes must be sought by problematizing, interesting, and enrolling new actants or by strengthening existing connections. By conceiving programme implementation as an expansion of a sociotechnical network, we can account for the continuous adjustment to changing or emerging situations that occurs in effective programmes (Bisset et al., 2009).

Finally, by distinguishing between stabilized and emerging networks (Callon, 1999), we can avoid predetermining the scale at which to analyse and understand a network. According to ANT, in a stabilized network—as opposed to an emerging network—as connections strengthen, individual identities become weaker. Once stabilized, the network forms a so-called 'black box' of stable and predictable elements. This increases its efficiency but at the price of weakened individual identities, particularly with respect to the capacity of individual entities to act independently of the role assigned to them through their identity within the network. Interests have become aligned within the network, and the actants have assumed the role of vehicle for conveying uncontested concerns and directions. The spokespersons can effectively displace the network at minimal cost. In our research, we examined networks at different scales: networks of networks, networks of organizations, and simply networks of individuals. Each entity within a network may itself be viewed as a stabilized network in that it contains few or no conflicts. There is no absolute scale for analysing networks. Nevertheless, a stabilized network becomes less effective with time and changing contextual conditions because it is usually devoid of controversy, and is consequently less able to innovate. In emerging networks, however, conflict is more liable to arise because the entities are still negotiating with each other.

The four operations of translation described above provide an appropriate framework for observing, analysing, and guiding what happens within networks that comprise different sets of actors and actants. Other authors have also used these four operations to make sense of innovation in the policy process—namely, in the process leading to the adoption of anti-smoking laws (Young et al., 2010) (see Box 5.1).

Box 5.1 ANT and policy innovation for smoke-free places

Young et al. (2010) used ANT to compare the process of creating policies for smoke-free places in different countries. They argue that ANT can describe all four stages of the creation of an innovation: autonomization of the issue, contesting of the issue, negotiation of a solution, and resolution. Applying ANT to each of those innovation stages, they showed how second-hand smoke was gradually built up as a problem requiring action (smoke-free places). Problem narratives were built around the academic literature, local policy issues and local cultural norms, and thus differed between countries. For instance, the problem in California was branded as an environmental problem under the jurisdiction of the Clean Air Act, thus eliciting the support of environmental groups and citizens. By contrast, in Australia it was an occupational health and safety problem, so worker and employer organizations were involved. This led to different narratives around the issue, which prompted different forms of contesting by social groups and, consequently, different alliance-building strategies on the part of the proponents of smoke-free places.

In the above study, the authors consider the whole policy-making process to be an innovation, starting with the creation of a public problem, agenda-setting, policy formulation, and even policy implementation. They look at the whole policy sub-system as a loose network drawn through existing relationships between the actors and their arguments. A limitation of this approach is that it may overlook absentees in the policy-making process because it follows policy in action. However, using ANT in conjunction with a theory of the policy process, such as the advocacy coalition framework or the multiple streams theory, can prove useful as a planning tool for policy-makers because it identifies the links where policy innovation can occur (Young et al., 2010).

Methodological innovations for the analysis and support of sociotechnical networks

When applying ANT to the study of sociotechnical networks, CACIS was faced with a lack of methodological guidelines for putting the theory into practice. Although Callon defined the translation operations of problematization, interestment, enrolment, and displacement, he did not propose any methods for carrying out these operations, nor define the associations between participants in a sociotechnical network (Callon, 1986). Methodological problems arise not only when identifying a posteriori the interactions between the participants in an intervention's sociotechnical network but also when prospectively guiding social actors engaged in intersectoral initiatives. A first objective, therefore, was to examine the translation process in order to identify relationship patterns and/or sets of practices that could be used to mitigate discrepancies among social actors in terms of power, legitimacy, and the capacity to act, and hence establish cooperative relationships among these actors.

In this spirit, some CACIS studies attempted to operationalize the translation terms and develop a formal, theory-based research method. This is the first methodological innovation. Bisset et al. (2009) proposed a coding procedure for activities associated with the two critical translation operations of problematization and interestment in order to track the work of nutritionists setting up a school intervention programme. In this case, the problematization was defined based on the identity of the actors in the sociotechnical network, including their qualities, qualifications, capacities, expertise, and roles, as well as the interests, objectives, and concerns of the actors (Bisset et al., 2009).

Using successive coding, the authors found that the nutritionists used three interestment strategies to build connections with the students: reinforcing existing connections with food, creating new connections between students and food, and expanding the students' interpersonal relationships. They also developed two interestment strategies to build connections with the schools: creating connections between the school and nutrition education, and adapting workshops to teachers' schedules. Through this operationalization of the translation categories, the authors showed that programme implementation is a dynamic process that results in an adjustment between predefined rules and the interests of programme stakeholders.

The second methodological innovation is a 'diagnostic tool' developed by Bilodeau et al. (2011) to assess the relevance and stability of partnerships and their actions. According to ANT, a partnership depends on the strength of the sociotechnical network and on the existence of continued translation among the actors present in the network. The tool is an 18-item questionnaire that assesses the four conditions that support successful partnerships.

1. The actors present in the partnership represent all the different perspectives on the issue at hand.

2. Beyond operational or tactical choices, partnership members are involved in strategic decision-making at an early stage in the project.

3. Partnership members are actually able to influence the decision-making process within the partnership—that is, their contribution reaches beyond mere consultation.

4. Key actors (without whom no action can be carried out) and strategic actors (who can displace other players) are actively involved in the partnership.

Tested and validated with community-based partnerships, this questionnaire is designed for use by partnership groups as part of their practice.

The governance of participatory initiatives

In our research, we have paid particular attention to a specific type of emerging network that develops within a participatory space. Insofar as our research programme required us to combine research protocols with interventions carried out by local actors, we sought to develop a coherent theoretical perspective to fully account for the governance processes of these spaces. The propositions presented in this section build upon ANT to raise new issues about the governance of participatory spaces—namely, multidirectional translations and translation practices that can also be applied to theorize the governance of intersectoral collaborations. We conclude with a discussion of power relationships in the context of ANT.

Proposition 3. The governance of intersectoral initiatives requires that actors participate in a multidirectional translation process

Our conceptualization of programmes as sociotechnical networks that are implemented and stabilized through a series of translation processes does not imply a specific type of governance. Translations are not the purview of a single designated committee or actor. They are, rather, practices that actors develop by interacting with other actants, regardless of official status. Within a qualified partnership management committee, it may happen that one actor is the sole translator of a programme's development and management. This occurs when either there is little uncertainty or there exist proven interestment devices that can be used by a translator with sufficient resources to apply these devices. However, even in this case, conflict inevitably arises, necessitating negotiations and adjustments. Given that the entities connected within the network are not passive, they may resist accepting the roles proposed by the problematization of the programme, and this requires adjustments and adaptations: that is, translation. In other words, translations take place even in a programme that is hierarchically managed and centralized in the hands of a single actor. Nevertheless, the presence of translation alone is insufficient to characterize the programme's governance (i.e. as hierarchical or participatory) (Potvin, 2007).

In our research, we have characterized the translation process in participatory programmes. We assume that participatory governance involves multidirectional translations among the network's actors through spokespersons representing each of the contributing and relevant networks: that is, a meta-network (Potvin, 2007). The presence of multiple translations indicates that none of the parties is able to, or wishes to, impose their particular problematization onto the others; that a diversity of problematizations proposed by the different networks must be considered; and that diverse interestment devices can be used to mobilize the diverse interests. In this kind of space, the identities of all participating networks come into play, and these identities are reshaped as the meta-network stabilizes. Of course, these multiple translations do not simultaneously involve all the entities that make up the networks: the situation would rapidly dissolve into unmanageable chaos. This is where spokespersons play a pivotal role. The greater the number of translators, the more unstable the arrangement, so the number of translators must be curtailed. At the same time, there must be enough legitimate translators to serve as effective spokespersons for all the participating networks. In a space of multiple translations within a network of networks, they speak for and promote the networks' interests through a translation process between the networks.

In addition to multiple translations, participatory spaces are characterized by translations that occur across levels of network organizations. Spokespersons from each of the networks that participate in a given initiative must not only represent the problematizations of their own networks through multiple translations but also displace their network of origin to support the overall cause. Participatory programmes, as well as intersectoral initiatives, are therefore characterized by governance structures in which spokespersons from the constituent networks translate the interests of their network of origin into the objectives of the meta-network. In return, they translate these negotiated objectives into the interests of their own network in order to mobilize it to support the meta-network's objectives. Thus, the multiple translations of participatory governance also require translation processes across levels of organizations. Cargo et al. (2008) studied a participatory intervention and research project to promote physical activities and reduce diabetes in schools within an indigenous community. They found that the various spokespersons for the participating networks—community elders, community organizations, and private sector and academic researchers—influenced the steering committee, necessitating multiple translations within the committee. In addition, the steering committee members, as spokespersons for the constituent networks, achieved reciprocal alignments between the interests of their networks and the interests of the steering committee. For instance, community members working for the research project increased their presence and involvement during the activities because they believed that the research should support the planning and implementation of activities, not just their evaluation. As such, they aligned the interests of the community and the steering committee, something that academic researchers were not able to do, given the constraints of their professional settings (Cargo et al., 2008).

Using ANT in conjunction with other theories, Jansen et al. (2012) have stressed similar conclusions in their study of knowledge transfer networks gathering academics, practitioners, and policy-makers. In a similar way to research done for CACIS, the authors used ANT to identify reconfigurations within the systems of actors involved. They observed how managers, academics, and practitioners developed a shared understanding of the situation and how they endorsed new roles as part of the process of building the knowledge transfer network. Most notably, Jansen et al. addressed the issue of multiple translations by using two additional sets of theories about how to act at the interface between research, practice, and policy. First, institutional re-design theories focus on how interactions between network participants lead to changes in the 'rules of the game' (de Leeuw et al., 2008: 9). Such changes have the potential to alter interactions between network participants in the long term—that is, beyond the life-span of the knowledge transfer network itself. Second, blurring the boundaries theories place emphasis on the contents of the exchange between network participants (de Leeuw et al., 2008). They recommend that each actor in the network has access to the values and cultures of other network participants. Based on these two sets of theories, Jansen et al. have shown the extent of the changes that followed the original agreement to build a network for knowledge transfer. For instance, the rules of the game were altered as far as material conditions went, but more permanent changes to how knowledge was to be produced did not spread beyond the original group of actors involved in the network. In sum, this combination of multiple sets of theories addressing different levels of collaboration provides another way to question the existence and extent of what we called multiple translations.

Intersectoral initiatives, like participatory projects, require a governance structure in which a limited number of spokespersons/translators operate multiple and cross-level translations in order to promote the interests of the networks/organizations they represent. These translators, therefore, become spokespersons for the compromises negotiated within this governance space on behalf of the networks they represent. They must continuously ensure interestment, enrolment, and mobilization of their originating network according to the roles and identities they have negotiated as compromises. Any lack of legitimacy on the part of the spokespersons creates conflict in the participating networks and prevents their mobilization. At the same time, if there are too many translators in the governance structure, the overall network becomes unstable, making it more difficult and costly to regulate.

Proposition 4. The regulation of these complex translation spaces requires specialized practices and tools.

It takes more than good intentions to be a translator. Above all, this role cannot be improvised. The current trend is to require an increasing number of actors to have both specialized expertise and a generalized perspective in order to communicate effectively with a variety of interest groups. In the research world, for example, researchers are increasingly being asked to reach out and disseminate their results to decision-makers and the general public, in addition to publishing articles in high-profile journals. To be relevant in these broader communication strategies, the research findings, which are also actants in the network, must be translated (Latour, 1999b). In fact, the diversity of actants within a network calls for the translation abilities of a professional 'inter-facer', 'boundary spanner', or 'policy entrepreneur' (de Leeuw et al., 2008; Skok, 1995; Williams, 2002). For instance, there are inherent problems in coordinating actions when the actors come from cultures as different as those of public institutions and community organizations, with their diverse and, to some degree, irreconcilable interests (Bilodeau et al., 2003). In addition to the good will of all actors involved, it takes expertise to align interests, apply interestment devices, and identify controversies and then find solutions. This expertise must be backed up by effective practices and competencies. According to Clavier (2010), partnerships are not consensus spaces that simply need to be adminis-trated. Rather, they are spaces for debate and negotiation, and this requires specialized know-how.

Combined with other literature on the sociology of intermediary actors, ANT has proven to be a practical approach for studying how key actors support the interactions taking place within sociotechnical networks (Clavier et al., 2012). Our case study was CACIS itself—namely, the participatory research spaces set up to carry out research projects on interventions to reduce social inequalities in health. These participatory research spaces involved academics as well as practitioners from community organiza-tions and public institutions. Professionals were hired by the research teams; they 'coor-dinated' these spaces and sustained interactions between the various partners. As part of our reflection on the Chair and its activities, we investigated the practices of these professionals. In essence, our question was: what does 'coordinating' actually mean in this context? Using ANT and translation as a theoretical framework, we identified three types of translation that characterize these spaces and that require specific practices and competencies: cognitive, strategic, and logistic translation (Clavier et al., 2012).

Cognitive translations are required to develop a shared vision of the situation and the actions to be taken. Whether for an intervention or a collaborative research project, the actors involved must have a common understanding of the problematization of the situ-ation and of the relevant actors and their roles. They must develop a shared language in order to express their views of the situation. To facilitate these translations, the practices applied must result in discussions in shared spaces, and must allow diverse stakehold-ers to deconstruct a shared discourse surrounding a situation or action. The translator's role, as a pivotal interfacer who is knowledgeable about the participating cultures, is to facilitate information-sharing between actors from different social spheres, each with their own values and professional norms. This generally means having the ability to sort, decontextualize, and recontextualize what is needed for the diverse networks to success-fully carry out the shared action. In projects related to CACIS, the translators very often had professional experience in both academia and health institutions, or had sat on the advisory committees of local health projects. This allowed them to speak both profes-sional jargons, to grasp the significance of empirical problems for the research, and to formulate research questions.

Strategic translation refers to balancing power among involved groups. A key aspect of variation among network actants is the power differential. Although it is flexible and relatively horizontal, the organization of a network still features the power issues and structures that characterize the relationships between the constituent social groups. In fact, such networks may bring together city institutions or public health authorities that have decision-making and financial authority, and community organizations whose projects in a large part depend on funding from these city and public health institutions. Power issues clearly exist between such actors, and they are part of the actors' identities (Mantoura et al., 2007). A key function of strategic translation is to develop and implement procedures that enable power, within the network, to be balanced. It is therefore important to identify differences in power and resources, and to implement devices and procedures to mitigate the effect of these differences. For instance, devices can be established to help the various actors to voice their expectations and assume their responsibilities. Other practices directly encourage participation by compensating for opportunity costs, which also vary between actors.

Finally, these two types of translation are supported by the wide array of logistic translations that are normally associated with routine management tasks—writing up and circulating notes from meetings, making phone calls to keep in touch with each partner, etc.—but which become vital in the complex space of multiple translations. In these spaces, communications must be fluid, comprehensive, open, and transparent. The actors must be convinced that their views are heard, regardless of their social position or the resources they contribute to the network. For each of these three forms of translation, the translators must act relatively autonomously, because most of the information is funnelled through the translators.

In this research, ANT has served as a basis for developing a model of the practices necessary to sustain sociotechnical networks. We have proposed a pyramid representing the interrelations between cognitive, strategic, and logistic translations (Clavier et al., 2012). In turn, this graphic representation of the types of translation can serve as a practical tool for the study of participatory or intersectoral spaces, or for actors involved in such spaces.

ANT and power relations: theoretical and practical challenges

The study of intervention programmes through the lens of ANT has some theoretical limitations. A shortcoming frequently mentioned in the literature is that this approach fails to consider the hierarchy and temporality of scientific debates. There are also considerable challenges related to methodological objectivation because the data are mostly mobile and transactional (Alcadipani and Hassard, 2010; Gingras, 1995; Grossetti, 2007; Whittle and Spicer, 2008).

In the study of intersectoral interventions and partnership research initiatives, the chief shortcoming of ANT is its failure to account for power relations. It is a particularly serious drawback when considering programmes to reduce social health inequalities, which are closely associated with power differentials (CSDH, 2008). This limitation stems from the principle whereby all human and non-human participants in a sociotechnical network must be considered equivalent, and is the result of the context in which the theory was originally developed.

When explaining the success or failure of an innovation, Callon and Latour (Callon, 1986; Latour, 2005) proposed that no distinction should be made between social actors and technical objects. In other words, no a priori causal power is attributed to either one. This a priori assumption is mostly methodological rather than epistemological or ontological. Based on the principle of symmetry in the sociology of science (Bloor, 1976), this premise means that success does not have to be attributed to the supposed technical superiority of a given innovation over another. Moreover, failures do not have to be explained in terms of social or political arguments (Callon and Latour, 1986). Once this principle was established, sociologists of science could enter into a debate with philosophers who advocated a positivist view of science, according to which the 'best' technical solution should necessarily prevail. By contrast, ANT proposes a diversity of social, economic, political, and technical influences on the innovation process. It offers a way of describing what happens, while emphasizing the fact that reasons other than endogenous causality can explain an innovation's success or failure (Gingras, 1995; Mol, 2010). Meanwhile, as this principle underwent some adaptive changes, notably by Latour, it tended to be understood as an obligation to consider social actors and material or technical objects on the same level—a view that denies the specificity of social actors whose identities are associated with power differences (Grossetti, 2007; Latour, 2005).

A literal application of this principle makes it difficult to account for the capacity to take action on the part of diverse social actors, or for the ways that actors strive to influence interactions so that their interests are served. The development and implementation of an intersectoral initiative, for example, brings together regional and local public health institutions, community actors, philanthropic organizations, and citizens. These actors may vary greatly in terms of legitimacy, resources, interests, and capacity to act. Consequently, their relationships to material objects and institutional regulations may also differ considerably.

However, there are other, more nuanced, interpretations of ANT that allow for a consideration of this diversity in social actors and the power relations that shape the sociotechnical network. For example, in one formulation, although the social, political, and technical entities in a sociotechnical network have distinct features, they are not organized according to a pre-established system of relationships. Instead, these relationships evolve as the situation evolves (Gingras, 1995). In other words, the relationships between the actors are not predetermined by a hierarchical structure or system of relations that depends entirely on the interests and capacity to act of the social actors. Their interactions with each other and with the diverse non-human actants, which are mobilized through these relationships, enable them to reconfigure these relationships in attempts to achieve a certain balance of power. Extending this interpretation, other authors have proposed that we consider non-human actants (including technical objects and written documents) as resources that social actors can mobilize to guide their interactions, balance power relations, and align their interests (Grossetti, 2007).

Our work for CACIS is closer in many respects to these nuanced interpretations than to a completely symmetric view of social actors and non-human actants. The point of departure for all our analyses was to highlight the identities of the actors concerned, thereby taking into consideration their separate resources, interests, and legitimacy. Our research, as underlined in proposition 4, has underscored the importance of the translator's role (usually assigned de facto to be a member of the sociotechnical network) in serving as an interface and mediator between the actors of the sociotechnical network and in calling attention to common points of interest to the different strategies. This role requires a clear acknowledgement of the power relations between actors: in research partnerships, the translators make sure that each partner can fully participate and has a voice, regardless of their influence in other spheres of action. For example, community representatives are financially compensated so that they can participate on the same level as representatives of public institutions. We have determined that these translators often use written documents (i.e. non-human actants) to establish common ground between the actors in a sociotechnical network. These actants were sometimes considered as support resources for the strategies and interests of the social actors.

In more proactive uses of ANT, CACIS has at times introduced material resources into the sociotechnical network in order to regulate interactions between the network's social actors. A telling example is the partnership agreement that was drawn up between academic, institutional, and community research partners within CACIS (Bernier et al., 2006). This tool, which was developed in the early stages of the Chair's existence, framed the respective contributions and mutual engagements of academics, community partners, and public administrations taking part in participatory research on local interventions to reduce social inequalities in health. Inspired by similar existing agreements, it had four parts. The first two comprised a statement of the mission, values, and principles underlying the partnership. Together, they helped to ensure that all partners had an equal voice. As Bernier et al explained, the agreement:

> sets out shared responsibility among the various partners to help ensure respect for all parties, to adhere to standards for the ethical conduct of research, and to find financial support to enable the participation of representatives of the community or local organizations.
>
> (Bernier et al., 2006: 340)

The list of respective roles and obligations of each category of partner, as well as the tools that help to guide the definition of research projects, clarify this even further, thereby ensuring that all contributed to an equal degree in the research. Notably, the agreement postulated that the research partners should all be given the opportunity to participate in data interpretation and, if no consensus was reached, to publicly dissent from the interpretation.

The Chair's partnership agreement has played a central role in counteracting discrepancies in the capacity to act, interests, and legitimacy of the various partners that have taken part and contributed to research under the Chair. By openly acknowledging the separate identities of partners, the Chair's partnership agreement has helped to regulate interactions between partners, establish a climate of cooperation, and provide the conditions for participative interpretations of research results (Aubry and Bernier, 2012).

Conclusion

Local, community-based action on the determinants of health that aims to reduce social health inequalities requires coordinated actions, mainly in the form of programmes that bring together actors from diverse spheres and with diverse interests. Drawing on the principles of ANT and our own research, we have defined these intersectoral initiatives as sociotechnical networks made up of human and non-human actants, where action is enabled through translation operations that create and strengthen connections between the intervention's stakeholders. Our studies have laid the theoretical groundwork for practices that are often described but rarely explained in articles on participatory research. These studies have also opened up a theoretical discussion on the nature of these programmes, an issue that is seldom problematized. Building upon ANT, we have also gained a deeper understanding of the notions of the sociotechnical network and translation by considering the interdependencies among multiple networks (and hence multiple, multidirectional translations) and by reflecting on the practices and tools required to regulate sociotechnical networks and effect translation operations. All the while, we have striven to resolve some inherent problems in applying the theory on the ground by objectifying methods and tools that are based on ANT and that can be used within existing intervention or research partnerships. In this sense, ANT becomes a practical tool for guiding and planning intersectoral or participatory action in policy and programme implementation.

No theory can completely account for the richness and complexity of the problems that arise in practice. Analysts who conceive of action as a knowledge object or project will invariably be waylaid by the need to make ad hoc theoretical adjustments or to redraw their picture of reality in order to accommodate theory after the fact. Thus, in order to understand action, theory must take its place in a dimension other than that defined by the two poles of sense: object and project. Action in practice shows up theoretical weaknesses, and ad hoc adjustments then become hypotheses to be verified by observations that are sharpened through practice. The inverse is also true—that theory makes sense of practice—and because theory is situated outside the action, it allows us to reflect on the practice.

Acknowledgement

This chapter is adapted with permission from Potvin, L. and Clavier, C. (2012). La théorie de l'acteur-réseau, in F. Aubry and L. Potvin (eds.) *Construire l'Espace Socio-sanitaire. Expériences et Pratiques de Recherche dans la Production Locale de la Santé*, pp. 75–98, Montréal: Presses de l'Université de Montréal, Copyright © 2012.

References

Agence de la santé et des services sociaux de Montréal (2011). *Les Inégalités Sociales de Santé à Montréal. Le Chemin Parcouru. Rapport du Directeur de Santé Publique 2011*. Montréal: Direction de la santé publique de l'Agence de la santé et des services sociaux de Montréal.

Alcadipani, R. and Hassard, J. (2010). Actor network theory, organizations and critique: towards a politics of organizing. *Organization*, **17** (4), 419–35.

Aubry, F. and Bernier, J. (2012). Les rencontres d'équipe comme espaces de réflexivité, in F. **Aubry** and L. **Potvin** (eds.) *L'espace Socio-sanitaire. Expériences et Pratiques de Recherche dans la Production Locale de la Santé*, pp. 163–177, Montréal: Presses de l'Université de Montréal.

Aubry, F. and Potvin, L. (eds.) (2012). *L'espace Socio-sanitaire. Expériences et Pratiques de Recherche dans la Production Locale de la Santé*. Montréal: Presses de l'Université de Montréal.

Berghmans, L. and Potvin, L. (2005). La promotion de la santé et les acteurs locorégionaux: les enseignements d'un colloque. *Promotion & Education*, **12** (Suppl. 3), 68–71.

Bernier, J., Rock, M., Roy, M., Bujold, R., and Potvin, L. (2006). Structuring an inter-sector research partnership: a negotiated zone. *Sozial- und Präventivmedizin/Social and Preventive Medicine*, **51** (6), 335–44.

Bilodeau, A., Lapierre, S., and Marchand, Y. (2003). *Le Partenariat: Comment ça Marche? Mieux s'Outiller pour Réussir*. Montréal: Direction de santé publique.

Bilodeau, A., Galarneau, M., Fournier, M., and Potvin, L. (2011). L'outil diagnostique de l'action en partenariat: fondements, élaboration et validation. *Revue Canadienne de Santé Publique*, **102** (4), 298–302.

Bisset, S. and Potvin, L. (2007). Expanding our conceptualization of program implementation: lessons from the genealogy of a school based nutrition program. *Health Education Research*, **22** (5), 737–46.

Bisset, S., Daniel, M., and Potvin, L. (2009). Exploring the intervention context interface: a case from a school-based nutrition intervention. *American Journal of Evaluation*, **30** (4), 554–71.

Bloor, D. (1976). *Knowledge and Social Imagery*. London: Sage.

Callon, M. (1986). Eléments pour une sociologie de la traduction: la domestication des coquilles Saint-Jacques et des pêcheurs dans la baie de Saint-Brieuc. *L'Année Sociologique*, **36**, 169–208.

Callon, M. (1999). Le réseau comme forme émergente et comme modalité de coordination: le cas des interactions stratégiques entre firmes industrielles et laboratoires académiques, in M. **Callon**, P. **Cohendet**, N. **Curien**, J.-M. **Dalle**, F. **Eymard-Duvernay**, D. **Doray**, and E. **Schenk** (eds.) *Réseau et Coordination*, pp. 13–64, Paris: Economica.

Callon, M. and Latour, B. (1986). Les paradoxes de la modernité. Comment concevoir les innovations? *Prospective et Santé*, **36**, 13–25.

Cargo, M. and Mercer, S. L. (2008). The value and challenges of participatory research: strengthening its practice. *Annual Review of Public Health*, **29**, 325–50.

Cargo, M., Delormier, T., Levesque, L., Horn-Miller, K., McComber, A., and Macaulay, A. C. (2008). Can the democratic ideal of participatory research be achieved? An inside look at an academic-indigenous community partnership. *Health Education Research*, **23** (5), 904–14.

Clavier, C. (2010). Les compétences des médiateurs dans les partenariats intersectoriels, in L. **Potvin**, M.-J. **Moquet**, and C. M. **Jones** (eds.) *Réduire les Inégalités Sociales de Santé*, pp. 326–34, Paris: Institut National de Prévention et d'Éducation à la Santé.

Clavier, C., Sénéchal, Y., Vibert, S., and Potvin, L. (2012). A theory-based model of translation in public health participatory research. *Sociology of Health and Illness*, **34** (5), 791–805.

CSDH (2008). *Closing the Gap in a Generation. Health Equity through Action on the Social Determinants of Health. Final Report of the Commission on Social Determinants of Health*. Geneva: World Health Organization.

de Leeuw, E., McNess, A., Crisp, B., and Stagnitti, K. (2008). Theoretical reflections on the nexus between research, policy and practice. *Critical Public Health*, **18** (1), 5–20.

Direction de santé publique de Montréal (1998). *Rapport Annuel 1998 sur la Santé de la Population Réduire les Inégalités Sociales de Santé*. Montréal: Direction de la santé publique de l'Agence de la santé et des services sociaux de Montréal.

Frohlich, K. L., Ross, N., and Richmond, C. (2006). Health disparities in Canada today: some evidence and a theoretical framework. *Health Policy*, **79**, 132–43.

Gingras, Y. (1995). Un air de radicalisme. Sur quelques tendances récentes en sociologie de la science et des technologies. *Actes de la Recherche en Sciences Sociales*, **108**, 3–17.

Grossetti, M. (2007). Les limites de la symétrie, *SociologieS [online]*. Available at: <http://sociologies. revues.org/712> (accessed 17 April 2012).

Hawe, P. and Stickney, E. K. (1997). Developing the effectiveness of an intersectoral food policy coalition through formative evaluation. *Health Education Research*, **12** (2), 213–25.

Hawe, P., Shiell, A., and Riley, T. (2009). Theorising interventions as events in systems. *American Journal of Community Psychology*, **43** (3–4), 267–76.

Jansen, M. W., de Leeuw, E., Hoeijmakers, M., and de Vries, N. S. (2012). Working at the nexus between public health policy, practice and research: dynamics of knowledge sharing in the Netherlands. *Health Research Policy and Systems*, **10** (33), 1–19.

Lascoumes, P. (1996). Rendre gouvernable: de la 'traduction' ou 'transcodage': L'analyse du changement dans les réseaux d'action publique, in CURAPP (ed.) *La Gouvernabilité*, pp. 325–338, Paris: PUF.

Lascoumes, P. (2004). Traduction, in **L. Boussaguet, S. Jacquot**, and **P. Ravinet** (eds.) *Dictionnaire des Politiques Publiques*, pp. 437–44, Paris: Presses de Sciences Po.

Latour, B. (1987). *Science in Action: how to Follow Scientists and Engineers through Society*. Cambridge, MA: Harvard University Press.

Latour, B. (1999a). On recalling ANT, in **J. Law** and **J. Hassard** (eds.) *Actor-Network Theory and After*, pp. 15–25, London: Wiley-Blackwell.

Latour, B. (1999b). *Pandora's Hope: Essays on the Reality of Science Studies*. Cambridge, MA: Harvard University Press.

Latour, B. (2005). *Re-assembling the Social. An Introduction to Actor-Network Theory*. Oxford: Oxford University Press.

Lendvai, N. and Stubbs, P. (2007). Policies as translation: situating trans-national social policies, in **S. M. Hodgson** and **Z. Irving** (eds.) *Policy Reconsidered: Meanings, Politics and Practices*, pp. 173–89, Bristol: Policy Press.

Lipp, A., Winters, T., and de Leeuw, E. (2012). Evaluation of partnership working in cities in phase IV of the WHO Healthy Cities network. *Journal of Urban Health* [online]. Available at: <http://bchealthycommunities.ca/res/download.php?id=433> (accessed 17 April 2012).

Mantoura, P., Gendron, S., and Potvin, L. (2007). Participatory research in public health: creating innovative alliance for health. *Health and Place*, **13** (2), 440–51.

Mol, A. (2010). Actor-network theory: sensitive terms and enduring tensions. *Kölner Zeitschrift für Soziologie und Sozialpsychologie*, **50** (1), 253–69.

Moore, M. H. (2000). Managing for value: organizational strategies in for-profit, nonprofit and governmental organizations. *Nonprofit and Voluntary Sector Quarterly*, **29** (Suppl. 1), 183–204.

Nay, O. and Smith, A. (2002). Les intermédiaires en politique. Médiation et jeux d'institutions, in **O. Nay** and **A. Smith** (eds.) *Le Gouvernement du Compromis. Courtiers et Généralistes dans l'Action Politique*, pp. 1–21, Paris: Economica.

Poland, B., Frohlich, K. L., and Cargo, M. (2008). Context as a fundamental dimension of health promotion program evaluation, in **L. Potvin** and **D. McQueen** (eds.) *Health Promotion Evaluation Practices in the Americas. Values and Research*, pp. 299–317, New York: Springer Science+Business Media, LLC.

Potvin, L. (2007). Managing uncertainty through participation, in **D. V. McQueen, I. Kickbusch, L. Potvin, J. M. Pelikan, L. Balbo**, and **T. Abel** (eds.) *Health and Modernity. The role of Theory in Health Promotion*, pp. 103–28, New York: Springer.

Potvin, L., Lessard, R., and Fournier, P. (2002). Inégalités sociales de santé. Un partenariat de recherche et de formation. *Canadian Journal of Public Health/Revue Canadienne de Santé Publique*, **93** (2), 134–7.

Rhodes, R. A. W. (1996). The new governance: governing without government. *Political Studies*, **44**, 652–67.

Skok, J. E. (1995). Policy issue networks and the public policy cycle: a structural-functional framework for public administration. *Public Administration Review*, **55** (4), 325–32.

Whittle, A. and Spicer, A. (2008). Is actor network theory critique? *Organization Studies*, **29** (04), 611–29.

WHO and Government of South Australia (2010). *Adelaide Statement on Health in All Policies: Moving Towards a Shared Governance for Health and Well-being*, Adelaide: World Health Organization and Government of South Australia.

Williams, P. (2002). The competent boundary spanner. *Public Administration*, **80** (1), 103–24.

Young, D., Borland, R., and Coghill, K. (2010). An actor-network theory analysis of policy innovation for smoke-free places: understanding change in complex systems. *American Journal of Public Health*, **100** (7), 1208–17.

Chapter 6

Emerging theoretical frameworks for global health governance

Evelyne de Leeuw, Belinda Townsend, Erik Martin, Catherine M. Jones, and Carole Clavier

Global health rises

The concept of 'global health' has become a mainstay of the scholarly discourse since the late 20th century. This has happened because governments and the aid industry abandoned the notion of 'international health', which was considered by many a limited infectious-diseases-in-countries-with-warm-climates approach. Global health appears to have larger appeal, greater urgency, and more forceful mobilization potential than its predecessors. Yet the use of the concept is somewhat equivocal. Some agencies and actors seem to use the term for the old wine of international health in the new bags of neo-liberal discourse. Others argue that global health is qualitatively different from international health.

We fall in the latter camp, with authors such as Kelley Lee, David Fidler, and Ilona Kickbusch. We see global health as the natural evolution and consequence of a world that is becoming ever more connected, be it in cognitive, spatial, or temporal terms (Lee and Dodgson, 2000). Other chapters in this volume describe the importance of policy networks for health, or actor–network theory to study health phenomena and parameters. Such a network perspective, in an increasingly connected world, uniquely sets global health apart from international health. Global health is characterized by the engagement of diverse, multilevel sets of stakeholders in the determinants and expressions of health that transcend the boundaries of the nation-state system established by the Treaty of Westphalia in 1648 (Fidler, 2003).

The Westphalian world order established the nation-state prerogative of non-interference in a state's internal affairs. The hermetic boundaries of nation states were increasingly reaffirmed in the two centuries following the signing of the Treaty. Where people could travel around the world without formal identity papers (stating, for instance, name and citizenship) in the 17th century, such a situation had become impossible by the end of the 19th century. Similar to the strengthening of nation-state regulations on individual mobility, states also increasingly codified their own mutual and reciprocal relationships over this period. With the growing numbers of parliamentary democracies in the 19th century, such relations went beyond the prerogative of the monarch and started to involve other interests and stakeholders. This can be observed in particular in the health field: the building of the Panama Canal added urgency to the series of international sanitary conferences that France had initiated in 1851, and the International Conference of American States convened a first public health conference in 1902.

> In hindsight, the immediate threat of yellow fever and other epidemic diseases may have been a necessary, although not entirely sufficient, condition for the early growth of inter-American cooperation in public health. Cultural factors likely also played a role. The first decade of the 20th century was one of exuberant belief in the infinite and universal possibilities of progress. In this belle époque, Pan-Americanism became a popular world view, and the early development of the Sanitary Bureau reflected that view.
>
> (Kiernan, 2002)

With the looming opening of the Panama Canal (eventually in 1914), commercial interests started to overlap more than ever before with state interests, cultural consideration, and human development (Missal, 2008). The Westphalian world order enabled a smooth integration of industry and state interests within the nation state. This world order, however, started to crumble after the Second World War.

First of all, industry interests and representations divorced themselves from what were often imperialist state interests. Where, for instance, Eisenhower's 'military-industrial complex' encompassed a state-sponsored amalgamate of financiers, the weapons industry, and state-sanctioned violence (Giddens, 1981; McNeill, 1982), and the oil industry's commercial interests seamlessly overlapped with national strategic interests (Mommer, 2002), the evolving service industries in banking, computing and software development, and health care delivery were much less unequivocally associated with a country's geopolitical priorities (Hadi, 2009). Second, those countries themselves engaged in a range of efforts towards closer collaboration and association, be they military (e.g. the North Atlantic Treaty Organization) or economic (e.g. the European Coal and Steel Community, then European Community, now European Union). Third, the emergence of social movements—such as the women's health movement (Boston Women's Health Book Collective, 1971, cited in Zola, 1991) or transnational non-governmental organizations (NGOs) such as Amnesty International—challenged the authority of the nation state. This has, in the health realm, led to a consumer health movement that is playing different roles in different contexts (Löfgren et al., 2011), but has certainly challenged the authoritarian professionalism that dominated the medical-industrial complex well into the 1980s. Fourth, in response to what were seen as the slow and bureaucratic bowel movements of both governmental and non-governmental (e.g. Red Cross and Red Crescent) actors, organizations such as Médecins sans Frontières (MSF) started to deploy their own crisis intervention teams. These 'rogue' health delivery efforts subsequently required a need for stronger legitimacy and argumentation, and MSF and others (like lawyers—Avocats sans Frontières—and IT specialists—Nerds without Borders) staunchly argue for aid and human rights activism that transcend traditional nation-state borders. Finally, the stock exchange internet bubble and capitalist boom of the 1990s led to massive, some would say obscene, wealth creation for a few transnational corporations and their individual executives. Some of these embarked on philanthropic endeavours on a grand scale, such as the Bill and Melinda Gates Foundation (with a financial injection by Warren Buffett of US$30.7 billion) and the Bloomberg Family Foundation, both of which dedicate substantial efforts towards 'global health'.

Partly as a result of these shifts towards a post-Westphalian world order, the nature and perceptions of health problems have changed as well. Where the ongoing series of cholera epidemics was considered an international issue that should be resolved through quarantine measures for over 150 years (Lee, 2001), the HIV/AIDS epidemic was explicitly framed as a global health problem (Parker, 2002). Where the Declaration of Alma-Ata on Primary Health Care of 1978 considered that meeting the basic health needs of all happened at the interface of government action and community development, the Commission on Social Determinants of Health (CSDH, 2008) considered that closing the health equity gap was possible within a generation through the concerted efforts of the many actors beyond national governments. Indeed, authors like Fidler (2003) have argued that global health threats such as SARS and the Mexican influenza H1N1 have ended the primacy of the Westphalian state, and that the boundaries of democracy have to be redefined beyond the nation state and public sector alone for effective future use.

There is also a widely held belief that we are witnessing a virtually tectonic shift in our perceptions of what constitutes health. The work by the CSDH, including the extensive range of detailed background papers developed by 'knowledge networks', suggests that traditional biomedical and micro-biological ideas of what determines population health now attain less prominence, and that perspectives that include political economies and sociodemographic issues gain ground. Such a shift would be fully commensurate with a new conceptualization of 'global health'. Positive health, or salutogenesis (Antonovsky, 1984) provides an alternative to the pathogenic paradigm of health (or rather, disease). The traditional biomedical model of health stipulates that pathogens such as microbes, toxins, and malfunctioning proteomics cause ill health. Many believe that the introduction of a 'social model of health' in the second half of the 20th century should have been a powerful counter-argument, dealing appropriately with the medical dominance alluded to above. Kelly and Charlton (1995), however, demonstrate that although the discourse and methods may differ between the two, the epistemology remains essentially the same: in the social model the pathogens are housing, poverty, literacy, etc. They show that both discourses are close modernist relatives.

Although Antonovsky acknowledges that salutogenesis is not totally abandoning the pathogenic paradigm, he claims that it may provide the perspective needed for citizen groups to position themselves more strongly in the policy discourse. By adopting salutogenesis—that is to say, by looking to strengthen health and make individuals and communities more resilient—he claims that individuals and citizen groups would free themselves from the professional dominance of health care providers, and would be liberated to advocate for their own health, not just individually but at the systems level. This would suggest that individuals and communities most affected by the new institutional arrangements that are being shaped by globalization processes do indeed have the potential to engage in shaping the determinants of health at 'glocal' levels.

Globalization and global health: an opportunity for governance

We started this chapter by observing the blurred and opportunistic boundaries between global and international health. Now that we have established the context and drivers of health in a new global world order, it seems prudent to attempt to arrive at an appropriate working definition. Koplan et al. state that '[w]e will all be best served (and best serve the health of others around the world) if we share a common definition of the specialty in which we work and to which we encourage others to lend their efforts' (2009: 1995). In describing the parameters of this 'specialty' and contrasting it with international health and public health they are remarkably apolitical (Table 6.1).

Table 6.1 Koplan et al.'s comparison of global, international, and public health

	Global health	**International health**	**Public health**
Geographical reach	Focuses on issues that directly or indirectly affect health but that can transcend national boundaries	Focuses on health issues of countries other than one's own, especially those of low income and middle income	Focuses on issues that affect the health of the population of a particular community or country
Level of cooperation	Development and implementation of solutions often requires global cooperation	Development and implementation of solutions usually requires binational cooperation	Development and implementation of solutions does not usually require global cooperation
Individuals or population	Embraces both prevention in populations and clinical care of individuals	Embraces both prevention in populations and clinical care of individuals	Mainly focused on prevention programmes for populations
Access to health	Health equity among nations and for all people is a major objective	Seeks to help people of other nations	Health equity within a nation or community is a major objective
Range of disciplines	Highly interdisciplinary and multidisciplinary within and beyond health sciences	Embraces a few disciplines but has not emphasized multidisciplinarity	Encourages multidisciplinary approaches, particularly within health sciences and with social sciences

In a four-part series in *PLoS Medicine* there is greater awareness of the sociopolitical context of global health (Szlezák et al., 2010; Frenk, 2010; Keusch et al., 2010; Moon et al., 2010). They define the global health *system* as:

> …the constellation of actors (individuals and/or organizations) 'whose primary purpose is to promote, restore or maintain health' and 'the persistent and connected sets of rules (formal or informal), that prescribe behavioral roles, constrain activity, and shape expectation among them'.
> (Szlezák et al., 2010: 2)

Although this definition does not prioritise certain actors over others, and there is explicit recognition in the Szlezák et al. (2010) paper that modern and emerging global health is about partnerships or networks, it is most interesting to observe that Frenk (2010) emphasizes the profound importance of national health systems, and that Moon et al. (2010) mention almost in passing the tension between the World Health Organization (WHO)'s role on the one hand as a global health leader, and on the other as an equal collaborator in very large institutional arrangements such as the Roll Back Malaria Partnership, consisting of more than 500 partners. Instead of applying, for instance, the network dynamics and theories that have been described elsewhere in this volume (de Leeuw et al., Chapter 8; Potvin and Clavier, Chapter 5) the *PLoS Medicine* series authors seem to find it difficult to abandon the nation-state governance perspective as the main driver for global health.

Neither the 'specialty' nor the 'system' definition addresses two further issues. First, a conceptualization of determinants of global health and what drives these towards health equity for all is absent. Second, neither definition is explicit on how particular governance perspectives would enable a more transparent operation of the global health system. Ruger (2012) contends that efforts towards better global health governance have failed, in particular because global health governance has lacked a sound and rigorous moral and value system or theoretical context that would include equity and justice considerations. Ruger considers the 'congested, chaotic and complex nature of the activities of various global health actors' and finds that there is little global health coordination: 'Public and private actors each pursue their own goals and preferences and not necessarily those of their "beneficiaries"' (Ruger, 2012: 653). She proffers the John Rawls-inspired provincial globalism perspective that would lead, through a theory of shared health governance, to a global health constitution that would complement the Constitution of WHO in acknowledging the complexities of a value-driven global health system.

Although Ruger's call for a morally just value base of shared health governance has great appeal, it is, in our view, too much a normative perspective that does not allow for constructive studies of global health issues. We therefore adopt a definition of global health that looks at health being determined and constructed by people and their institutions at every (glocal) level of human activity, and acknowledge that there are no longer predetermined institutional arrangements for the governance of health at the glocal level. Governments may be as powerful in driving global health as individuals, industries, or NGOs. It may well be that individuals are more powerful than any other actor: Bill Gates is known to have telephoned presidents and major media outlets personally arguing for continued (global) health funding (Anon, 2012). Although such a non-normative or less ideologically grounded view may admittedly appear to be a cynical perspective, it does allow for a range of different global health analyses, theories, and methodologies.

An eclectic but complementary multitheoretical approach to the study of global health governance builds on the work by Stuckler and McKee (2008) and Lee (2009). Stuckler and McKee (2008) propose five metaphors to describe the different dimensions of global health policy: it can be construed as an international foreign policy agenda grounded in trade and diplomacy; as global security, responding to global (bio)terrorist threats and massive new and re-emergent disease epidemics; as a philanthropic endeavour to invest in the nexus between health, poverty, and development; as an economic approach to maximize global development; or as a public health strategy at the international level. Clearly, each of these metaphors is firmly grounded in a particular political and disciplinary treatise, with often incommensurate research and practice paradigms. Similarly, Lee (2009) argues that the global health discourse follows the lines of biomedical, economic, human rights, and security paradigms—and we could observe for these (like Ruger, above) that particular political-philosophical approaches could pervade and connect each. Such approaches would include social justice philosophies and neo-marxist thought, to name but two, but also—possibly most dominantly—the current neo-liberalism agenda (Kay and Williams, 2009).

To us, this denotes that global health can be studied through programmes and initiatives addressing the health needs of people across many countries, rather than through the concerns of particular nations (Townsend et al., 2012). This perspective concurs with studies of governance: like these, studies of global health may place emphasis both on the institutions, norms, and other arrangements that allow for the regulation of global health issues and on the legitimacy of these collective regulations. We believe that such an approach holds greater opportunities for describing the potential and the challenges of global health.

Governance in policy studies

In our view, as explained above, the shift from an international to a global world order has substantially transformed how health is produced at the global level and, consequently, how health can be regulated at the global level. If individuals, NGOs, and national governments, as well as international organizations, can drive the global governance of health, then traditional theories of international relations alone cannot predict how this governance will work. This means that analysts need new sets of theoretical tools to analyse global health governance. To this end, we propose to pay attention to the concept of 'governance' as defined in policy studies.

Broadly construed, governance can be defined as the process of coordinating actors, groups, and institutions across levels of decision and intervention in view of a common goal or concern. The term has lent itself to normative uses by institutions seeking to impose good governance practices (generally aiming at increased economic efficiency) and to analytical uses by scholars striving to capture changes in the policy-making process (Dodgson et al., 2002; Rhodes, 1996). In this vein, governance has been used to point out three main issues. First, in many areas of society, governments cannot make policy on their own but increasingly need to interact with other levels of government and to include private and civil society actors in the policy-making process and in the provision of 'public' services (Rhodes, 1996). The term 'governance' has often been used to capture such transformations in the modes of urban government, though it also applies to other levels of policy-making. Second, related concepts such as multilevel governance (Hooghe and Marks, 2003) and multiple governance (Hill and Hupe, 2006) have also been coined to insist on the increased interdependencies between policy-making levels. Examples where this conception of governance applies are the decentralization of public health policy-making to municipalities and their local communities (Jansson et al., 2011) or the creation of intermediate-level institutions to manage the decentralization of health services (Touati et al., 2007). Policy-making within the European Union is another classic example of multilevel governance. Third, both transformations call into question the democratic legitimacy of governing and policy-making arrangements involving a broad range of actors across levels (Papadopoulos, 2003). This implies the need to grant attention to power relationships and inequalities between the different actors involved in governance processes, including the ability of all actors effectively to influence these arrangements. For instance, White (2009) questions the relationship between governance and democracy, investigating the influence of grassroots organizations on government within a network elaborating a national policy for the support of community organizations. In sum, studies of governance place emphasis on the institutions, networks, norms, and other arrangements that allow for the regulation of a society or the regulation of a given issue (for instance, health) across levels, and on the legitimacy of this collective regulation.

It follows that governance is not a theory proposing a set of falsifiable hypotheses that would allow the making of pronouncements on how to act (Dodgson et al., 2002; Le Galès, 2004). It is, however, a heuristic device that describes and raises questions about regulatory transformations within societies. It is the combination of governance with other concepts and theories on the actors, institutions, interests, and ideas involved in governance processes that give it its explanatory value. These can be theories on democracy and public participation as in White's paper, theories on decision-making, or theories on policy transfer and the circulation of ideas for instance.

Insights from policy studies on the concept of governance strongly echo contemporary issues of health and health policy-making (Dodgson et al., 2002). As mentioned above, the shift from international health to global health calls for governance processes that include not only nation states but also a whole range of non-governmental, private, and community actors. Besides, the need to act on a variety of social determinants of health across policy sectors calls for fluid forms of regulation that make way for a broad range of actors with different expertise. Finally, the concept of governance also encompasses the increased cooperation and negotiations between institutions across levels within health systems and policies. In other words, the advent of global health fits into broader political changes captured under the concept of governance.

Three case studies

The following case studies of global health deal with major governance issues: the opening of policy-making processes to 'new' private, community, and non-governmental actors; the increased interdependencies and negotiations between levels of decision and intervention; and the legitimacy of global health governance processes. Each draws on different theoretical perspectives to make sense of new developments with global health governance. Implementation theory is brought in to our first case study to shed light on small Pacific islands' dealings with the Framework Convention for Tobacco Control. Our case study on access to medicines within the parameters of the Doha declaration provides a constructivist perspective on the governance of treaties, with a particular focus on the role of those most affected (individuals, groups, and communities depending on equitable access to affordable pharmaceuticals), thus shedding light on power imbalances between the actors involved in those governance processes. Our third case study outlines an idea-based perspective on the circulation of concepts and policies that have led nation states to address global health from a diplomatic angle, applying a suite of theories taking the epistemic communities notions as a starting point.

I: Making sense of global commitments to 'access to medicines': rhetoric, discourse and conflict

In the mid-1990s the World Trade Organization's (WTO) Agreement on Trade-Related Aspects of Intellectual Property Rights (TRIPS) (1994) came into being as the first binding agreement that extended intellectual property law into the multilateral trading system. Signed by all members of the WTO, the Agreement extended patent protection 'in all fields of technology', including extending intellectual property rights in the form of twenty-year patent protection in all areas (encompassing pharmaceutical processes and products). This placed a constraining and limiting medicines policy on developing countries in particular, many of which did not at the time provide pharmaceutical product and/or process patents and relied on generic production for lower-cost medicines. Concerned for the negative health impact this Agreement would have, in particular on developing countries, a global civil society network emerged, calling for universal 'access to medicines'. At the time, attention to the HIV/AIDS epidemic and the prohibitively expensive cost of treatment for HIV/AIDS was a key demonstration of the impact of patent monopolies for essential medicines (MSF, 2011a). In coordination with developing countries, and in the context of global attention to the HIV/AIDS epidemic, this network succeeded in bringing the public health concerns over TRIPS onto the global agenda, where they have remained ever since. In 2001 an amendment—the Doha Declaration on the TRIPS Agreement and Public Health—reaffirmed safeguards in the Agreement to protect public health, such as issuing compulsory licenses or parallel imports for medicines (WTO, 2001). Article 4 of Doha states:

> The TRIPS Agreement does not and should not prevent Members from taking measures to protect public health....we affirm that the Agreement can and should be interpreted and implemented in a manner supportive of WTO Members' right to protect public health and, in particular, to promote access to medicines for all.

Global attention to the problem of 'access to medicines' has served as a catalyst for the proliferation of a number of global actors that form the present ad hoc and often conflicting global health architecture.

However, despite unprecedented resources and commitments, access to medicines is still out of reach for many (MDG Gap Task Force, 2009). While there are many downstream factors, such as procurement, domestic supply chains, and health worker training, upstream factors at the global governance level are also limiting access. Many of the leading causes of death in developing countries are preventable, but medicines and technologies have not been adapted for country needs—including paediatric formulations, easy-to-use forms (such as fixed dose combinations rather than multiple pills per day), and forms suitable in settings of limited resources (such as those without refrigeration capacity and with low availability of funds for equipment) (MDG Gap Task Force, 2009: 53). Further, many products are not developed to address disease strains affecting developing countries. The debate over how best to address this issue and the actions taken by various actors is a revealing case that highlights the globalized and political nature of health in the 21st century.

Theoretical perspectives

A critical research agenda must investigate 'how other perspectives on global health issues emphasise and de-emphasise different agendas, concerns and policies; and how this can engage different actors, facilitate or inhibit effective governance, and shape the modalities through which it operates' (McInnes and Lee, 2009: 2). This inquiry rests on the contention that the way that we reconstruct, interpret, and analyse global health has consequences in how we address global health issues. The study undertakes a critical analysis of the competing discourses that actors espouse while interacting with and challenging each other in the debate over 'access to medicines'. This theoretical framework has been selected as it encourages a reflexive study of the policy-making of global health. As Deborah Stone argues:

> to become fluent in these languages is to learn how to see problems from multiple perspectives and to identify the assumptions about both facts and values that political definitions don't usually make explicit...with multiple perspectives, one can achieve an understanding of problems that is more comprehensive and more self-conscious and explicit about the values and interests any definition promotes.
>
> (2002: 135)

In this critical account, international institutions such as WHO are 'not simply social collectives where shared meaning is produced but rather...sites of struggle where different groups compete to shape the social reality of organizations in ways that serve their own interest' (Mumby and Clair, 1997: 182). This requires an investigation of the political processes and strategies of various actors who influence governance arrangements—not just states and multilateral organizations, but also civil society actors, the pharmaceutical industry, and philanthropic donors.

A critical discourse approach enables this study to reveal and make explicit the often implicit perspectives that inform the behaviour and strategies of different actors. Discourses frame health and its governance differently, generating tensions over what is to be considered the appropriate role of state, market, and democracy in the provision of 'good governance'. Most importantly, discourses have a power to shape and change how we understand and respond to global health issues. This gives a fuller picture to the political debates and governance proposals pursued or not pursued in the name of 'access to medicines'. Box 6.1 provides a brief practical demonstration that outlines competing views of appropriate governance for 'access to medicines' between actors over the current proposals for a European Union—India Free Trade Agreement.

Box 6.1 European Union–India Free Trade Agreement— practical application of theoretical approach

India is often invoked as the 'pharmacy of the developing world' because 80% of the antiretrovirals procured by MSF and 91% of the generic antiretrovirals approved by the US Food and Drug Administration for the President's Emergency Plan for Aid Relief (PEPFAR) come from India (MSF, 2011b: 1). Furthermore, 70% of the antiretroviral treatment purchased by UNICEF, the International Development Association, the Global Fund and the Clinton Foundation since July 2005 have come from Indian suppliers (MSF, 2011b: 1). In 2005, India revised its Patent Act to align with the TRIPS Agreement. As part of this, India introduced a safeguard under Section 3(d), which states that a 'new use for a known substance' is not an invention and therefore not patentable, in an attempt to prevent companies from seeking 'unjustified' patents (Basheer, 2006: 230). India was supported by NGOs such as MSF and the Delhi Network of Positive People (DNP+), who view this as a safeguard that 'secures the way for generic competition which IS the most effective and sustainable way of bringing drug prices down' (Loon Gangte in MSF, 2010a).

The negotiations of a European Union–India Free Trade Agreement have been underway for some time. The European Union claims that 'nothing in this Agreement shall be construed as to impair the capacity of the Parties to promote access to medicines' (De Gucht, 2010: 1), but nonetheless reaffirms its commitment to protecting the current intellectual property regime, stating that 'an adequate protection on intellectual property in India is crucial to incite innovative industry for the development of

(Continued)

Box 6.1 (Continued)

new medicines and to enable EU generic companies to compete with Indian companies on a level playing field' (De Gucht, 2010: 1). Based on leaked draft texts, MSF has raised concerns that the Agreement will negatively impact on 'access to medicines' (MSF, 2010b). It is joined by the Indian coalition of the People's Health Movement (Jan Swasthya Abhiyan) and DNP+, among others, who argue that the Agreement will 'have a grave impact on generic production of medicines and ultimately access to medicines for patients in the developing world', and 'request India to NOT TRADE AWAY OUR LIVES and right to health in the name of another trade agreement' (DNP+, 2010: 3).

This brief description reveals that, despite all actors openly expressing a rhetorical commitment to 'access to medicines', behind the rhetoric is a range of diverse competing interests, where the discourses espoused by actors seek to protect, transform, or do away with the intellectual property rights system. In addition, discourses of human rights and state and human security are invoked. It is important that we unmask the interests of competing actors and identify the discursive strategies used, as the discourse that comes to dominate the finalized European Union–India Free Trade Agreement will be likely to set the terms of future bilateral agreements.

II. Studying the implementation of the Framework Convention on Tobacco Control

According to WHO, the global tobacco epidemic is one of the largest public health threats the world has ever faced, killing nearly six million people each year (WHO, 2012). Unlike more traditional health threats such as malaria, polio, and HIV/AIDS, the tobacco epidemic is not facilitated by a transmissible pathogen, but is a man-made creation. The uptake in global tobacco use has been driven by the increase in tobacco trade through trade liberalization, direct foreign investment, global marketing, transnational advertising, promotion and sponsorship, and the international movement of contraband and counterfeit cigarettes (WHO, 2005). The Tobacco Atlas suggests that in 2008 just five tobacco companies contributed to 81% of market share in tobacco (their share had also increased significantly in preceding years), the largest of which is the government-owned China National Tobacco Corporation (Eriksen et al., 2012). Despite it being almost 60 years since the relationship between tobacco use and lung cancer was proven through evidence such as the Doll and Hill (1954) study of British doctors (not to mention its association with many other diseases, proven in subsequent decades), global tobacco use is still increasing to this day, largely due to the increased uptake in developing countries such as China and Indonesia (Eriksen et al., 2012; Hurt et al., 2012). This increase has been spurred on by the tobacco industry targeting markets in the developing world, as cigarette sales in developed countries have been in decline (WHO, 2004). Empirical evidence on the health burden of tobacco use alone cannot be viewed as the solution to the global tobacco epidemic, as otherwise global consumption should have decreased since the 1950s. Furthermore, the tobacco industry has been widely known to fund lobby groups, legal challenges, and media campaigns, and to obfuscate scientific evidence (Assunta, 2012; Francis et al., 2006; Trochim et al., 2003; Yach and Bettcher, 2000). Such activities, of course, do not occur in other health threats like communicable diseases. Health promotion professionals must therefore embrace the political process as a key tool for addressing the global tobacco epidemic. WHO also suggests that the medical model alone is not enough, and states that 'tobacco control requires a comprehensive approach, using a mix of policies, legislation and program interventions' (WHO, 2004: 39) with the involvement of various stakeholders in society. Hence, controlling the tobacco epidemic is dependent on a political process involving a multitude of actors, institutions and interests.

The first international public health treaty, the Framework Convention on Tobacco Control (FCTC), was negotiated under the auspices of WHO. It was developed in response to the globalization of the tobacco epidemic. The provisions within the FCTC—such as raising taxes on tobacco; enabling smoke-free environments; mandating health warnings on cigarette packaging; and banning tobacco advertising, promotion, and sponsorship (as well as many others)—are evidence-based and policy-oriented approaches designed to curb the tobacco epidemic. It is evident that FCTC implementation requires a multisectoral approach with no undue influence from tobacco industry interests. After entering into force in 2005, the FCTC has now been ratified by 176 parties, representing 88% of the world's population (Framework Convention Alliance, 2012). The key focus of the FCTC is now on implementation, as many nations have recently drafted and passed national tobacco control policies including provisions such as those already mentioned. The FCTC has been met with some success. Countries generally reported high implementation rates of smoke-free environments; packaging and labelling; sales to and by minors; and education, communication, and public awareness (though implementation rates were low for some other provisions) (WHO, 2010). In 2011, 42 parties out of the 144 that have reported at least once have adopted national legislation after ratifying the FCTC, and of those that already had legislation at the time of ratification, 83% reported that they had since strengthened their legislation (WHO, 2011). However, this does not go without a significant challenge in many developing countries, which may lack the capacity to implement and enforce the FCTC (Albuja and Daynard, 2009; Owusu-Dabo et al., 2010; Sussman et al., 2007; Townsend et al., 2012), particularly as they often have to stretch already scarce resources to implement the FCTC, and may have competing issues such as access to primary health care and the Millennium Development Goals (Lin, 2010). Furthermore, the FCTC (and WHO) is reliant on private sector funding in increasingly difficult economic times, and the tobacco industry is still able to influence national implementation of the FCTC (Townsend et al., 2012). In certain cases like China, its government also runs its tobacco industry monopoly, highlighting a stark conflict of interest (Lv et al., 2011). Other global mechanisms such as WTO may also serve to undermine national tobacco control efforts (Townsend et al., 2012).

Theoretical perspectives

We used a theory-based evaluation approach to explore this issue in the multiple-case study of FCTC implementation in small Pacific island nations. This primarily qualitative study explored the variables that affect the implementation of the FCTC in such countries and how these ultimately influence its success or failure. It held a strong emphasis on policy implementation—an issue that political scientists have long grappled with, and where significant lessons can be learned in terms of implementing policies for health. Policy implementation can be viewed as highly complex: Ferman concisely, but aptly, defines it as 'what happens between policy expectations and (perceived) policy results' (1990: 39). However, implementation is not a clear-cut, linear process where intentions correlate directly with results. 'The content of the policy and its impact on those affected, may be substantially modified, elaborated or even negated during the implementation stage' (Anderson, 1975, cited in Hill and Hupe, 2003: 7).

Key perspectives in implementation theory consist of top-down, bottom-up and synthesized approaches (Hill and Hupe, 2003). A top-down approach involves policies made and implemented under the direction of senior policy-makers (in this case it would be the FCTC Secretariat and Conference of Parties), whereby the policy is the hierarchical execution of centrally defined policy intentions (Pülzl and Treib, 2006). A model of variables affecting the implementation process by Mazmanian and Sabatier (1989) is a noteworthy top-down theoretical framework, which has been used by numerous scholars. For the purposes of this study, it was seen as somewhat rigid and had less recognition of the bottom-up and developing country perspectives.

The bottom-up approach emerged as a critical response to the top-down approach, whereby instead of policies being defined at a central level, discretion is allowed closer to where the policy is delivered, as local bureaucrats are much nearer the real problems than central policy-makers (Pülzl and Treib, 2006). Bottom-up theories such as Lipsky's (1980) concept of street-level bureaucracy argue that the dynamics of policy implementation cannot be fully grasped until one focuses at the level where it comes into contact with those it is intended to influence. Many theorists have since recognized the importance of both top-down and bottom-up approaches, and have embraced a synthesized approach, which integrates aspects of both. While the FCTC can be considered significantly top-down, in this study it was important to acknowledge the small developing island environments in which the policy is sought to be implemented in the Pacific. The bottom-up approach was also seen as critical here (and would be important for analysing developing countries in general).

Najam (1995), while considering the domestic adoption of international environmental policy in developing countries, developed the '5C Protocol', which was applied in this case study. This protocol was also developed utilizing a synthesized perspective in which both top-down and bottom-up models for policy implementation are embraced. Najam explains that implementation is determined by five interrelated clusters of variables that affect one another: the content of the policy itself; the institutional context through which the policy travels; the commitment and capacity of those entrusted to carry out its implementation; and the clients (those affected by the policy) and coalitions (those who have an influence on the policy's implementation). Furthermore, Najam views 'implementation as a dynamic process of negotiation between multiple actors, operating at multiple levels, within and between multiple organizations' (1995: 5). This is a view that is pertinent to FCTC implementation and what is required to counter the global tobacco epidemic.

In using this theoretical framework, it was possible to conduct research on FCTC implementation in small developing Pacific island nations with a solid conceptual framework built on political theory. Its synthesized perspective was particularly useful in recognizing the demands of the FCTC-based policies at both the international and local community levels; the impact of coalition groups, whereby pro-health and pro-tobacco interests are often highly polarized; and also the specific (and somewhat challenging) implementation environments of small developing Pacific island nations. This case study provides a number of important lessons. First, while global FCTC governance was important, how the FCTC is transferred to the coalface where it actually reaches the people it intends to change was more critical. Second, governance in this scenario was multisectoral, to some degree. However, the fundamentals of FCTC implementation and the institutional mechanisms to combat the global tobacco epidemic are still very state-centric (though it is increasingly privately funded). This may vary in other health issues and in other contexts. Last, this case study does not imply that Najam's theoretical framework is superior to analyse the implementation of all policies in all situations. It is believed that this is neither desirable nor achievable. Rather, it serves as an example of one of a plethora of political theories that can be applied to key issues in public health and health promotion, each of which may have some suitability under certain circumstances.

III. Understanding the emergence of global health as foreign policy

As argued above, global health is a way of understanding the global interdependence of the determinants of health and the processes that distribute them. Global health is as much a facet of globalization processes as it is a product of them. The transnational nature and interconnectedness of health problems and their solutions has been subject to examination by the CSDH (2008), which underlines how the inequitable distribution of power, money, and resources has influenced global health. Global health in this regard becomes a worldwide concern permeating national and continental boundaries, and a global health perspective implies that the health of all populations is intertwined with the policies, practices, and programmes of their respective jurisdictions and those of others. This perspective calls for a collaborative approach to the governance of health at the global scale.

The leadership and authority for health at the global scale has conventionally been the responsibility of international organizations specializing in health, such as WHO.

However, the rationale of governance at the global scale has created the opportunity for a range of other actors, and in particular those not specialized in health, to participate in the establishment of health priorities, to engage in discussions on collaborative action, to identify resources, and to develop recommendations for policy. International organizations, multilateral organizations, and donors are bodies that house debates and interest in improving health equity globally (Braveman and Tarimo, 2002; Walt, 1998). This is part of the shift towards global collaboration that is stressed in many definitions of global health, based on the recognition that global problems call for global solutions. Global health governance involves diverse actors—such the World Economic Forum, the European Commission, and the General Assembly of the United Nations—in dialogue for the identification of resources, policies, technical support, and research that may be useful to address global health issues; this serves as a mechanism for organizing collective action on these issues. Global health governance provides internationally agreed norms, practices, and institutions.

In addition to the proliferation of global health governance, a salient development in the field of global health is that it has emerged as an object of interest for national public policy. In particular, health at the global scale is being dealt with as an object of foreign policy. Foreign policy is 'the totality of a state's external behavior toward other states and non-state actors' (Shimko, 2008: 169), or rather 'the sum of the official external relations conducted by an independent actor (usually a state) in international relations' (Hill, 2003: 3). Authors have acknowledged the importance of health promotion in the scaling up of public health as part of foreign policy (Fidler, 2006; Labonte, 2008). The links between health and foreign policy are the subject of considerable discussion in the literature (Bustreo and Doebbler, 2010; Davies, 2010; Feldbaum et al., 2010; Harris, 2004; Kickbusch, 2011; Labonte and Gagnon, 2010; Møgedal and Alveberg, 2010; Owen and Roberts, 2005). The Oslo Ministerial Declaration in 2006, founding the Global Health and Foreign Policy Initiative, recognizes that 'health as a foreign policy issue needs a stronger strategic focus international agenda' (Ministers of Foreign Affairs, 2007: 1373), and this is echoed by the UN General Assembly Resolution on Global Health and Foreign Policy (United Nations, 2009) and the ensuing global health and foreign policy agenda within the United Nations (Davies, 2010).

Global health governance and national policies for global health are not unrelated. In fact, the literature suggests that global health governance has played a role in introducing health at the global scale to national policy agendas by transforming global health into a new field of action for foreign policy. In particular, it provides international norms embedded in global networks to which national policies can refer for legitimacy (Gostin et al., 2010; Nie and Li, 2010). National policies on global health can be understood as part of the response of nation states to the claims generated and commitments produced by global health governance processes.

Examples of policies from Switzerland (FDFA and FDHA, 2012; FDHA, FDFA and FOPH, 2006) and the United Kingdom (HM Government, 2008)—the first countries formally to adopt such policies—will serve as the basis for this case study to explore how global health becomes an object of foreign policy. Recognizing the links and the points of convergence between the domains of global health and foreign policy is but a starting point for exploring the problem of how global health governance may influence and forge such connections. In the context of increasing expectations for intersectoral action and the momentum for a Health in All Polices approach as a policy practice, this case will benefit from the use of theories from the policy sciences to explore how intersectoral policy is formulated at the national level with regard to foreign policy on global health.

Theoretical perspectives

As a starting point for our research, we rely on existing analyses of the relationships between global health and foreign policy (Feldbaum et al., 2010; Feldbaum and Michaud, 2010; Fidler, 2005). Acknowledging the increasingly prominent role for health in foreign policy and international relations, Fidler (2005) proposes three theoretical perspectives to characterize the relationships between health and foreign policy. Fidler's analytical focus is on the direction of influence, 'whether [it] reflects a transformation of foreign policy for the benefit of health, or a transformation of health for the benefit of foreign policy' (2005: 179). The first perspective is ideological and presents health as a value that influences the substance of foreign policy. The second perspective is set within power politics and considers that foreign policy transforms how we conceptualize health: health has become another issue with which traditional approaches to foreign policy must grapple. The third perspective is set within the dynamic between science (i.e. the production of knowledge about health) and politics (i.e. foreign policy-making). It considers that health's rise as an international relations issue has created a relationship between health and foreign policy in which neither completely transforms the other. While the first two perspectives postulate a direction of influence, the third is less normative and offers interesting opportunities for exploring how such a dynamic operates in practice, the processes by which these relationships are constructed and transformed, and the mechanisms or ways by which ideas circulate within those relationships. This is what we propose to explore in the case described above.

We propose that there are two important features of the problem regarding the processes that construct global health as an object of foreign policy: that of scale and that of intersectorality. The first, scale, has been critically discussed by geographers identifying issues concerning politics of scale (Brenner, 2001; Swyngedouw, 2004) with respect to the importance of scalar considerations for social and political action and for the redefinition of power relationships (Leitner and Miller, 2007). In the case of foreign policy on global health, scale refers to the relationship of the mutual exchanges between global health governance and national policy on global health as different scales of policy formulation. This case presents an exploration of the flow of policy ideas between the global and the national policy-making scales.

The second, intersectorality, is related to ideas about intersectoral action for health and healthy public policies that were developed under the auspices of the WHO as part of its Health for All agenda in the 1980s (Sihto, Ollila and Koivusalo, 2006). Intersectorality in this case refers to the multiple government sectors and ministries involved in for-eign policy on global health. For instance, in this comparative case, the policy from Switzerland (FDFA and FDHA, 2012; FDHA, FDFA and FOPH, 2006) involves the Federal Department of Home Affairs, the Federal Department of Foreign Affairs and the Federal Office of Public Health. Similarly, an interministerial group including but not limited to the Department of Health, the Department for International Development and the Foreign and Commonwealth Office led the development of the UK government-wide strategy (HM Government, 2008). We would argue that foreign policy on global health is a case of 'policy for health' (see de Leeuw et al., Chapter 8 in this volume). Policy for health provides an encompassing framework under which healthy public policy—emphasizing intersectoral action—and Health in All Policies—emphasizing horizontal governance—can be incorporated to address policy-making processes in a more sys-temic manner.

Both scale and intersectorality point to critical issues for the problem of how global health becomes an object of foreign policy: actors, institutions, networks, and ideas. We suggest that theoretical frameworks from policy studies can be useful to under-stand these processes and add substance to the claim that global health as foreign policy results from dynamic interactions between politics and science. Concepts such as epis-temic communities (Haas, 1992) and policy transfer (Dolowitz and Marsh, 1996) pro-pose ways in which we may look at this problem.

Epistemic communities are broadly defined as 'networks of knowledge-based experts' and more specifically as a network 'of professionals with recognized expertise and com-petence in a particular domain and authoritative claim to policy-relevant knowledge within that domain' (Haas, 1992: 2–3). They produce and circulate knowledge and ideas that can frame issues, interests, and policies, such as the framing of global health as an object of foreign policy. Also understood as scientific communities, the expan-sion of these specialized networks accommodates international membership, allowing knowledge-based expertise to cut across jurisdictional boundaries; this makes the epis-temic communities approach useful for exploring scalar considerations in a transna-tional level of analysis of policy change that includes both state and international actors (Haas, 1992). Epistemic communities are international actors that can influence inter-national relations (Alder and Haas, 1992).

The concept of policy transfer has been defined by Dolowitz and Marsh as a 'pro-cess in which knowledge about policies, administrative arrangements, institutions etc. in one time and/or place is used in the development of policies, administrative arrangements and institutions in another time and/or place' (1996: 344). This con-cept is a useful complement to that of epistemic community in that it addresses the transnational circulation of ideas, paying attention, among other things, to the actors who circulate policy ideas and to the transformations that ideas undergo via their transfer in various contexts (Clavier, 2010). It also relates to the idea of scale: by dis-tinguishing various levels and pathways of policy transfer, Evans and Davies's (1999) three-dimensional model underscores the importance of scalar considerations, in particular global and transnational systems. Today, within the context of a rise in reflexive governance, the concept of policy mobility has emerged, whereby policy ideas, practices, and techniques may be modified and mutated as part of policy mobilization that is increasingly transnational, cross-scalar and relational in nature (Peck and Theodore, 2010).

Therefore, to understand the dynamic relationship between global health and foreign policy, we propose to consider issues of scale and intersectorality in the emergence of national policies on global health. The concepts of epistemic communities and policy transfer will enable the identification of actors involved in global health and foreign policy at the global and national levels, and will allow questioning of the circulation of ideas between these two levels. While our research is in its infancy, we think that the use of public policy theories such as those discussed here will be valuable to our exploration of the processes underlying the relationships between health and foreign policy characterized by Fidler (2005), in particular for the more in-depth investigation of how the dynamic between science and politics operates.

Towards managed complexity in global health governance

Hill (2011) argues that the problem of global health governance requires a research lens that applies complexity *theory*. His argument is that the global health landscape, and the governance parameters that are constantly emerging from it, would benefit from the application of complexity notions in order to better understand the relationships between stakeholders and structures, and the influence of their interactions on the evolution of global health governance. Proponents of complexity theory acknowledge that many systems are continuously shifting, adaptive networks. However, in our conceptualization of 'theory' we cannot accept such a statement as allowing for the framing of testable propositions; the complexity perspective, in our mind, is a heuristic device or model linking a range of notions that describe the ever-changing multilevel and incremental adjustments systems make to self-organize and maintain order from chaos. Thus, Hill (2011) explains the field of global health and its governance as a complex adaptive system. For each of the metaphorical perspectives offered by Stuckler and McKee (2008), the discourses outlined by Lee (2009) and the full political-philosophical array of perspectives offered (among others) in the remainder of this volume, unique theoretical frameworks will offer complementary insights on the structuring and functioning of the systems' relationships.

Research in global health has predominately focused on the role of specific institutions, specific disease interventions, and the role of states in implementing policy. This research has failed to adequately grasp more fundamental reasons why there is a disjuncture between global health needs and governance responses (McInnes et al., 2012). We seek to promote a critical reflexive turn in the research of global health governance that reflects the nature and the mechanisms of global health governance, which McInnes and Lee (2009) argue are currently narrowly defined and poorly understood.

The concept of global governance in the political science and international relations literature is referred to as 'the arrangements that prevail in the lacunae between regimes and, more importantly, to the principles, norms, rules, and procedures that come into play between competing interests' (Rosenau and Czempiel,1992: 9). This concept is both prescriptive and analytical: 'who rules? In whose interests? By what mechanisms? For what purposes?' (Held and McGrew 2002: 8). Attention to this is important in order to reveal often implicit assumptions that protect interests, include, or exclude actors and ideas, and proscribe governance outcomes. The literature on global health governance tends to focus on the prescriptive aspects of these questions. The research that contributes to this literature is, in fact, preoccupied with global governance as a way to improve global health, hence the prescriptive approach. What we suggest in this chapter is that this objective can also be served by focusing on political science-analytical aspects of global health governance.

Policy studies on global governance question interests and power relationships between the different kinds of actors involved in such processes (such as global health governance). They also address issues of policy-making across levels and issues of legitimacy and democratic accountability of governance processes. The three case studies in this chapter have illustrated the centrality of such questions for global health issues—namely, the political interactions and inequities between the participants in the TRIPS Agreement, the local implementation of the global FCTC, and the legitimacy of state interventions in global processes. Adopting a policy studies point of view on the processes of global health governance enables the incorporation of a more political view of governance processes for global health; a more nuanced understanding of how governance processes operate across levels of health systems and policies; and a more critical look at the (global) politics of governance.

The other point raised in this chapter is that political studies of global governance do not refer to a single, unified theory of governance. On the contrary, they call for a broad range of conceptualizations and theoretical frameworks that each shed light on a different dimension of the global governance phenomenon. The case studies all highlight a different way the processes of governance are conceptualized, how they operate and why they are important by using different theoretical lenses (constructivist theories, implementation theories, epistemic communities, and theories on policy transfer and the circulation of ideas). Similarly, we argue that the field of global health governance research would benefit from studying governance processes from a variety of theoretical points of view. The complexity and diversity of the global governance—and in our case of the global *health* governance—challenge merits a multilevel and multidisciplinary approach. Based on Hill and Hupe's typology of multiple governance (2006), we tentatively suggest the following way to make sense of global health governance research (see Table 6.2).

Hill and Hupe suggest that policy processes are nested across three levels of governance: constitutive governance (the 'decisions about the contents of the policy and about the organisational arrangements for its delivery'); directive governance ('the formulation of and decision making about collectively desired outcomes'); and operational governance, which 'concerns the actual managing of that realisation process' (Hill and Hupe, 2006: 560–1). Their argument is that these three dimensions of the policy process are not tied to a particular scale and nested locus of action; rather, they may each take place at

Table 6.2 An application of Hill and Hupe's multiple governance framework to phenomena, research questions, and theories in global health governance

		Constitutive Governance (structure)	Directive Governance (content)	Operational Governance (process)
System (*world*)	Phenomenon	◆ The World Health Assembly, WHO Executive Board, and Regional Committees, driven by WHO Constitution ◆ Framework Convention on Tobacco Control ◆ Trade Related Aspects of Intellectual Property Rights	◆ United Nations Summit on Non-Communicable Diseases ◆ Framework Convention on Tobacco Control Conference of Parties	◆ International Health Regulations ◆ Global Alliance for Vaccines and Immunisation
	Question	◆ How do industrial interests impact on state capacity to structure implementation?	◆ How does civil society respond to ritualistic or symbolic priority setting?	◆ How do institutional parameters structure responses to new and re-emergent disease?
	Theory	◆ International relations (e.g., 'Balance of Power' theories)	◆ Policy network theories ◆ Agenda-setting theories	◆ Compliance and quality assurance 'theories' ◆ Theories on knowledge building and transfer
Organization (*nation-state, industry, NGO*)	Phenomenon	◆ North American Free-Trade Agreement ◆ European Union	◆ World Trade Organization ◆ Global health in national foreign policy ◆ The Bill and Melinda Gates Foundation Grand Challenges	◆ Westphalian world order ◆ Trade Related Aspects of Intellectual Property Rights
	Question	◆ How do economic policies structure political participation in international governance arrangements? ◆ How have European Union institutions and treaties shaped the European Union's policy on health in the past 30 years?	◆ How does a 'health diplomacy' approach influence the discourse between actors? ◆ How is health integrated within the objectives of foreign or economic policies? ◆ How do international and intersectoral networks contribute to the facilitation of Health in All Policies in 'beyond health' organisational structures?	◆ How is nation-state sovereignty challenged by changes in procedural and scholarly analyses of epidemiological evidence? ◆ How does an international legal instrument such as TRIPS influence the health policymaking process within a developing country (i.e. influence on the health issues under discussion, on the balance of power between coalitions of actors, etc.)?
	Theory	◆ Political economy theories (e.g., neo-Marxism) ◆ Historical neo-institutionalism	◆ Critical theory ◆ Theories on inter-sectoral policymaking ◆ Policy learning theories	◆ Implementation theories (political science) ◆ Inter-organisational work (management) theories ◆ Theories on policy instruments

(Continued)

Table 6.2 (Continued)

		Constitutive Governance (structure)	Directive Governance (content)	Operational Governance (process)
Individual *(actor, client, stakeholder)*	Phenomenon	◆ People's Health Movement advocacy	◆ Aid and humanitarian relief	◆ Health diplomacy ◆ Global Alliance for Vaccines and Immunisation
	Question	◆ What strategies can 'clients' deploy for integrating their role in global health?	◆ How can health equity considerations structure global health responses?	◆ How does a future generation of health diplomats generate leverage for policy change? ◆ How do national policies on border crossing regarding the travel practices of individuals living at or near borders fit within the strategy of the Global Alliance for Vaccines and Immunisation?
	Theory	◆ Critical theory ◆ Social movement/ collective action theories	◆ Social justice theories ◆ Agenda-setting theories (from the perspective of the role of individual actors)	◆ Policy transfer theories (e.g., epistemic communities) ◆ Policy learning theories ◆ Theories on the politics of frontiers ◆ Implementation theories (behaviourist)

From Hill, M. and Hupe P., Analysing policy processes as multiple governance: accountability in social policy, *Policy and Politics*, Volume 34, Issue 3, pp. 557–573, Copyright © 2006. Reproduced by permission of The Policy Press.

any or all of the individual, organizational, and system loci of action. The intersection of each level of governance with a locus of action raises a different issue about governance processes. For instance, directive governance at the system level directs attention towards the definition of general rules and objectives of a policy. In other words, Hill and Hupe's framework offers a way to identify variables for the study of public policy processes.

Our adaptation of this framework to the specific case of global health governance similarly directs attention to different issues about global health governance. We also suggest a few theoretical frameworks that could be used in the study of these phenomena. The examples in the matrix are obviously not exhaustive, as the research questions addressed to each of the issues may command different theoretical approaches.

The Global Alliance for Vaccines and Immunisation can be studied from a system perspective—for instance, asking how the institutional parameters of this institution structure responses to new and re-emergent diseases. Compliance and quality assurance 'theories' or theories on knowledge building and transfer could shed light on the procedures involved to respond to epidemics or on the institution's ability to react to epidemics. At the individual level, examining the national management of travel practices of individuals living at or near the borders in epidemic-prone areas using theories on the politics of frontiers would provide information about the local governance of the Global Alliance for Vaccines and Immunisation. Looking at the organizational level tends to shift the research focus to the effects of institutions on governance arrangements or policy-making processes. For instance, historical neo-institutionalism would be appropriate to study how institutions of the European Union—whether the European Commission, the Directorates-General or the European Parliament—and treaties have shaped the European Union's ability to develop a health policy (constitutive governance) or the health issues that it could deal with (directive governance).

Perhaps the most compelling example of phenomena playing out across the cells of the matrix (demonstrating the delicate intertwined nature of its individual, organizational, and system parameters) relates to the existence, roles, and visions of the People's Health Movement (PHM). On the one hand the self-declared grassroots counterpart of the WHO bureaucracy strongly opposes singularly profit-driven (public) private partnerships and the dominance of neo-liberal 'charity' (e.g. the Bill and Melinda Gates Foundation); on the other hand PHM is a loose conglomerate of individuals and advocacy groups advocating the rights and interests of 'those affected' (on philosophical grounds we may reject, in this case, the use of 'clients' or 'consumers', as this would suggest an unwarranted supply–demand relationship). While PHM is exploring new forms of governance in taking advantage of the largely untapped power of networks, it is also playing the game of global scholarship and peer-reviewed publishing really well. The Movement advances high-level advocacy pleas for equity and social justice, and can back these up with hugely successful coalface action involving women, children, and people with disabilities.

The PHM appears to occupy the different spaces in our analytical approach of Table 6.2 with strategic insight, not because there are cunning leaders (alone), but precisely *because* it is a networked organization with global reach, different from many other actors in the global health governance sphere. The Movement's success also substantiates the idea that studying the politics and policy dimensions of governance is important for global health governance because it is part of a wider set of political issues. Hill (2011: 601) actually posits that '[t]he evidence suggests, however, that consistent with the model of complex adaptive systems, the "main game" will be played out beyond the constraints of a defined global architecture'.

With this chapter we hope to have demonstrated that practical theories for understanding global health policy and governance issues can, and perhaps must, be both rigorous and eclectic: there will be no 'unified field theory' for global health governance. But the field must be driven by innovative, value-conscious, politics-relevant scholarly and policy activism that deliberately links individuals, organizations, and systems. We think that in our historical overview, three case studies, and proposed governance-research matrix we have started such an approach.

References

Albuja, S. and Daynard, R. A. (2009). The Framework Convention on Tobacco Control and the adoption of domestic tobacco control policies: the Ecuadorian experience. *Tobacco Control*, **18**, 18–21.

Alder, E. and Haas, P. M. (1992). Epistemic communities, world order, and the creation of a reflective research program. *International Organisation*, **46** (1), 367–90.

Anderson, J. E. (1975). *Public Policy-Making*. New York: Praeger. Cited by **Hill, M. and Hupe, P.** (2003). *Implementing Public Policy*. London/Thousand Oaks/New Delhi: Sage Publications.

Anon. (2012). Bill Gates vreest Nederlandse bezuinigingen op hulp (Bill Gates fears Dutch aid cuts). *De Volkskrant*, 23 March 2012, p. 1. Available at: <http://www.volkskrant.nl/vk/nl/9824/De-zoektocht-naar-miljarden/article/detail/3230239/2012/03/23/Bill-Gates-vreest-Nederlandse-bezuinigingen-op-hulp.dhtml> (accessed 15 June 2012).

Antonovsky, A. (1984). The sense of coherence as a determinant of health, in **J. D. Matarazzo** (ed.) *Behavioral Health. A Handbook of Health Enhancement and Disease Prevention,* pp. 114–29, New York: Wiley.

Assunta, M. (2012). Tobacco industry's ITGA fights FCTC implementation in the Uruguay negotiations. *Tobacco Control*, **21** (6), 563–8.

Basheer, S. (2006). India's tryst with TRIPS: The Patents (Amendment) Act 2005. *The Indian Journal of Law and Technology*, **1**, 15–46.

Braveman, P. and Tarimo, E. (2002). Social inequalities in health within countries: not only an issue for affluent nations. *Social Science & Medicine*, **54** (11), 1621–35.

Brenner, N. (2001). The limits to scale? Methodological reflections on scalar structuration. *Progress in Human Geography*, **25** (4), 591–614.

Bustreo, F. and Doebbler, C. (2010). Making health an imperative of foreign policy: the value of a human rights approach. *Health and Human Rights*, **12** (1), 47–59.

Clavier, C. (2010). Bottom-up policy convergence: a sociology of the reception of policy transfer in public health policies in Europe. *Journal of Comparative Policy Analysis*, **12** (5), 451–66.

CSDH (2008). *Closing the Gap in a Generation. Health Equity through Action on the Social Determinants of Health. Final Report of the Commission on Social Determinants of Health*. Geneva: World Health Organization.

Davies, S. (2010). What contribution can international relations make to the evolving global health agenda? *International Affairs*, **86** (5), 1167–90.

De Gucht, K. (2010). *Letter to Executive Director MSF Mr. von Schoen–Angerer*. Available at: <http://msfaccess.org/sites/default/files/MSF_assets/Access/Docs/ACCESS_letter_ECTradeCommisioner_Gucht_ENG_2010.pdf> (accessed 12 September 2011).

DNP+ (2010). *Open Letter to Hon Prime Minister of India: Don't Trade Away our Lives*, 28 September 2010. Available at: <http://donttradeourlivesaway.files.wordpress.com/2010/10/letter-to-pmo.pdf> (accessed 3 July 2012).

Dodgson, R., Lee, K., and Drager, N. (2002). *Global Health Governance. A Conceptual Review*. London: Centre on Global Change and Health, London School of Hygiene and Tropical Medicine; Department of Health and Development, World Health Organization.

Doll, R. and Hill, A. B. (1954). The mortality of doctors in relation to their smoking habits. *British Medical Journal*, **1 (4877)**, 1451–5.

Dolowitz, D. and Marsh, D. (1996). Who learns what from whom: a review of the policy transfer literature. *Political Studies*, **44 (2)**, 343–57.

Eriksen, M., Mackay, J., and Ross, H. (2012). *'The Tobacco Atlas', American Cancer Society and World Lung Foundation*. Available at: <http://www.tobaccoatlas.org/uploads/Files/pdfs/products/cigarette_consumption/cigarette_consumption_pdf.pdf> (accessed 22 June 2012).

Evans, M. and Davies, J. (1999). Understanding policy transfer: a multi-level, multi-disciplinary perspective. *Public Administration*, **77** (2), 361–85.

FDFA and FDHA (2012). *Swiss Health Foreign Policy*. Available at: <http://www.bag.admin.ch/themen/internationales/13102/index.html?lang=en> (accessed 10 August 2012).

FDHA, FDFA and FOPH (2006). *Swiss Health Foreign Policy: Agreement on Health Foreign Policy Objectives*. Available at: <http://www.bag.admin.ch/themen/internationales/07416/index.html?lang=en> (accessed 28 October 2010).

Feldbaum, H. and Michaud, J. (2010). Health diplomacy and the enduring relevance of foreign policy interests. *PLoS Medicine*, **7** (4), e1000226.

Feldbaum, H., Lee, K., and Michaud, J. (2010). Global health and foreign policy. *Epidemiologic Reviews*, **32** (1), 82–92.

Ferman, B. (1990). When failure is success: implementation and Madisonian government, in **D. J. Palumbo** and **D. J. Calista** (eds.) *Implementation and the Policy Process: Opening Up the Black Box*, pp. 39–50, New York: Greenwood Press.

Fidler, D. (2003). SARS: Political pathology of the first post-Westphalian pathogen. *The Journal of Law, Medicine & Ethics*, **31** (4), 485–505.

Fidler, D. (2005). Health as foreign policy: between principle and power. *The Whitehead Journal of Diplomacy and International Relations*, **6** (2), 179–94.

Fidler, D. (2006). Health as foreign policy: harnessing globalisation for health. *Health Promotion International*, **21** (Suppl. 1), 51–8.

Framework Convention Alliance (2012). *Status of the WHO Framework Convention on Tobacco Control (FCTC)*. Available at: <http://fctc.org/images/stories/FCTC_ratification_latest_010612.pdf> (accessed 15 November 2012).

Francis, J. A., Shea, A. K., and Samet, J. M. (2006). Challenging the epidemiologic evidence on passive smoking: tactics of tobacco industry expert witnesses. *Tobacco Control*, **15** (Suppl. 4), 68–76.

Frenk, J. (2010). The global health system: strengthening national health systems as the next step for global progress. *PLoS Medicine*, **7** (1), e1000089.

Giddens, A. (1981). *A Contemporary Critique of Historical Materialism*. Berkeley, CA: University of California Press.

Gostin, L.O., Heywood, M., Ooms, G., Grover, A., Røttingen, J.-A., and Chenguang, W. (2010). National and global responsibilities for health. *Bulletin of the World Health Organization*, **88** (10), 719–20.

Haas, P.M. (1992). Introduction: epistemic communities and international policy coordination. *International Organization*, **46** (1), 1–35.

Hadi, A. (2009). *Globalization, medical tourism and health equity. Proceedings of the Symposium on Implications of Medical Tourism for Canadian Health and Health Policy*, Nov. 13. Ottawa, Canada: Institute of Population Health, pp. 1–28.

Harris, S. (2004). Marrying foreign policy and health: feasible or doomed to fail? *Medical Journal of Australia*, **180** (4), 171–3.

Held, D. and McGrew, A. (2002). *Governing Globalization: Power, Authority and Global Governance*. Malden, MA: Wiley.

Hill, C. (2003). *The Changing Politics of Foreign Policy*. New York: Palgrave Macmillan.

Hill, M. and Hupe, P. (2003). *Implementing Public Policy*. London/Thousand Oaks/New Delhi: Sage Publications.

Hill, M. and Hupe, P. (2006). Analysing policy processes as multiple governance: accountability in social policy. *Policy & Politics*, **34 (3)**, 557–73.

Hill, P. S. (2011). Understanding global health governance as a complex adaptive system. *Global Public Health: An International Journal for Research, Policy and Practice*, **6** (6), 593–605.

Hooghe, L. and Marks, G. (2003). Unraveling the central state, but how? Types of multi-level governance. *American Political Science Review*, **97** (2), 233–43.

HM Government (2008). *Health is Global: A UK Government Strategy 2008–13*. Available at: <http://www.dh.gov.uk/en/Publicationsandstatistics/Publications/PublicationsPolicyAndGuidance> (accessed 28 October 2010).

Hurt, R. D., Ebbert, J. O., Achadi, A., and Croghan, I. T. (2012). Roadmap to a tobacco epidemic: transnational tobacco companies invade Indonesia. *Tobacco Control*, **21** (3), 306–12.

Jansson, E., Fosse, E., and Tillgren, P. (2011). National public health policy in a local context—implementation in two Swedish municipalities. *Health Policy*, **103** (2–3), 219–27.

Kay, A. and Williams, O. (2009). Introduction: The international political economy of global health governance, in A. Kay and O. Williams (eds.), *Global Health Governance: Crisis, Institutions, and Political Economy*, pp. 1–24, Basingstoke: Palgrave Macmillan.

Kelly, M. P. and Charlton, B. (1995). The modern and the postmodern in health promotion, in R. Bunton, S. Nettleton, and R. Burrows (eds.) *The Sociology of Health Promotion*, pp. 77–89, London: Routledge.

Keusch, G. T., Kilama, W. L., Moon, S., Szlezák, N. A., and Michaud, C. M. (2010). The global health system: linking knowledge with action—learning from malaria. *PLoS Medicine*, **7** (1), e1000179.

Kickbusch, I. (2011). Global health diplomacy: how foreign policy can influence health. *BMJ*, **342**, d3154.

Kiernan, J. P. (2002). 100 years of Pan-Americanism, 1902–2002. *Perspectives in Health*, **6** (2), 1–4. Available at: <http://www.paho.org/english/dpi/Number12_article3_5.htm> (accessed 14 November 2012).

Koplan, J. P., Bond, T. C., Merson, M. H., Reddy, K. S., Rodriguez, M. H., Sewankambo, N. K., Wasserheit, J. N., and Consortium of Universities for Global Health Executive Board (2009). Towards a common definition of global health. *The Lancet*, **373** (9679), 1993–1995.

Labonte, R. (2008). Global health in public policy: finding the right frame? *Critical Public Health*, **18** (4), 467–82.

Labonte, R. and Gagnon, M. (2010). Framing health and foreign policy: lessons for global health diplomacy. *Globalization and Health*, **6** (14), 1–19.

Le Galès, P. (2004). Gouvernance, in L. Boussaguet, S. Jacquot, and P. Ravinet (eds.), *Dictionnaire des Politiques Publiques*, pp. 242–50, Paris: Presses de Science Po.

Lee, K. (2001). The global dimension of cholera. *Global Change & Human Health*, **2** (1), 6–17.

Lee, K. (2009). Understandings of global health governance: the contested landscape, in A. Kay and D. O. Williams (eds.) *Global Health Governance: Crisis, Institutions, and Political Economy*, pp. 27–41, Basingstoke: Palgrave Macmillan.

Lee, K. and Dodgson, R. (2000). Globalisation and cholera: implications for global governance. *Global Governance*, **6** (2), 213–36.

Leitner, H. and Miller, B. (2007). Scale and the limitations of ontological debate: a commentary on Marston, Jones and Woodward. *Transactions of the Institute of British Geographers*, **32** (1), 116–25.

Lin, V. (2010). The Framework Convention on Tobacco Control and health promotion: strengthening the ties. *Global Health Promotion*, **17** (Suppl. 1), 76–80.

Lipsky, M. (1980). *Street-Level Bureaucracy: Dilemmas of the Individual in Public Services*. New York: Russell Sage Foundation.

Löfgren, H., de Leeuw, E., and Leahy, M. (ed.) (2011). *Democratising Health: Consumer Groups in the Policy Process*. Cheltenham: Edward Elgar Publishing.

Lv, J., Su, M., Hong, Z., Zhang, T., Huang, X., Wang, B., and Li, L. (2011). Implementation of the WHO Framework Convention on Tobacco Control in mainland China. *Tobacco Control*, **20** (4), 309–14.

McInnes, C. and Lee, K. (2009). *The Transformation of Global Health Governance: Competing Worldviews and Crises: Project Synopsis*. Available at: <http://www.aber.ac.uk/en/media/GHG-Synopsis.pdf> (accessed 20 November 2012).

McInnes, C., Kamradt-Scott, A., Lee, K., Reubi, D., Roemer-Mahler, A., Rushton, S., Williams, O. D., and Woodling, M. (2012). Framing global health: the governance challenge. *Global Public Health: An International Journal for Research, Policy and Practice*, **7** (Suppl. 2), S83–S94.

McNeill, W. (1982). *The Pursuit of Power: Technology, Armed Force and Society since AD1000*. Chicago: University of Chicago Press.

Mazmanian, D. A. and Sabatier, P. A. (1989). *Implementation and Public Policy* (2nd edn.). Lanham/New York/London: University Press of America.

MDG Gap Task Force (2009). *Strengthening the Global Partnership for Development in a Time of Crisis.* New York: United Nations.

MSF (2010a). *Victory for Access to Medicines as Valganciclovir Patent is Rejected in India.* Available at: <http://www.doctorswithoutborders.org/press/release.cfm?id=4432&cat=press-release> (accessed 20 November 2012).

MSF (2010b). *EU–India Free Trade Agreement: Last Chance to Remove Provisions that Block Access to Medicines.* Available at: <http://www.doctorswithoutborders.org/press/release.cfm?id=4388&cat=press-release> (accessed 20 November 2012).

MSF (2011a). *Background: Access to Antiretrovirals, Untangling the Web of ARV Price Reductions.* Available at: <http://utw.msfaccess.org/background> (accessed 3 July 2012).

MSF (2011b). *Examples of the Importance of India as the 'Pharmacy of the Developing World'.* Available at: <http://www.doctorswithoutborders.org/news/access/background_paper_indian_generics.pdf> (accessed 16 November 2012).

Ministers of Foreign Affairs of Brazil, France, Indonesia, Norway, Senegal, South Africa, and Thailand (2007). Oslo Ministerial Declaration – global health: a pressing foreign policy issue of our time. *The Lancet*, **369** (9570), 1373–8.

Missal, A. (2008). *Seaway to the Future: American Social Visions and the Construction of the Panama Canal.* Madison, Wis.: University of Wisconsin Press.

Møgedal, S. and Alveberg, B. (2010). Can foreign policy make a difference to health? *PLoS Medicine*, **7** (5), e1000274.

Mommer, B. (2002). *Global Oil and the Nation State.* Oxford: Oxford University Press.

Moon, S., Szlezák, N. A., Michaud, C. M., Jamison, D. T., Keusch, G. T., Clark, W. C., and Bloom, B. R. (2010). The global health system: lessons for a stronger institutional framework. *PLoS Medicine*, **7** (1), e1000193.

Mumby, D. K. and Clair, R. P. (1997). Organizational discourse, in T. A. van Dijk (ed.) *Discourse as Social Interaction. Discourse Studies. A Multidisciplinary Introduction, volume 1*, pp. 181–205, London: Sage.

Najam, A. (1995). *Learning from the Literature on Policy Implementation: A Synthesis Perspective.* Laxenburg, Austria: International Institute for Applied Systems Analysis.

Nie, J. G. and Li, J. (2010). Globalized health and its governance. *Chinese Medical Journal*, **123** (13), 1796–9.

Owen, J. W. and Roberts, O. (2005). Globalisation, health and foreign policy: emerging linkages and interests. *Globalization and Health*, **1** (12), 1–5.

Owusu-Dabo, E., McNeill, A., Lewis, S., Gilmore, A., and Britton, J. (2010). Status of implementation of the Framework Convention on Tobacco Control in Ghana: a qualitative study. *BMC Public Health*, **10** (1). Available at: <http://www.biomedcentral.com/1471-2458/10/1> (accessed 17 April 2013).

Papadopoulos, Y. (2003). Cooperative forms of governance: problems of democratic accountability in complex environments. *European Journal of Political Research,* **42** (4), 473–501.

Parker, R. (2002). The global HIV/AIDS pandemic, structural inequalities, and the politics of international health. *American Journal of Public Health*, **92** (3), 343–7.

Peck, J. and Theodore, N. (2010). Mobilizing policy: models, methods, and mutations. *Geoforum*, **41** (2), 169–74.

Pülzl, H. and Treib, O. (2006). Implementing public policy, in F. Fischer, G. J. Miller, and M. S. Sidney (eds.) *Handbook of Public Policy Analysis*, pp. 89–107, Boca Raton, FL: CRC Press/Taylor and Francis Group.

Rhodes, R. A. W. (1996). The new governance: governing without government. *Political Studies*, **44** (4), 652–67.

Rosenau, J. N. and Czempiel, E.-O. (1992). *Governance without Government: Order and Change in World Politics.* Cambridge: Cambridge University Press.

Ruger, J. P. (2012). Global health governance as shared health governance. *Journal of Epidemiology & Community Health*, **66** (7), 653–61.

Shimko, K. (2008). Foreign policy, in W. A. Darity (ed.) *International Encyclopedia of the Social Sciences, volume 3,* pp. 169–72, Detroit, MI: McMillan Reference.

Sihto, M., Ollila, E., and Koivusalo, M. (2006). Principles and challenges of Health in All Policies, in T. Ståhl, M. Wismar, E. Ollia, E. Lahtinen, and K. Leppo (eds.) *Health in all Policies: Prospects and Proposals,* pp 3–20, Helsinki: Ministry of Social Affairs and Health.

Stone, D. A. (2002). *Policy Paradox: The Art of Political Decision Making.* New York: Norton.

Stuckler, D. and McKee, M. (2008). Five metaphors about global health policy. *The Lancet,* **372** (9633), 95–7.

Sussman, S., Pokhrel, P., Black, D., Kohrman, M., Hamann, S., Vateesatokit, P., and Nsimba, S. E. D. (2007). Tobacco control in developing countries: Tanzania, Nepal, China and Thailand as examples. *Nicotine and Tobacco Research,* **9** (Suppl. 3), S447–S457.

Swyngedouw, E. (2004). Globalisation or 'glocalisation'? Networks, territories and rescaling. *Cambridge Review of International Affairs,* **17** (1), 25–48.

Szlezák, N. A., Bloom, B. R., Jamison, D. T., Keusch, G. T., Michaud, C. M., Moon, S., and Clark, W. C. (2010). The global health system: actors, norms, and expectations in transition. *PLoS Medicine,* **7** (1), e1000183.

Touati, N., Roberge, D., Denis, J.-L., Pineault, R., Cazale, L., and Tremblay, D. (2007). Governance, health policy implementation and the added value of regionalization. *Health Policy,* **2** (3), 97–114.

Townsend, B., Martin, E., Löfgren, H., and de Leeuw, E. (2012). Global health governance: Framework Convention on Tobacco Control (FCTC), the Doha Declaration, and democratisation. *Administrative Sciences,* **2** (2), 186–202.

Trochim, W. M. K., Stillman, F. A., Clark, P. I., and Schmitt, C. L. (2003). The development of a model of the tobacco industry's interference with tobacco control programmes. *Tobacco Control,* **12** (2), 140–7.

United Nations (2009). *Resolution adopted by the General Assembly: 63/33. Global Health and Foreign Policy.* Sixty-third session, Agenda item 44. New York:United Nations. Available at: <http://www.undemocracy.com/A-RES-63-33.pdf> (accessed 14 November 2010).

Walt, G. (1998). Globalisation of international health. *The Lancet,* **351** (9100), 434–7.

White, D. (2009). *Network Governance and Democracy: Can Grassroots Participation Influence National Policy Orientation?* Paper presented at the annual meeting of RC 19 of the International Sociological Association, Montreal.

WHO (2004). *Building Blocks for Tobacco Control: A Handbook,* Geneva: World Health Organization.

WHO (2005). *WHO Framework Convention on Tobacco Control.* Geneva: World Health Organization.

WHO (2010). *2010 Global Progress Report on Implementation of the WHO Framework Convention on Tobacco Control,* Geneva: World Health Organization.

WHO (2011). *Global Implementation of the WHO Framework Convention on Tobacco Control—progress note.* Available at: <http://www.who.int/entity/fctc/reporting/Progress_note_September2011.pdf> (accessed 2 July 2012).

WHO (2012). *Fact Sheets: Tobacco.* Geneva: World Health Organization. Available at: <http://www.who.int/mediacentre/factsheets/fs339/en/index.html> (accessed 22 June 2012).

WTO (1994). *Agreement on Trade-Related Aspects of Intellectual Property Rights.* Geneva: World Trade Organization. Available at: <http://www.wto.org/english/tratop_e/trips_e/t_agm0_e.htm> (accessed 3 July 2012).

WTO (2001). *Declaration on the TRIPS Agreement and Public Health. Geneva: World Trade Organization.* Available at: <http://www.wto.org/english/thewto_e/minist_e/min01_e/mindecl_trips_e.htm> (accessed September 2010).

Yach, D. and Bettcher, D. (2000). Globalisation of tobacco industry influence and new global responses. *Tobacco Control,* **9** (2), 206–16.

Zola, I. K. (1991). Bringing our bodies and ourselves back in: reflections on a past, present, and future 'medical sociology'. *Journal of Health and Social Behaviour,* **32** (1), 1–16.

Chapter 7

Getting knowledge on 'wicked problems' in health promotion into action

David Hunter

Introduction

This chapter describes a collaborative research initiative bringing together academics and practitioners interested in how those engaged in policy and practice use, misuse, or fail to use knowledge on health promotion to modify and improve their work. It starts from the premise that health promotion is a 'wicked problem' and draws on theories of knowledge exchange and translation in an effort better to tackle complex problems. The collaborative research initiative which is the focus of the chapter is known as Fuse— the Centre for Translational Research in Public Health—and the author is its deputy director. One of five centres for public health excellence supported by the UK Clinical Research Collaboration, Fuse's particular focus is on translational research. Although all five centres have concerned themselves with this agenda, arguably Fuse has made it a particular priority.

The starting point for Fuse's work programme is an acknowledgement that getting research evidence into practice is difficult for a complex set of reasons; these are explored in more detail in later sections. A key task for Fuse and its health system partners, therefore, is to help to facilitate and nurture a culture that is receptive and responsive to the acquisition and application of knowledge and evidence. Apart from producing knowledge in a variety of ways that are appropriate and that fit particular circumstances, Fuse is also committed to undertaking research on how that knowledge is used and implemented, or why it may not be.

The case study material used to illustrate the issues and themes covered in the chapter draws on two very different initiatives in which the author has been directly involved. The first is an evaluation of a series of special workshops designed to explore the use and nature of evidence on a range of health promotion topics with policy-makers and practitioners working in health, local government, and third sector agencies. The topics were chosen because of their importance to the work of these organizations, and the workshops were designed to promote interaction between researchers and practitioners in the hope that a deeper understanding of the value of, and limits to, evidence and knowledge would be forthcoming. The series of workshops—known as the Research to

Reality (R2R) programme—was independently evaluated and this section of the chapter draws on that research.

The second example comes from work with the World Health Organization (WHO) Regional Office for Europe and results from a commission to develop a European action plan (EAP) for strengthening public health capacities and services. The EAP accompanies the Regional Office's policy framework and strategy, Health 2020, launched in September 2012. The content of the EAP is unexceptional but the journey embarked upon in its production is revealing and demonstrates some of the complex organizational, procedural, professional, and political factors that can arise and have a decisive influence on how knowledge is used and presented.

The chapter is divided into four main sections. In the first, the theoretical basis of the chapter's topic is described. It draws on work on the existence of 'wicked problems', on the relevance of systems thinking in understanding such issues and how to tackle the policy and practice challenges they pose, and on what is understood by the term 'knowledge translation' and its off-shoots—knowledge transfer, knowledge exchange, and knowledge brokerage. The second section then examines how the theories associated with knowledge and practice can be combined and applied in practice by reviewing a typology of policy-making models and the role research plays, and its differential use, in each of them. The third section examines the implications of the conclusions from the first and second sections for health promotion research, practice, and policy. The issues are illustrated with reference to the aims and purpose of Fuse and how it is pursuing its mission, including the factors either facilitating or impeding its progress. These concerns are illustrated with the two contrasting examples briefly described above. The final section considers key learning points from these two examples, and their implications for Fuse and, more broadly, for wider discussions about knowledge exchange and its importance.

Theoretical considerations

Three theoretical strands underpin the topics that are the subject of this chapter. First, the nature of wicked problems and the factors that comprise them; second, the insights provided by systems thinking into how wicked problems might be understood and tackled; and third, the notion of knowledge translation, which in fact is often used as a form of short-hand to include related terms such as knowledge transfer, knowledge exchange, and knowledge brokerage. What is important about these different terms is the position they adopt in respect of what constitutes knowledge, its generation, and its application in policy and practice. It is therefore desirable to have some clarity about their respective meanings.

Wicked problems

The notion of wicked problems is not new, but only fairly recently has it been applied to the complex challenges presented by public policy including health promotion (Australian

Public Service, 2007; Kickbusch and Gleicher, 2011). Wicked problems share a number of defining features, some or all of which may be present in a particular case (Rittel and Webber, 1973). For example, there may be difficulty in defining the issue; it may have multiple causes and interdependencies; wicked problems often lead to unforeseen consequences; they tend to evolve and mutate and are unstable; wicked problems are rarely confined to one organization but are cross-cutting in nature; there are usually no clear solutions available, and those which exist are likely to offer better or worse rather than right or wrong alternatives; and wicked problems involve changing behaviour.

Examples of wicked problems in public policy are climate change, health inequalities, obesity, and alcohol misuse. In each case there are disputes over the precise nature of the problem, including whether there is one at all, its causes, and the appropriate solutions to them. But whatever the merits or otherwise of particular solutions, what is clear is that action is required on multiple fronts, which demands a whole-systems approach (Lang and Rayner, 2012). For example, tackling alcohol misuse through raising the minimum unit price might be effective, but on its own is unlikely to tackle the growing problem of excessive drinking in many countries. Attention simultaneously to cultural and behavioural factors is also required. Solutions therefore require whole-of-government and whole-of-society approaches, which lie at the heart of the WHO Regional Office for Europe's new health strategy, Health 2020 (WHO, 2012a).

Systems thinking

The link between wicked problems and systems thinking is in many ways an obvious one, but is often not made explicit. A rational, linear approach to problem-solving is not an appropriate response to wicked problems, whereas viewing organizational and policy systems as complex adaptive systems is far more likely to be suitable. Rational thinking views organizations and systems as resembling machines—they are predictable and can be planned and controlled accordingly. Ideas to tackle perceived problems are generated by experts and specialists, and implementation of agreed interventions that have worked elsewhere is seen to be straightforward and unproblematic. In this context, the issue of evidence is viewed as uncontroversial and a matter of effective collection and dissemination. Finally, organizations are regarded as being largely similar and not affected much by context, so it is possible to adopt a generic approach.

The adoption of a systems approach views organizations and policy arenas as complex adaptive systems (CAS) (Plsek and Greenhalgh, 2001; Best, 2011). Plsek and Greenhalgh define a CAS as 'a collection of individual agents with freedom to act in ways that are not always totally predictable, and whose actions are interconnected so that one agent's actions changes [sic] the context for other agents' (2001: 626). CASs invariably have fuzzy boundaries, with changing membership and members who simultaneously belong to several other systems or subsystems. In such contexts, tension, paradox, and ambiguity are natural phenomena and cannot necessarily or always be resolved or avoided. More often than not, they need to be acknowledged and managed (Hunter et al., 2010).

In CASs, organizations are not regarded as machine-like but as organisms that are able to adapt to their environment. Learning and adapting are therefore key characteristics, and in such settings ideas for tackling problems may emerge from anyone and are encouraged. These ideas may be informed by what has worked elsewhere, but crucially they must be adapted to the local context rather than seek to ignore or deny it. Evidence in complex systems is not simply a matter of off-the-shelf dissemination and application but of sharing knowledge through nurturing and cultivating relationships and then reframing the evidence to suit the local context (Hunter, 2003). Health promotion interventions are good examples of both wicked problems and complex systems (Best, 2011; Leischow et al., 2008). The point can be illustrated by a recent research study examining the impact of the UK government's health prevention policies in four areas—smoking, excessive drinking, poor diet, and lack of exercise—in the period between 2003 and 2008 (Buck and Forsini, 2012). These behaviours account for around 50% of the disease burden in developed countries. The study found that the proportion of the population engaging in three or four of these behaviours fell by 8% (from 33 to 25%) over the period, which suggests remarkable success in terms of the policy interventions and their impact. However, the study also found that the number of manual workers and people with no qualifications engaging in all four behaviours remained unchanged. This served to widen health inequalities between social groups rather than reduce them, thereby failing to implement the government's policy of improving the health status of the poorest sections of the population at a faster rate than those which are better off. The report concluded by recommending that health promotion professionals and others need to adopt a whole-systems approach to the problem and tackle multiple behaviours together rather than separately in silos. There was also a recommendation to target the lower socioeconomic groups if the health gap was not to become wider. The example is pertinent because, as Best (2011) observes, most of those active in health promotion or public health do not think in such ways when it comes to the design of interventions and the types of knowledge that are required and need to be mobilized.

Knowledge translation

The application of a systems approach necessitates viewing evidence as a socially constructed reality in which various types of knowledge might be relevant depending on the issue, the context, and the state of the evidence base. Typical practice change from knowledge translation activities has been estimated to be only about 8–15% (Best and Holmes, 2010). This would seem to suggest that if we want more evidence-informed practice then we need more practice-informed evidence. If health promotion policy and practice problems are embedded in complex systems, these need to be understood if the problems are to be tackled and solved, even if only partially.

Since such systems for the most part remain little understood, it should come as no surprise to discover that knowledge transfer and adopt processes are likewise little understood. Many factors can intervene in how research is used, or even if it is used at all. For example, Phil Davies, an academic and former senior policy adviser to the UK

Box 7.1 Policy-makers' sources of evidence

- ◆ Experts' evidence (including consultants and think tanks)
- ◆ Evidence from professional associations
- ◆ Opinion-based evidence (including lobbyists and pressure groups)
- ◆ Ideological evidence (including party think tanks, manifestoes)
- ◆ Media evidence
- ◆ Internet evidence
- ◆ Lay evidence (including constituents' and citizens' experiences)
- ◆ 'Street' evidence (including urban myths, conventional wisdom)
- ◆ Research evidence

Reproduced with permission of the author Philip Davies.

government, identified nine sources of evidence that policy-makers usually rely on (see Box 7.1). Out of these nine, research comes last.

Although we still know too little about what makes research use happen or not happen, some of the factors that might explain the reasons are being captured in studies. One of the emerging issues is that there is an increased chance of research findings being found to be useful if there is evidence of close interaction between researchers and end users. This relationship appears to be crucial, and there is therefore a case to be made for building capacity for evidence-informed decision-making and practice-informed evidence.

Until quite recently, knowledge transfer was assumed to follow a rational linear model with a number of characteristics, including the views that knowledge is a product to be acquired and applied; that there is a uni-directional flow from the producers of knowledge to end users; and that knowledge is generalizable across contexts. Underpinning these assumptions is a view of knowledge as a commodity to be packaged and presented to those who may be seen to benefit from access to it. It is a largely passive view of the relationship between knowledge producers and users. But other models take a very different view of knowledge—both its production and take-up. Two that draw on the work of Best and colleagues (Best et al., 2009) are considered here.

First is the relationship model of knowledge exchange, which starts from the assumption that knowledge can be acquired from multiple sources, including research, theory, and practice (i.e. tacit knowledge). Social relationships are key to the transmission and exchange of knowledge; networks of research producers and consumers are established, which collaborate through the production, synthesis, and integration cycles of research. Relationships are seen as being of vital importance because knowledge is regarded as context-specific and adaptive rather than as static and of a 'one size fits all' variety.

Furthermore, the use and application of knowledge is a function of effective relationships and processes. In essence, knowledge exchange is a function of not only the science but also the degree to which the purveyor of that knowledge is viewed as a credible witness who can win over and convince an audience, especially a sceptical one.

The second model is known as the systems model of knowledge co-production and has a number of characteristics, many of which overlap, or are shared, with the relationship model. Knowledge is linked to priorities, culture, and context; it comprises and respects both explicit and tacit knowledge to inform decision-making; relationships are mediated through the cycle; and the degree to which knowledge is used is a function of effective integration with the organizations and systems to which it is directed.

The appeal of both these models is that they more accurately reflect the messy complexity of the real world in which knowledge, of whatever type, is likely to be one among many factors that influence policy and practice. Another way of conceptualizing the way knowledge is generated and used is to refer to the distinction made between Mode I and Mode II research (Greenhalgh and Wieringa, 2011). Those seeking to strengthen the take-up and impact of research wish to see a shift from Mode I to Mode II. Mode I represents the rational linear model of research production and use mentioned above. Here, the focus is on knowledge generation, with the researcher as expert dispensing knowledge that has been produced using clear standards. In contrast, Mode II research starts with a focus on problem-solving, on learning by doing, with knowledge being co-created and its precise type and configuration dependent on context. The methods adopted are flexible and there is no fixed quality standard—there are only general guidelines for quality.

Van de Ven and Johnson (2006) argue in their classic paper that there are three ways in which the gap between theory and practice may be framed. The first approach, echoing the rational model of knowledge transfer described above, is typically framed as a knowledge transfer problem. The assumption here is that practice knowledge concerning how to do things derives at least in part from research knowledge that has been acquired through scientific study. The problem, therefore, is one of translating research knowledge into practice. The second approach sees knowledge of theory and practice as separate and distinct kinds of knowledge. They may be complementary but they reflect different ontologies and methods. The third view holds that the gap between theory and practice is a knowledge production problem and is akin to Mode II thinking as described above. Van de Ven and Johnson therefore propose what they term 'a method of engaged scholarship in which researchers and practitioners coproduce knowledge that can advance theory and practice in a given domain'. They go on to define engaged scholarship 'as a collaborative form of inquiry in which academics and practitioners leverage their different perspectives and competencies to coproduce knowledge about a complex problem or phenomenon that exists under conditions of uncertainty found in the world' (Van de Ven and Johnson, 2006: 803). Engaged scholarship is not only aimed at enhancing the value and relevance of research for practice, as much collaborative research seeks to do; it also advances research knowledge through improved understanding. As a later section shows, Fuse's modus operandi (or maybe modus vivendi would be more accurate) is being modelled along these lines.

For engaged scholarship to occur meaningfully, the relationship between researchers and practitioners becomes one of 'negotiated order' (Strauss et al., 1964) as they respectively explore and seek to understand each other's domains, from which they then move to nurture and sustain a relationship that is mutually rewarding for both groups, thereby demonstrating a form of reciprocity. From such a coming together of different views of the world in order to try and improve it, the aim is the production of knowledge that is relevant not only for theory but also for practice in a given context (Pettigrew, 2001).

Arguably, life in the real world for researchers and practitioners is even more complex and variegated, with research providing a political currency to advance (or conversely terminate) particular interests. The next section therefore examines a range of policy-making models that engage with and use research for different purposes in the pursuit of their goals.

Policy-making models

If it is accepted that there is a need for a new type of 'engaged scholarship' (Van de Ven and Johnson, 2006: 809) then the challenge is one of how to achieve this in a given context. Moreover, there might conceivably be variants of what the term actually means and what level of engagement and of scholarship is sought. In their review of policy-making models and the role of research in respect of each of them, Bowen and Zwi (2005: 602) describe six models:

◆ knowledge-driven
◆ problem-solving
◆ interactive
◆ political
◆ enlightenment
◆ tactical.

Both the knowledge-driven and problem-solving models resemble Van de Ven and Johnson's first approach, whereby emergent research about a given problem will lead to direct application to policy. If it does not, the argument goes, it is because of a knowledge transfer problem. The interactive model begins to engage with the complexity of policy and practice, suggesting that the search for knowledge moves beyond evidence, as conceived of in the previous two models, and includes a variety of sources including politics and stakeholder interests. It aims to reflect the complexity of the policy and practice as described in the previous section. The political model offers a more selective and opportunistic perspective, with decision-makers paying scant regard to research unless it serves their political purposes. Here, evidence is used to justify the problem and/or the solution to it. Under the enlightenment model, which is in keeping with Weiss's (1979) interpretation, research over time may shape thinking and permeate the policy process, thereby influencing how decision-makers view issues. Finally, the tactical model is related to the political model insofar as it may be invoked to justify delay or inaction when it comes to policy formation or implementation.

What this typology shows is that many of the models in good currency, while providing useful insights and perspectives, risk suggesting or implying—even if unintentionally—that policy-making is a logical, rational, and linear process. But as we have seen, and as the next section of the chapter will demonstrate with examples, it is difficult for evidence to remain intact and unsullied through the process from conception to completion, given the existence of messy policy contexts and the realities of decision-making that require evidence to be adapted and moulded to particular situations and circumstances that themselves are often in a state of constant flux. The conclusion to be drawn is that evidence and context need to intermingle, and far from this being a heretical thought to be disregarded or hastily dismissed, it offers perhaps the only hope that research evidence might have value in promoting health and improving health and well-being.

We can therefore conclude that if knowledge is going to be of value in policy and practice settings, the chances are it is not going to be a one-off, uni-directional event or process. More likely, as Bowen and Zwi argue, it is going to be 'a powerful and continuous process in which knowledge accumulates and influences thinking over time' (2005: 603). But the construction of the evidence itself, as well as who participates in that undertaking, is also an important part of getting evidence and context to interact in new and different ways. Making progress in respect of bringing together the theory and practice of evidence use is the challenge taken up in the next section.

New directions for acquiring and using knowledge in policy and practice

This section describes a recent venture to explore new ways of putting academic researchers together with policy and practice partners for the mutual benefit of all. In 2008, as mentioned at the start of the chapter, the UK Clinical Research Collaboration invested in establishing five centres for research in public health excellence with funding for an initial period of five years, although it has recently been agreed that a second injection of funds tapering over a further five years will be available to be administered through the Medical Research Council. This will allow the initial investment in staff and new ways of working to continue and become more fully embedded, which was always the intention behind the initiative.

The centres were expressly designed to be capacity-building entities to strengthen the public health research community in England and Wales (Scotland made separate arrangements) and invest in the infrastructure to increase not only the volume of high-quality research being undertaken but also, as importantly, the potential for research findings to have an impact on policy and practice. One of the centres, known as Fuse—the Centre for Translational Research in Public Health—took the form of a partnership between the five universities in the north-east region of England, together with involvement from the National Health Service (NHS) and local government. It sought to complement the work of the other four centres by focusing on knowledge exchange and how this might be developed in terms of both advancing the theory of getting knowledge into action and illuminating—and deepening an understanding of— how action occurs in policy and practice.

In its approach, Fuse has eschewed a traditional rational linear and uni-directional approach to knowledge translation, including related terms like 'knowledge transfer', and instead has adopted an approach more in keeping with the Canadian Institutes of Health Research definition (CIHR, 2004), which regards knowledge translation in terms of exchange, synthesis, dialogue, and interaction between researchers and users. In keeping with the earlier discussion of wicked problems and complex systems, and the various policy-making models which endeavour to capture these concerns, the Canadian Institutes of Health Research definition has greater real-world relevance than a narrow reductionist approach that has more in common with evidence-based medicine. As others have acknowledged, the evidence-based medicine paradigm does not in any case adequately reflect the complex reality of the public health environment (Ogilvie et al., 2009). It is not, as Greenhalgh points out, that evidence-based medicine is inherently wrong, but that it has exceeded its terms of reference and 'plays to a vision of science that is characterised by predictive certainty' (Greenhalgh, 2012: 96). The evidence-based medicine paradigm, and the rationalistic assumptions on which it draws, which entail reducing complexity and uncertainty, is not 'fit for purpose' in respect of comprehending and transforming complex systems that require engagement with 'the personal, political and institutional context' (Greenhalgh, 2012: 97).

In pursuing its mission, Fuse has undertaken various initiatives to raise awareness of the issues and to begin to work out how it can best support its policy and practice partners to meet their needs. Such ground-clearing has been an essential feature of Fuse's work, and while it is time-consuming and may seem to be going over very basic and familiar ground, it is also essential. It became clear early on that even those academic members of Fuse who had signed up to its mission remained vague and often confused about what exactly knowledge exchange entailed. Some saw the role as one of knowledge transfer—i.e. sharing research findings and making them known more widely. Others were more inclined to favour a knowledge translation approach, which required research findings to be represented and repackaged in a language and format that would be more readily accessible to, and understood by, policy-makers, practitioners, and the public. But there was also a small group of researchers who saw the need for a more radical departure from the basic acceptance of a uni-directional, rational model, whereby the challenge lay in communicating an assembled body of knowledge or evidence in such a way that it would have an impact on policy and practice. This group of Fuse staff introduced a new language, adopting terms like 'knowledge exchange', 'knowledge mobilization', 'knowledge brokerage', and 'the co-creation and co-production of knowledge' to describe what Fuse ought to be doing in fulfilment of its knowledge-to-action mission.

These terms demanded a quite different approach and a rebalancing of the relationship between those doing research and those who are potential users of it. Rather than policy and practice partners being viewed as receptacles into which knowledge could be poured by experts with the answers, they were to be seen as co-equals in the research endeavour. Rebalancing the relationship and power structure in this way takes time to embed and Fuse has some way to go before it can claim success.

In the remainder of this section, two examples are offered of ways in which Fuse academics are engaging with policy and practice partners. The examples are very different—intentionally so—to reflect the diverse nature of public health. The first concerns the R2R programme, which entailed the running and evaluation of a series of workshops designed to raise awareness of the evidence available in regard to selected public health topics, with a view to exploring the issues around its use and/or non-use. The workshops were confined to the north-east region of England and were focused on local policy-makers and practitioners.

The second example describes work undertaken for the WHO Regional Office for Europe as part of its new health policy framework and strategy, Health 2020 (WHO, 2012a). The Regional Office covers 53 member states and around 900 million people, resulting in considerable variety and diversity, with countries at very different stages of development in respect of health promotion. The specific assignment on which academics based at Durham University were engaged was the production of an EAP to accompany the Health 2020 policy framework (WHO, 2012b). Its purpose is to serve as one of the main pillars to assist with the implementation of the strategy through a focus on strengthening public health services across Europe.

Both examples encountered some similar challenges and obstacles in applying knowledge and evidence, but they also displayed significant differences. These were perhaps not so surprising when consideration is given to the very different contexts and levels framing each of the examples. Following brief descriptions of the two examples, the next and final section offers an analysis of them in an attempt to draw out some lesson-learning for Fuse and others engaged in similar work.

Research to Reality (R2R): the story of a knowledge-to-action initiative

One of the early initiatives undertaken by Fuse was in response to a commission from the North East Improvement and Efficiency Partnership (NEIEP). Between 2008 and 2011, when the Partnership was abolished, it worked with local authorities and other agencies in the north-east region, with the aim of delivering outcomes to improve the well-being of local communities through better and more efficient services. Part of its interest in holding a series of what were called R2R workshops was in trying to improve the use of evidence in the efficient running of services. There were eight workshops in the series, the last of which drew on the preceding seven in order to raise more general issues that had emerged about getting knowledge into action. The other workshops were topic based. The topics were selected by NEIEP following consultation with those working in health and well-being in local authorities in order to ensure that they reflected local concerns and priorities.

The topics covered were wide-ranging and included all the major concerns in public health and health promotion: stopping smoking; alcohol misuse; teenage pregnancy; work and incapacity; obesity; young people not in education, employment, or training; public perception of local services; and the engagement of the public in service design and delivery. The seven half-day workshops were delivered over the period of a year, 2009–10, with the eighth and final workshop taking place in early 2011.

Each workshop had the same purpose and followed the same format. They had the specific aim of facilitating a two-way knowledge transfer between academics and practitioners. The design and format were intended to enable the sharing of innovative practice, to encourage improved networks between practitioners from different organizations, and to help participants consider the implications of the evidence for their current and future practice and policy needs. Delegates from a wide range of organizations—but principally local authorities, the health sector, and third (or social) sector—attended most of the workshops. Attendees to each workshop were circulated in advance, with a research digest prepared by a leading academic in that particular field. The digests were around eight pages in length and written in an accessible style. Their purpose was to update delegates on the latest state of research on that topic and to point to any gaps or issues arising from the research. At each workshop there were brief presentations from the academic who had prepared the digest and a senior policy or practice person. But the emphasis of the workshops was on round-table facilitated discussion about the evidence that had been presented, and any particular obstacles or barriers that seemed to exist to prevent its uptake. Each workshop ended with action planning, including a written pledge completed by each delegate committing them to doing something different in their practice as a result of having attended the workshop. Finally, a full report on the workshop presentations and discussion was produced shortly after each event and put up on the NEIEP website.

In addition to being members of the planning team that oversaw and organized the workshops, a team of researchers who were part of Fuse and based at Durham and Northumbria Universities were commissioned to evaluate the initiative (Rushmer et al., 2011). The following review of the R2R initiative draws heavily on the research findings.

The evaluation sought to explore what activity took place as a result of the programme, either on the day of the workshop or as follow-up action. A realist evaluation approach was adopted to ask questions about what worked, where, for whom, and under what conditions. Data collection methods included observation of the workshops (this took the form of observing delegates' use of, and responses to, group discussions and other workshop material and activities: two researchers took field notes and compared findings to ensure consistency); documentary analysis of written workshop material (this comprised action plans, summaries of round-table discussions, and flip charts); and interviews with a purposive sample of delegates in the weeks following the workshop (short term) and again a few months later (medium term). Interviews were audio recorded and transcribed.

The evaluation team employed a modified participatory action approach, working with the steering group as the programme proceeded, sharing data and jointly interpreting these, while at the same time drawing on members' knowledge and experience to inform the research findings. This ensured ownership of the evaluation and its findings by the steering group, but also allowed for timely changes to be made to the programme of workshops as the evaluation unfolded and particular issues were picked up by the research team. The initial findings were presented at the final workshop in the series.

The study was a small one, so over-generalizing from its findings should be avoided. It also took place against a turbulent background in respect of policy and organizational change as a result of a switch of government in May 2010, which promptly set about introducing several major change initiatives affecting public services. Many of these had a direct impact on public health and health promotion services and on staff, who were subjected to unforeseen pressures. Context was therefore a critically important factor in terms of who attended the workshops (the drop-out rate was quite high) and also what they expected and/or wanted from them.

On the positive side, the research digests were well received, as were the workshop presentations, but there was still a tendency to regard these as a one-way flow of information and knowledge from the academic expert to the practitioner rather than as enabling a two-way dialogue or flow of knowledge. The workshop discussions were also welcomed for a variety of reasons and offered delegates an opportunity to contribute to multiple flows of knowledge between them from various parts of the health system. The opportunity the workshops gave delegates to reflect upon their practice and engage in more in-depth conversation, especially with the session leads, was especially valued.

On the negative side, delegates believed the workshop discussions did not work where they were dominated by particular groups or organizations, or where the thinking was viewed as too parochial and blinkered when set against wider issues. Several delegates felt that the wide mix of experience and seniority across delegates stunted discussion and kept it at too basic a level. This reflected a more general problem with the workshops as a whole, whose intended target audience was strategic policy-makers locally rather than front-line practitioners. But in practice the audiences for the workshops tended to be dominated by front-line practitioners, despite repeated attempts—and huge effort invested in trying—to secure attendance by senior policy-makers. Even when they signed up to attend these tended to be the ones who failed to show on the day, often without so much as an apology to the organizers. The other failure was over the action planning. The follow-up actions to which delegates committed themselves on the day were of two different types. The first comprised modest, low-level, mainly individually focused commitments, such as making a phone call and connecting with another policy or practitioner delegate or an academic contact made at the workshop. The second type of follow-up action was more ambitious but still rather vague and non-specific, giving little detail of how it would be achieved. An action of this type might include feeding research findings into a wider arena.

The third negative finding was arguably the most significant in terms of the primary purpose of the workshop series. It concerned working with academics and the nature of the evidence, about which a number of issues were raised by delegates. Many, if not most, delegates simply wanted existing evidence identified and made available to them in formats they could use and in a language they could understand. They wanted such manageable packages to be delivered automatically to them (perhaps electronically) or be available in clear 'one-stop' places. The principal message coming through was to 'tell us what works', or does not work, backed up by a call for 'clear messages'. When asked how academics could assist in achieving these ends, delegates often saw them as having the ability to bridge, translate, and interpret for the various knowledge contexts present at the workshop, including practitioner, commissioner, researcher, and so on.

There was some acknowledgement that different forms of knowledge, data, and information exist, but also frustration that whereas research tended to answer the questions 'What is happening? And why?', delegates often felt they knew enough about the causes of issues and were looking more for answers and clear pointers on what to do about them in order to inform their decision-making. It was widely perceived that research was far less able to provide easy or unambiguous answers here. Delegates did express a desire to work closely with academics to address local questions and to build research capacity, but creating such opportunities and knowing how to go about this task seemed to defeat many. There was also a feeling that research evidence was used in particular ways in delegates' organizations; for example, that it was cherry-picked to support planned activity and largely ignored if not. This perception echoes the policy-making models reviewed in the previous section, in particular the appeal of the political and tactical models (Bowen and Zwi, 2005).

When all is said and done, a clear finding from the evaluation is that for the majority of delegates nothing of significance or great import changed as a result of attending any of the workshops. Latent learning (or a process similar to the enlightenment model mentioned earlier) could perhaps be a consequence of workshop attendance, whereby seeds planted at the event might pop up and connect later with a particular problem or issue the delegate happened to be struggling with. But, more commonly, delegates had difficulty remembering the workshop when interviewed some weeks after it had taken place. Apart from a few ongoing discussions and maintenance of some connections that had been forged or rekindled at the workshops, by and large the workshop series did not result in any lasting or noteworthy change. One or two delegates claimed that workshop attendance had given them the impetus or confidence they needed to advance things, but they were very much the exception.

On closer inspection, the delegates' comments revealed a complex set of contextual conditions and factors that clearly militated against change and acted as a considerable barrier to using research evidence effectively. The reasons given included lack of time and capacity; the negative impact of national targets in driving certain behaviours and agendas while at the same time precluding others; and wider system instability and financial pressures, all of which they had to juggle. Other reasons advanced referred to the cultural backdrop of delegates' organizations, revealing a reluctance to use research evidence; and historical reasons—or what might be termed 'mind traps'—were given, which acted to prevent delegates thinking differently or creatively.

A theme which came through strongly was the notion of passivity. None of the practitioners attending the workshops saw themselves as having an active or leading role in shaping and modifying the evidence to suit their needs. Rather, they sought the help of others in such work. It is possible that such passivity is learned behaviour—a coping strategy within a wider system that does not encourage evidence use, or value innovation, or provide mechanisms to encourage it. A culture of disempowerment may also account for passivity where delegates were discouraged from stepping outside their specific roles and responsibilities. Showing initiative was not applauded. Perhaps of greater significance, the workplace culture was a 'can do' one of '(s)he who does, knows'. For all the rhetoric and good intentions, seeking out evidence was not in practice seen to matter and was not valued.

It is, of course, difficult to know if the contextual reasons given for lack of follow-up or impact are genuine reasons or convenient excuses that let the delegates off the hook of accepting personal responsibility for such a negative outcome. Some delegates were clearly embarrassed when talking about lack of follow-up, so resorting to factors beyond their immediate control could hold appeal to absolve them from blame. On the other hand, perhaps this is being overly harsh and judgemental and placing too much responsibility on individual discretion. It may be that academics still enjoy a degree of space and freedom of manoeuvre in their work that is denied others employed in the health system. Taking such employees out of their routine work and giving them an opportunity to stand outside their comfort zone and learn about and share possibly new and innovative ways of working on larger remits, before returning them to their work settings where nothing has changed, might well give rise to a context that is hostile and unreceptive to change, making lack of follow-up both understandable and a perfectly reasonable coping mechanism.

A recurrent theme, related to what has just been described, was the difficulty of securing changes without senior leader commitment and buy-in. As noted, very few senior leaders attended the workshops, and their absence was noted and commented upon by many delegates. The absence of leaders could therefore well be a factor in accounting for why so little changed post-workshop. The workshops were targeted at such senior staff and provided ample opportunity to engage and hopefully get some take-away messages which could be used back in the workplace. If there was a failure it was in an inability to get such individuals to commit to the initiative despite their initial enthusiasm, which had prompted NEIEP to invest in it.

In conclusion, the R2R series of workshops largely succeeded in its aims of allowing and facilitating knowledge transfer (knowledge flowing to a targeted audience) from academics to practitioners, and knowledge translation (interpretation, synthesis, and presentation) through the research digests and presentations. The workshop discussions also facilitated knowledge exchange to a degree between participants. Yet, despite these positive and worthwhile features and experiences, the researchers could find no evidence that any of these useful outcomes or gains were either maintained or embedded post-workshop. Any lasting impact has been impossible to capture and any planned input was not sustained or followed through. Therefore, the R2R programme largely failed to secure any knowledge-to-action results. Nor did it succeed in offering a milieu to co-create and co-produce knowledge in new and different ways involving academics and practitioners working as partners in addressing their respective needs. As the evaluation report concluded: 'as a mechanism to prompt change the R2R workshops succeeded in initiating enthusiasm about research evidence and its potential to impact positively on practice but could not on their own sustain that interest or facilitate changes to practice' (Rushmer et al., 2011: 6). While serving a useful purpose, on their own the workshops were unable and/or insufficient to achieve the type and range of changes desired against a context of policy churn and system upheaval, and a culture that could be sceptical of the value of evidence and knowledge, especially if it questioned or even threatened accepted or cherished ways of working. Moreover, in the absence of senior leaders to engage in the dialogue it made it doubly difficult to envisage ways of mobilizing evidence and knowledge to achieve deeper and lasting changes in ways of working and their outcomes.

Reflecting on some of the suggestions made by delegates as to how the R2R programme could have been more effective is something to which the section below returns.

Working with WHO

The second example describes an attempt made by academics to engage with high-level policy and strategy development and centres on the WHO Regional Office for Europe's development of its new policy framework and strategy, Health 2020 (WHO, 2012a). It was a very different experience in both scope and scale from the R2R example, which was confined to a single region of England. In contrast, the new health strategy has to win the support of, and be formally endorsed by, all 53 member states represented on WHO's Regional Committee. These countries have little in common and operate very different health systems in respect of their financing and organization, and display different priorities as far as health promotion and public health are concerned.

The assignment from the Regional Office was given to two Durham University-based academics, one of whom is also active in Fuse and committed to its knowledge exchange mission. The background to the assignment is described in Marks et al. (2011), and Hunter (2012). The following section is different from the description of the R2R programme because it is not based on an independent evaluation or assessment of the work. Rather, it is based on the author's personal reflections on the process over the 18 months or so during which the work took place.

The commission required the production of an EAP to strengthen public health systems and capacities (WHO, 2012b). Designed to be one of the main pillars for implementing Health 2020, its genesis was in part a response to concerns that while having a strategy was all well and good, it would be of little practical use if countries lacked a proper functioning infrastructure when it came to health promotion and public health. Health 2020 was WHO's first attempt at a health strategy since Health for All and Health 21, published in the 1980s. Although these were welcomed and widely cited, there remained a sense that they had little traction on countries' governments and their priorities for health. Therefore, it is hoped that by accompanying Health 2020, and being linked directly to it, the EAP will provide a useful resource and access to tools that will enable countries to make up any gap or shortfall in their health promotion policies and services.

The production of the EAP and its content are unexceptional in themselves. What proved to be of far greater interest from the perspective of this chapter and Fuse's knowledge exchange mission is just how complex, messy, unexpected, and unpredictable is the business of bringing knowledge to bear on policy especially at a transnational level. Parallels exist between the WHO example and the R2R programme described earlier insofar as both reflected particular contexts, cultures, and histories, which acted to shape, guide, and influence what ultimately emerged, or failed to emerge. But in the case of the WHO example, such factors took on a significance that at times seemed to put at risk the very purpose of the EAP and its original design. At the same time, there were moments when having seemingly reached a dead-end or cul-de-sac from which there appeared to be no escape or return, something unexpected would happen to unblock the impasse and allow the work to proceed as planned. It is not certain if such difficulties arose from internal politics within the Regional Office or from external pressures coming from particular member states. While some countries did seem to be able to exert more influence than others on shaping the focus and content of the new health policy framework and strategy, it is also the case that senior members of staff within WHO were not always in complete agreement about how to define key terms like public health and health promotion. While some seemed more comfortable with a narrower, more biomedical focus located primarily within the health and health care system, others favoured a broader whole-systems approach, with an emphasis on whole-of-government and whole-of-society perspectives. In their view, improving health and well-being and tackling health inequalities required action far beyond the health system and ministries of health.

As a sometimes uncomprehending outsider, one simply had to accept these internal differences, which would work themselves out in the end, giving rise on occasion to sudden and unexpected course corrections. An outsider asking questions and seeking an explanation often met with feigned surprise. In any case, and somewhat paradoxically, officials at WHO, while never forgetting its history—marked by a series of landmark achievements, including the Alma-Ata Declaration, the Ottawa Charter, Health for All and the more recent Tallinn Charter—also seemed to thrive on, and live for, the moment. They existed in a state of perpetual motion—often in a literal sense as they moved relentlessly and seamlessly from one meeting to another between countries across the region. On occasion, officials were juggling, and dipping into and out of, several meetings that were occurring simultaneously in different parts of the building! The existence and application of sound robust knowledge and evidence in such highly charged circumstances was largely taken for granted. What took up much more attention—and was a source of constant preoccupation—was ensuring that agreed deadlines were met, since these were set to fit in with important meetings involving high-level government officials and health ministers, and also with the needs of the translators charged with the task of getting documents ready for distribution in four languages. As a consequence, many of the deadlines were very short (almost unrealistically so), which did not leave a great deal of time for in-depth evidence-gathering, analysis, or reflection. It was assumed that any contracted experts had instant access to the appropriate knowledge bank and were on top of it, and therefore able to extract from it what was needed to meet the brief.

What is also striking is how few people ultimately determine the outcome of a stream of work. In the case of the EAP reported here, it came down to a maximum of four or five senior WHO staffers and advisers, including the Regional Director who got engaged from time to time at crucial stages. Various drafts and redrafts of the EAP were prompted not by anything produced by the academics at Durham but by the views expressed at meetings or during the consultation process by some member states. Not all members are equal, and some are more equal than others. For example, and doubtless reflecting the different stages of their development, several countries had divergent views about the causes of ill health and about how these, and health inequalities more generally, should be tackled. One country in particular did not support the social determinants of health stance, which is assumed to be a central plank of WHO's approach, but wanted the emphasis placed on encouraging individuals to take more responsibility for their health and lifestyles. Another member state took precisely the opposite view, thereby posing a dilemma for WHO, which has always operated by navigating or negotiating a path through such disagreements in order to arrive at a position, and document, that has the unanimous support of all member states. It is not enough to achieve a consensus among most though not all countries, since each can exercise a right of veto that would vitiate the issue in question.

In such turbulent and ever-shifting political waters it is perhaps not surprising that a great deal of effort in WHO is placed on words and on word-smithing. Knowledge and evidence are secondary (or last, to pick up on Davies's sources of evidence—see Box 7.1), or at least so it would seem, to getting the right form of words that can then be supported by a spectrum of political voices. It is not easy work and credulity can be stretched, especially at a time when many governments across Europe are of a neo-liberal persuasion, in contrast to WHO's human rights-based approach to health and its social determinants. When it comes to health policy and those interventions favoured by policy-makers, the emphasis is heavily on individual behaviour change rather than on actions that governments can take at a population level (see Chapter 4 by Bryant in this volume, which discusses the influence of neo-liberalism on politicians' preferences for individual lifestyles). Unless those working for WHO as advisers contributing to the production of policy papers are able to comprehend and operate in such an asymmetrical and highly politicized setting, in which different conceptions of rationality prevail, then they should probably not consider doing so. Returning to the paradox noted earlier, while history weighs heavily with WHO, stretching back to the Declaration of Alma-Ata, the Ottawa Charter, and more recently Health for All, as well as its commitment to health as a human right arising from its UN status, a curious opportunism is also evident, borne out of a desperate need for WHO to be seen as both relevant to and needed by member states of different political persuasions. It is a dilemma that Navarro's critique of the World Health Report 2000 captures nicely (Navarro, 2000). He accuses WHO of subscribing to faith-based dogmas arising from the growing marketization of health policy with its emphasis on public–private partnerships and a weakening of the public service ethos. He concludes that it is wrong for WHO to reproduce this thinking uncritically. Echoes of this dilemma were evident in the work on Health 2020 and the EAP. For example, the fact that a large number of European governments are politically right-of-centre (although following events in France, the Netherlands and Greece there are signs that the balance of political forces may be shifting) has required WHO to acknowledge that not all countries subscribe to the view that tackling deficits should not be undertaken at the expense of the health of their citizens. Some countries believe that this is an inevitable sacrifice.

To end this personal reflection on working for WHO on a knowledge exchange venture, what emerged clearly was the political context in which the work was undertaken and the constant need to be attentive to this and its changing nuances. To this extent, much of what emerged came down to personal relationships and being able to work with a group of committed officers and advisers. It proved possible rapidly to build up high-trust relations and establish a modus vivendi. But to function in this way meant moving some way from being a traditional academic who stands apart from the action and does not engage with the messy reality that seemed to engulf all WHO did. WHO was certainly motivated by knowledge, but this did not all come from research or evidence. It came from multiple sources both within the Regional Office and outside it in member states and elsewhere. Performing as a knowledge broker might most accurately capture the nature of the role, but there was also an element of co-creating and co-producing knowledge. There was certainly no evidence of straightforward knowledge transfer or translation.

Perhaps the most intriguing paradox encountered in working for WHO is that for all the emphasis on its being an organization providing knowledge and technical support in the pursuit of improved health and well-being, how in reality it prosecutes this mission is intensely political.

Discussion: implications for health promotion research, practice, and policy

From the foregoing review of getting knowledge in health promotion into action, and the two examples presented of quite different attempts to advance such an agenda, some lesson-learning and pointers for next steps in developing Fuse's knowledge exchange agenda have emerged. Both examples illustrate the importance of context and culture. In the case of the R2R programme, these were largely non-receptive, if not hostile. How far these were reasons or excuses for inaction—or for not taking advantage of the opportunities the workshops afforded—is unclear, but conceivably both interpretations may be correct: two sides of the same phenomenon. The culture itself is ambivalent about the place of evidence. On the one hand, great emphasis is placed on evidence-based medicine and making evidence-based policy. But on the other, the complex reality and nature of the wicked problems overwhelms practitioners and induces a feeling of helplessness. Faced with this sense of disempowerment, practitioners collude, perhaps unwittingly, and conclude somewhat nihilistically that it is all just too difficult and that nothing or no one can make a difference to their lot.

Whatever failure there is among individuals in being able to break out of this miasma, there is a deeper systemic malaise, which requires attention if there is to be significant progress in switching from a Mode I (conventional scientific research that produces evidence to be taken up and applied) to a Mode II (research that emerges from two-way partnerships between researchers and decision-makers from various stakeholders) position. Rather than relying on individuals to take action, there needs to be a cultural shift that results in systems and processes being put in place which encourage practitioners actively to participate in knowledge inquiry. For this to happen there is a need for much closer dialogue and linkage between researchers and practitioners/ decision-makers. Indeed, many of the suggestions put forward by delegates to the R2R workshops were along these lines. They asked for a regular, rolling programme that over time allows participants to develop trust and ways of working together based on mutuality and shared interests. They felt this would help to create and maintain a sense of momentum. Challenging content was welcomed as long as it had a clear purpose and aim. The right people had also to be present, and this included many of those who had been absent, or had absented themselves, from the workshops. The discussions had also to be programmed to align with decision-making processes, with a view to influencing budget setting and resource allocation decisions. What format would best meet such requirements remains uncertain. It may not be a series of workshops or may need to comprise a mix of formats. In this sense, the topic workshops served a purpose. They demonstrated that a one-off intervention of this type is always likely to fall short of what is needed. Change will not occur from such a one-off event. What is needed is a process which allows for an ongoing flexible conversation that can be adjusted as and when necessary.

The WHO example of knowledge transfer, exchange or mobilization demonstrates how even in a setting where the culture is ostensibly favourably disposed towards evidence, and the currency of the organization is about evidence-based policy and rational linear policy-making, the reality is infinitely more complex and highly politicized, with multiple conceptions of rationality competing for attention. This is evident to such a degree that sometimes a position adopted at one point of the process may get completely overturned at a subsequent point, only to be reinstated at a later stage following a further development. This can all happen suddenly and without anyone seemingly being aware of the reversal in position. What is important and matters most is what is needed at that particular moment in time and how it can be massaged or made to fit into a coherent narrative with what has preceded it. In respect of such manipulations and machinations, knowledge is infinitely malleable, has many sources, and can serve many purposes.

To be able to work in such a setting requires a particular set of boundary-spanning skills and awareness of, and sensitive antennae to, political situations that may not be present in, or come naturally to, academic researchers. Such soft skills are not always present or easy to acquire, but they are critical in getting results. They are also a salutary reminder that scientific evidence alone or knowledge of a particular type is not in itself a sufficient basis for health policy (Greenhalgh, 2012). Progress in health promotion and public health generally 'has been as much driven by politics as by scientific and techno-logical innovation' (Humphreys and Piot, 2012: 1316). In some respects, WHO acts as a pivot between the worlds of science on the one hand and politics and values on the other. Probably more often than not politics will trump scientific evidence, and a combination of values, tacit or experiential knowledge, pragmatism, and standard operating proce-dures will prevail. But often the politics will change as well, so that what may be accept-able at one point in time may shift, often with great rapidity. Being well-attuned to such shifts, which can open up opportunities as well as closing them down, is a skill, or state of mind, more of us working to strengthen the knowledge base of decision-making need to acquire. Catching the tide when opportunities present themselves, and being ready to exploit them as they do, may provide the best hope of making progress to promote and improve health using evidence at judicious stages in the policy-making process. Above all, the best that can be expected and hoped for is that evidence can inform policy rather than determine it. Value judgements will remain important, and that is probably as it should be, especially when those producing knowledge and evidence are not themselves value-free.

The two examples afford other lessons for getting knowledge into action in respect of health promotion policy and practice. Four merit listing:

- there needs to be much closer dialogue and linkage between researchers and practi-tioners/decision-makers when it comes to planning research, from its initial concep-tion through to its design and execution, and finally to its successful dissemination;

- the design, selection, and framing of research questions must speak to the needs and priorities of practitioners;

- the passive dissemination of research findings through traditional academic channels is insufficient—the outlets used to convey important messages must fit the audience, and novel, attractive ways of communicating the key messages through story-telling and other means need to be found;

- developing knowledge brokerage is a necessary adjunct to ensure that getting knowl-edge into action may occur, while offering no guarantees that it will.

Above all, knowledge transfer is not a one-off isolated event—rather, it is a continuous process in which knowledge accumulates, is continuously revised and modified as circumstances change, and influences and shapes thinking over time.

Returning to an issue which runs through the chapter, it is desirable that academic researchers should be able to engage in getting knowledge into action at least to a degree, if only because research impact is of growing importance in assessing the value of research and whether or not it should receive funding. Of course, there will be some academics who are more drawn to such activity than others and who are better at it. They will either already possess the requisite skills or be able to acquire them. Such diversity among researchers should not pose a problem as long as research teams possess some members who have knowledge-to-action expertise. There is another issue about how far academic researchers should stray from their core business in undertaking research, and how far they should go in becoming change agents. However, it is inappropriate to be prescriptive about such matters and perhaps it should be left up to individual researchers to decide where they are comfortable in drawing the boundary—or not.

Finally, and this brings us back to where we began, working in real-life settings of the type described in the two examples presented is likely to make more sense and become possible if reference is made to the theoretical considerations introduced at the start of the chapter. These centre on the existence of wicked problems and complex systems and on being sensitive to different models of policy-making in order to maximize opportunities for knowledge and evidence to inform policy. Armed with this knowledge and understanding, academics who venture out of their comfort zone may be better equipped to cope with the messy and complex realities of decision-making and implementation. What is unlikely to work is retaining a stubborn adherence to notions of rationality and linear thinking (what Klein (1996) calls 'the new scientism'), which bear little relation to how knowledge is conceived and used in practice. That way lies disillusionment.

Conclusion

For Fuse, situated for the most part in a fairly traditional and orthodox academic research setting and having to manage the various tensions and conflicting demands arising from this, these issues go to the heart of what it is seeking to achieve, and how. The journey is far from over, although the destination it wishes to reach is becoming clearer. Fuse has moved away from the knowledge-driven and problem-solving models as representing the best means of achieving the goal of improved take-up of what works in health promotion and public health. They may occasionally be relevant and appropriate, but the interactive model, combined with the enlightenment model, probably offers a better prospect of making progress, provided the requisite channels of communication exist and there is real buy-in from all sides. And it will be accepted that at the end of the day both the political and tactical models may continue to shape and influence, and perhaps even determine, what outcomes emerge.

Conceivably, Fuse will never reach its destination because it will doubtless be required to change direction and shape as the changing environment it inhabits demands. Indeed, this is already the case in England, as the lead role for public health and much health promotion moves out of the NHS and returns to local government, from where it was removed in 1974. Having faced the NHS, Fuse will now need to face local government and build new relationships and networks. Critical for Fuse's success is that the processes and opportunities for continuous dialogue among all the relevant parties in which it is investing will prove sufficiently resilient and sustainable to withstand and survive the multiple and unforeseen vicissitudes associated with wicked problems, and that the attempt to develop healthy public policy is, as far as possible, based on what works and is effective. The difference is that what works and is seen to be effective will be achieved through this new type of dialogue between researchers and end users. In future, as Van de Ven and Johnson conclude, high-quality research that has an impact will emerge from implementation of four instructions:

> (1) confront questions and anomalies existing in reality, (2) organise the research project as a collaborative learning community of scholars and practitioners with diverse perspectives, (3) conduct research that systematically examines not only alternative models and theories but alternative practical formulations of the question of interest, and (4) frame the research and its findings to contribute knowledge to academic disciplines and to one or more domains of practice.
>
> (2006: 815)

These actions constitute a working agenda for Fuse as it enters its second term.

References

Australian Public Service (2007). *Tackling Wicked Problems: a Public Policy Perspective.* Canberra: Commonwealth of Australia.

Best, A. (2011). Systems thinking and health promotion. *American Journal of Health Promotion,* **25** (4), eix–ex.

Best, A. and Holmes, B. (2010). Systems thinking, knowledge and action: towards better models and methods. *Evidence & Policy,* **6** (2), 145–59.

Best, A., Terpstra, J. L., Moor, G., Riley, B., Norman, C. D., and Glasgow, R. E. (2009). Building knowledge-integration systems for evidence-informed decisions. *Journal of Health Organisation and Management,* **23** (6), 627–41.

Bowen, S. and Zwi, A. B. (2005). Pathways to 'evidence-informed' policy and practice: a framework for action. *PLoS Medicine.* **2** (7), 600–5.

Buck, D. and Forsini, F. (2012). *Clustering on Unhealthy Behaviours over Time: Implication for Policy and Practice.* London: King's Fund.

CIHR (2004). *Knowledge Translation Strategy 2004–2009.* Ottawa: Canadian Institutes of Health Research. Available at: <http://www.cihr-irsc.gc.ca/e/26574.html> (accessed 11 May 2013).

Greenhalgh, T. (2012). Guest editorial: why do we always end up here? Evidence-based medicine's conceptual cul-de-sacs and some off-road alternative routes. *Journal of Primary Health Care,* **4** (2), 92–7.

Greenhalgh, T. and Wieringa, S. (2011). Is it time to drop the 'knowledge translation' metaphor? A critical literature review. *Journal of the Royal Society of Medicine,* **104**, 501–9.

Humphreys, K. and Piot, P. (2012). Scientific evidence alone is not sufficient basis for health policy, *British Medical Journal,* **344**, e1316.

Hunter, D. J. (2003). *Public Health Policy.* Cambridge: Polity.

Hunter, D. J. (2012). Tackling the health divide in Europe: the role of the World Health Organization. *Journal of Health Politics, Policy and Law,* **37** (5), 867–82.

Hunter. D. J., Marks, L., and Smith, K. E. (2010). *The Public Health System in England.* Bristol: Policy Press.

Kickbusch, I. and Gleicher, D. (2011). *Governance for Health in the 21st Century.* Copenhagen: WHO Regional Office for Europe.

Klein, R. (1996). The NHS and the new scientism: solution or delusion? *Quarterly Journal of Medicine,* **89** (4), 85–87.

Lang, T. and Rayner, G. (2012). Ecological public health: the 21st century's big idea? *British Medical Journal,* **345**, e5466.

Leischow, S. J., Best, A., Trochim, W. M., Clark, P. I., Gallagher, R. S., Marcus, S. E., and Matthews, E. (2008). Systems thinking to improve the public's health. *American Journal of Preventive Medicine,* **35** (2S), S196–S203.

Marks, L., Hunter, D. L., and Alderslade, R. (2011). *Strengthening Public Health Capacity and Services in Europe. A Concept Paper.* Copenhagen: WHO Regional Office for Europe.

Navarro, V. (2000). Assessment of the World Health Report 2000. *The Lancet,* **356** (4), 1598–601.

Ogilvie, D., Craig, P., Griffin, S., Macintyre, S., and Wareham, N. J. (2009). A translational framework for public health research. *BMC Public Health,* **9**, 116.

Pettigrew, A. M. (2001). Management research after modernism. *British Journal of Management,* **12** (Special Issue), S61–S70.

Plsek, P. E. and Greenhalgh, T. (2001). The challenge of complexity in health care. *British Medical Journal,* **323**, 625–8.

Rittel, H. W. J. and Webber, M. M. (1973). Dilemmas in a general theory of planning. *Policy Sciences,* **4** (2), 155–69.

Rushmer, R., Steven, A., and Hunter, D. J. (2011). *'Hearing what Other People are Doing is Always Interesting…' From Research to Reality: a Realist Evaluation of a Knowledge to Action Initiative.* Newcastle: North East Improvement and Efficiency Partnership. Available at: <http://www.fuse. ac.uk/news.php?nid=1526> (accessed 25 November 2012).

Strauss, A., Schatzman, L., Bucher, R., Ehrlich, D., and Sabshin, M. (1964). *Psychiatric Ideologies and Institutions.* New York: Free Press.

Van de Ven, A. H., and Johnson, P. E. (2006). Knowledge for theory and practice. *Academy of Management Review,* **31** (4), 802–21.

Weiss, C. H. (1979). The many meanings of research utilisation. *Public Administration Review,* **39**, 426–31.

WHO (2012a). *Health 2020: Policy Framework and Strategy.* Working document EUR/RC62/8. Copenhagen: WHO Regional Office for Europe. Available at: <http://www.euro.who.int/en/ who-we-are/governance/regional-committee-for-europe/sixty-second-session/documenta-tion/working-documents/eurrc628-health-2020-policy-framework-and-strategy> (accessed 5 February 2013).

WHO (2012b). *European Action Plan for Strengthening Public Health Capacities and Services.* Working document EUR/RC62/12. Copenhagen: WHO Regional Office for Europe. Available at: <http:// www.euro.who.int/en/who-we-are/governance/regional-committee-for-europe/sixty-second-ses-sion/documentation/working-documents/eurrc6212-rev.1-european-action-plan-for-strengthening-public-health-capacities-and-services> (accessed 5 February 2013).

Chapter 8

Health policy networks: connecting the disconnected

Evelyne de Leeuw, Michael Keizer,
and Marjan Hoeijmakers

Introduction

Health is created outside the health (or rather sick care) sector. While this assertion has now been evidenced and substantiated time and again by scholars (e.g. Blum, 1974; Laframboise, 1973; Navarro, 1986) and reputable national and global fora (Lalonde, 1974; CSDH, 2008) a problem remains: if health is not created by the sick care sector, why should the sick care sector manage policy development for health? It would make much more sense if policy development for health were managed across those socioeconomic realms where health is made.

In our research on Healthy Cities, in fact, we discovered as much: staff units for (positive) health development directly connected to the municipal executive were found to have a greater impact on policies on the determinants of health than line units in a public health (or sick care) directorate (de Leeuw, 1999; de Leeuw et al., 1998). This finding emerged from several studies in which we applied John Kingdon's multiple streams theory to local health policy development.

Ideologically, the character of true policies for health has been established since the early 1980s. The Declaration of Alma-Ata on Primary Health Care (International Conference on Primary Healthcare, 1978) and the Ottawa Charter for Health Promotion (WHO, 1986) recognized that broad and integrated policies would support and sustain the conditions for good health across individuals, groups, communities, and populations. Rhetorically, however, this is a troubled area. We would prefer the simple designation 'policy for health'. Such policy consists of different subsets of sector or issue-driven policies, jointly addressing the broad determinants of health. The Ottawa Charter adopted the rhetoric of 'healthy public policy' (Milio, 1981; Hancock, 1985), which has now morphed into Health in All Policies. The practice in many health agencies the world over, however, is to refer variously and opaquely to 'public health policy', 'health policy', 'population health policy', 'health promotion policy', and many other permutations. In Figure 8.1 we attempt to provide some conceptual clarification and consistency to these terms. The total field in the figure should be labelled 'policy for health', as each of these arenas contributes to healthful conditions. 'Health policy', in this perspective, is

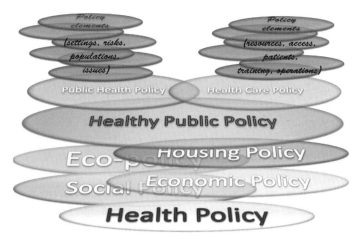

Figure 8.1 Policy for health and its subsets.

conceptually and ideologically on a par with any other sectoral policy, whether housing policy, social policy, or economic policy. We recognize, of course, that each of these by their very nature already is *inter*sectoral: for instance, housing policy may be the dedicated domain and prerogative of an agency charged with urban planning, but its remit is to take into account economic, transport, education, natural, and social capital, among others. Any housing policy that would not take these parameters into account is doomed to fail (e.g. Hasselaar, 2006).

The notion of healthy public policy (a subset of policy for health, and interchangeably used with Health in All Policies) endeavours explicitly to introduce health considerations in each of the underlying policy sectors, thus building momentum for change of all these policies towards health development. Traditionally, health agencies (ministries and public health services) have 'owned' health policy and, to a lesser extent, healthy public policy. In very operational terms they have been charged through traditional governance arrangements to develop two distinctive subsets of policies for health: public health policy and health care policy. In their very nature these two are qualitatively different from each other; this becomes obvious when we look at the policy elements each is supposed to address. Traditionally, health care policy deals with operations, access to services, individual patients, and resource allocations. Public health policy, on the other hand, is driven by notions of risk, populations, settings (such as workplaces or schools), and particular risk areas. It seems that, because of the diverging nature of the policy elements, policy development parameters that are deployed in one may be ineffective in another subset. Making policy for health, therefore, is certainly not a case of 'one size fits all': it needs to take into account the unique conditions of each policy domain.

To further strengthen this point it is helpful to apply two theoretical lenses. This first has been proposed by sociologist Joseph Gusfield (1981). Gusfield found that in the primordial, unstructured soup of social problems (an image very much applicable, too, to

Kingdon's work which we will review later) a social discourse will play out. This discourse attempts to attribute policy ownership to one of the many potential stakeholders in the game. The example Gusfield is best known for is the issue of drink–driving. Although in most countries it is now accepted that this is a public policy problem that should be addressed through law enforcement aimed at individual offenders, the ownership of this public problem might as well have been attributed to innkeepers and publicans (made accountable for responsible alcohol consumption), the alcohol industry (limiting availability), the automotive industry (making cars inherently safe, no matter the condition of the driver), transportation infrastructure (building roads in such a way that psychotropically induced accidents would only harm the intoxicated person), etc. Similarly, the social construction and ownership of health problems can go many ways, and the assumption that only one stakeholder is entitled to ownership has in fact consistently been challenged; for instance, elsewhere (de Leeuw and Clavier, 2011) we have argued that policies for health may fail because those affected are not (co-)owning the problem.

The second lens is Mazmanian and Sabatier's (1989) policy implementation theory (Figure 8.2). Mazmanian and Sabatier highlight a number of categories of variables they empirically determined important to policy implementation processes. These include the nature of the problem and the extent to which a policy intends to change it (for example, 'ending poverty' or 'eradication of polio' are policy implementation issues on a radically different scale from 'maintaining regular garbage collection'). They also recognize

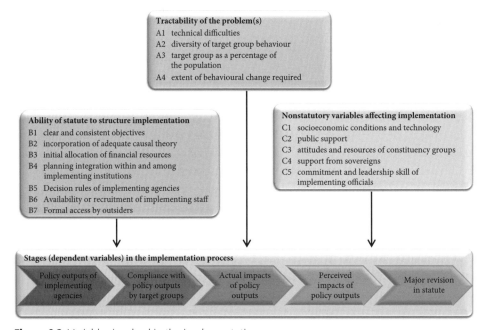

Figure 8.2 Variables involved in the implementation process.

Adapted with permission from Mazmanian, D. A. and Sabatier, P. A., *Implementation and Public Policy* (2nd edn.). University Press of America, Lanham, New York and London, Copyright © 1989.

that there is a range of capabilities and resources that needs to be put in place for effective implementation (e.g. the World Health Organization (WHO) on its own will not eradicate polio; among many other variables it requires the existence and commitment of national, regional, and local health agents trained in vaccination procedures). Finally, there is a set of variables that is external or peripheral to the core policy process but required for its implementation success (for instance, if there is massive opposition—for instance from religious groups—to vaccination programmes they are bound to fail).

The Mazmanian and Sabatier implementation model is useful for its description of the variables involved in policy implementation: they have a high degree of 'face validity'—they make sense. But Sabatier (2007) was among the first to criticize the 'stages heuristic' that had taken hold of the political sciences in the 1970s and 1980s. This simple, unilinear, causal approach to policy processes was deemed insufficient. For the Mazmanian and Sabatier model, for instance, it is obvious that 'tractability of the problem' has all sorts of immediate but intricate connections to 'non-statutory variables affecting implementation'. Ignoring the dynamic, multidimensional and reciprocal relationship between variables may in fact lead to ineffective implementation action. We would suggest that a multidimensional, or rather more networked, perspective for appreciating these variables has been proposed by Hill and Hupe (2006). They find that at different levels of the policy system different types of governance play out in the management of relations in the network (see Figure 8.3). Effective policy development and implementation, in their view, requires a 'whole-of-governance' approach. This requires a dynamic and continuous monitoring of the structures and agencies of the various actors in the policy system.

As stated before, however, it is the sheer nature of the policy problem which determines to a large extent what policy development options exist. Also, 'simple' problems are more easily addressed through effective (i.e. implementable, cf. de Leeuw, 2007) policies; however, it has been asserted—also in this volume—that many health problems (and in particular those that fall in the realm of health promotion and healthy public policy) are by their very nature 'wicked' (Blackman et al., 2006; de Leeuw, 1989; Kickbusch, 2010).

	Constitutive governance	Directive governance	Operational governance
System	Institutional design	General rule setting	Managing trajectories
Organization	Developing contextual relations	Context maintenance	Managing trajectories
Individual	Developing professional norms	Situation-bound rule application	Managing contacts

Figure 8.3 Hill and Hupe's multiple governance framework.

From Hill, M. and Hupe P., Analysing policy processes as multiple governance: accountability in social policy, *Policy and Politics*, Volume 34, Issue 3, pp. 557–573, Copyright © 2006. Reproduced by permission of The Policy Press.

Studying the complexities of the development of local policies for health would therefore benefit from stronger conceptual scaffolding.

Policy entrepreneurs opening a window

One such framework is John Kingdon's multiple streams theory (1995). In its simplest terms, this theory claims that there exist three continuously evolving streams around issues in society. Some of these issues become problems, and the nature of these problems is constantly evolving, on and off the agendas of those participants who feel engaged with the issue. Some of these participants are 'visible'—that is, legitimate problem stream actors, such as special interest groups, academics, and the media. Others, however, are 'invisible' and are called upon to provide, or volunteer, their under-the-radar services and capacities to contribute to problem framing. An invisible participant may be a lobbyist or a political staffer. Their invisibility relates not to their legitimacy to act, but to the formal role attributed to them. Visible and invisible participants similarly play roles in the other two streams: those of politics and policies. But an actor visible in one stream may well be invisible in another. In the politics stream the essential phenomenon is the raw nature of politics, as determined by Lasswell (1936): who gets what, when and how? The dynamic nature of the politics stream is determined by a degree of seasonality (terms of parliament, election periods, etc.), the political preferences of those in power and those in opposition, and the shifting sands of 'what's hot and what's not'. Finally, the policies stream is characterized by the existence and engagement of public policies in their social context. Some of these policies are only symbolic (as, for instance, in the case of most public health mass media campaigns), while some are truly redistributive in nature. (Perceived) incremental change to existing policy is often more easily argued for than radical policy shifts.

The participants in each of these streams all play their visible and invisible roles, either trying to maintain the status quo or trying to fuel arguments for change. Those most successful at doing so have been described by Kingdon as 'policy entrepreneurs', although Skok (1995: 326) has described such a role also as the 'social entrepreneur', 'issue initiator', 'policy broker', 'strategist', or 'caretaker'. In Kingdon's empirical view these policy entrepreneurs endeavour to link participants and issues across streams in order to open 'windows of opportunities' for policy change. In Figure 8.4 we endeavour to map some of the events that can take place in and between the three streams. It is obvious that the creation of windows of opportunity, and resulting policy change, happens in a complex networked environment.

In earlier research (Hoeijmakers et al., 2007; de Leeuw, 1999) we looked at the question of whether social or policy entrepreneurs were present in this environment, and if so, what they did in order to open windows of opportunity for local health policy development. Similar research in the health promotion domain has been published more recently (Harting et al., 2011). The key message from this body of work is that the very nature of the health domain represents a very dense network, and that effective entrepreneurs need to have the tools to engage in shaping the nodes and connections in it. Laumann and Knoke in their seminal *The Organisational State* (1987) effectively mapped health care and energy domains in the United States, and found that the most

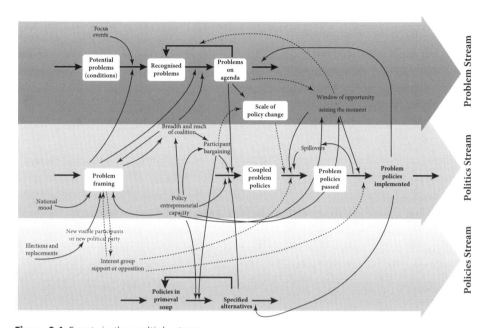

Figure 8.4 Events in the multiple streams.
Solid connections indicate a positive impact; dotted ones may also have negative impact.
Source: Data from Kingdon, J. W., *Agendas, Alternatives, and Public Policies*, Harper Collins College Publishers, Michigan, USA, Copyright © 1995.

effective players have allocated substantive resources to monitor the actions of the other actors in the network. It seems that some initial lessons can be learned for the development of policy for health (and, perhaps, the entrepreneurship of those engaged in policy development and health promotion). First, stakeholders may be assisted in structuring and aiming their health promotion (policy-making) actions by acquiring insight into their position in these networks relative to the positions of others. Second, stakeholders would be supported in their actions if these were tactically and strategically informed by appropriate knowledge of actions of others in the network.

Networking for health

Policy network theory is still very much a developing field. Policy network theoreticians and analysts have been challenged to 'deliver' and to show the benefits of a network perspective to policy development. Börzel (1998) describes how two perspectives have taken hold of the policy network discourse: an American/Anglo-Saxon one, where networks are being mapped on particular policy issues (such as 'health' or 'energy'), and a German/North-European one, where policy networks are used as theoretical models describing new forms of governance. Neither, Börzel ascertains, is capable of demonstrating its relevance to policy-making. In other words, she claims that the current state of play in both policy network perspectives yields explanatory yet no predictive power.

Further theoretical advances are required to generate this policy-making relevance. Kenis and Raab (2003) propose a course of action to develop a sound policy network theory, whereas Howlett (2002) finds that further theorizing on the nature of the policy problem and characteristics of network participants would yield demonstrable insight into the impact of network configurations on policy outcomes. These challenges were taken up by a research and policy development project which we carried out in a group of small municipalities in the southern province of Limburg, in the Netherlands (Hoeijmakers et al., 2007).

Under Dutch collective prevention legislation, municipalities in the Netherlands are required to develop and implement local health policies. These were supposed to be policies for health, inspired by the national Dutch government's efforts in the 1980s through what was called 'Nota 2000', a programme in itself directly related to the WHO European Region's 'health for all by the year 2000' strategies (de Leeuw and Polman, 1995). Such a broad perspective was reaffirmed in the first iteration of the legislation, and was specified in its background documents and evaluations of its predecessors (Lemstra, 1996; Ministerie van VWS, 2000; Ministerie van VWS et al., 2001). Explicitly and expressly, these local health policies aimed at the promotion of health across sectors, with strong community involvement, based on available epidemiological information. However, in the successive Public Health Law (2008), the broad understanding of local health policy was narrowed down by prescribing more precisely its (public health) policy elements. Similar policy requirements are found elsewhere—for instance, in Victoria, Australia (Department of Human Services, 2001), where an extensive evidence support package is in place to support municipal public health planning (the 'environments for health' framework). Similar support to policy development in the Netherlands has been delineated as being the statutory remit of the public health service. However, the fact of the matter is that since the adoption of the legislation virtually every stakeholder in this policy network has been challenged in driving this process forward, or even in assuming appropriate ownership and responsibility (de Goede et al., 2010; Jansen et al., 2010; Harting et al., 2011).

In terms of Gusfield's theory, no one at the local level has assumed ownership of broadly defined health. Hoeijmakers et al. (2007), applying social network theory, concluded the same in studying local health policy-making. This is no surprise, as in the local discourse few actors advocate health; rather, they advocate absence of disease (e.g. via the public health service), access to and efficiency of services (health care and social work providers), or patient interests (via quangos such as local chapters of Cancer Council, or the Patient and Consumer Platform). All stakeholders feel only partly responsible for the health perspective they have carved out for themselves. Therefore, responsibility for policies for broadly defined health has fallen to the default-by-law municipality. Municipalities, however, report that they are ill-equipped and professionally insufficiently resourced to formulate these policies (Jansen et al., 2010). In desperate quests for 'health' advice they end up in the preventive care realm and focus on healthy lifestyle issues; these belong more to public health policy as a subset of policy for health.

This notion that 'health' is an intangible, fluid and orphaned policy issue is mirrored by the findings of Putland et al., who investigated lay understandings of (the causes of) health inequity. The authors conclude that:

> ...the findings in this study are evocative of a kind of collective inertia within the public health field. The lack of congruence between explanations and public policy responses suggests that public health arguments directed at addressing the social determinants of health have not become absorbed into bodies of lay knowledge.
>
> (2011: 67)

The problem that no one owns health (and hence no one can be mobilized for its advocacy) cannot simply be attributed to a lack of resource or political will in the (public) policy-making environment, but seems reciprocally unsupported by a similar lack of commitment among the public.

Earlier research (Commers, 2002; Commers et al., 2000), however, demonstrated that the pitfalls of the disease care conundrum were not as serious as some might have construed them. This research showed that with careful and appropriate prompting, members of the community would be more than capable of defining, describing, and prioritising various determinants of individual and population health, and would in fact attribute considerable weight to social determinants of health. The research therefore concluded that there is sufficient potential constituent support for local policies for health. The Limburg small municipalities study (Hoeijmakers et al., 2007) sought to demonstrate what local networks for health policy looked like, and found that network configurations shifted, and in a sense seemed to be more amenable to developments in the direction of policies for health.

The foundation work for our inquiry was stakeholder analysis; this is popular in organizational analysis, policy analysis and programme development (Brugha and Varvasovszky, 2000). Stakeholders may include individuals, organizations, and different individuals within an organization, as well as networks of individuals and/or organizations. Stakeholder analysis is used as a tool to map the actors who have a stake in a policy, organization, or programme, and to describe the characteristics of these actors. For example, stakeholder analysis in policy-making is used to create support for policy decisions and commitment for the implementation of policy.

This inquiry looked at several characteristics of identified stakeholders: their ideas about local health policy, interests, collaboration with other actors in public health, influence, and contribution towards policy development. These attributes formed the principal constituents of the annual interviews with stakeholders; they also structured our approach to participatory observation. Over three years, we monitored the change or stability of the characteristics of stakeholders. We were interested in knowing how these characteristics related to the policy development process and whether stakeholders engaged in entrepreneurial activities for policy change. With a very small initial sample, we used 'snowball sampling' to reach a stable research population (cf. Salganik and Heckathorn, 2004) and subsequently one Delphi round to identify the most important stakeholders in the issue of 'broadly defined health' policy-making in the municipal cases under study. We were particularly eager to know whether citizen groups, neighbourhood committees, resident associations, and similar would be included in the list. Our interest was generated because—ever since Winslow (1920) originally defined public health as including 'social machinery' for the betterment of health and longevity (as a birth right!)—communities have, at least rhetorically, been at the centre of the health discourse. This was only reinforced by community development and empowerment advances in the 1960s and 1970s, culminating for the health promotion field in the Ottawa Charter in 1986. But even when communities are symbolically at the centre of the health argument, they may be absent from the policy game (e.g. de Leeuw and Clavier, 2011; Löfgren et al., 2011). Our results showed that community groups were indeed included as important stakeholders, and from here we adopted a normative approach to monitor explicitly the participation of these groups in the policy-making process and their position and connectedness in the policy networks. We found that their role and position were peripheral.

Whereas stakeholder analysis provides information on the set of actors who (should) have a stake in a certain issue, social network analysis, on the other hand, provides information on the interactions between these actors. In other words, stakeholder analysis describes the actor differentiation, whereas network analysis describes the actor integration related to a certain issue. Network analysis is a tool to describe and analyse the interactions between a defined set of actors. It considers the presence and absence of relations among actors (individuals, work units, or organizations); these are more powerful in explaining social phenomena than the attributes of these actors (see, for example, Brass et al. (2004) for an overview). Consequently, actors are embedded within a network of interconnected relationships that provide opportunities for and constraints on their behaviour.

The first thing to do in network analysis is to demarcate the network at hand. This is to define the subject of interaction (such as communication or exchange of resources) for a specific set of actors—in other words, to specify the in- and exclusion criteria (in our case, the stakeholders identified). Subsequently, structural characteristics of the actors, as well as characteristics of the overall network, can be calculated and described. The most commonly calculated characteristics of the overall network are the density (given a value between 0 and 1)—describing the extent to which all actors in the network are linked to each other, referring to a level of cohesion and integration of the network—and the centralization of the network—the extent to which the network is centralized around the actor(s) most densely connected to others. The most commonly calculated characteristic of an actor in a network is its prominence centrality (0–100%). This describes the extent to which an actor is important within a network through direct and indirect ties to other actors in the network (Scott, 2000). Actor centrality indicates the importance of an individual actor in the network.

As stated earlier, the most central tenet of network mapping is that networks exist around certain issues: the same set of actors involved in the implementation of vaccination programmes may display an entirely different network configuration when mapped for their annual Mardi Gras participation. In the exploratory phase of our research, therefore, we reviewed whether 'local policy for health' was in fact such an issue (cf. Laumann et al., 1989). Stakeholders informed us that this was not the case, and that they felt that they interacted differently, and on different dimensions, with others stakeholders in the environment. From this feedback we decided to map three networks for all four municipalities: communication for health policy development, involvement in public health action, and strategic (or opportunistic: some actors more proficiently than others adopted the first rule of politics—'be there'—see Chapman and Wakefield, 2001: 277) collaboration. The data on interaction between stakeholders in these domains were obtained from a structured questionnaire filled out during interviews. We calculated the density, centralization, and actor centrality of these networks. We found that all networks described were (to apply a term used by Putland et al. (2011)) relatively inert, without discernible policy entrepreneurial activity, with policy ownership attributed to (and possibly reluctantly accepted by) local government, and generally unaware of the potential and capacity for the development of local health policy.

Similar findings have been found repeatedly in follow-up studies. Most of these have started from the premise that something is going wrong at the nexus between research, policy, and practice (de Goede et al., 2010; Jansen et al., 2010). Such studies have, for instance, endeavoured to develop and validate local health reports for policy-making (van Bon-Martens et al., 2011), similar to the health profiles that have been part of Healthy City efforts in Europe and elsewhere (Waddell, 1995). Others have taken this idea a step further by exploring the utility of such reports as perceived by institutional actors (that is, the public sector stakeholders formally mentioned in the relevant legislation) in the local health domain (de Goede et al., 2012). A third perspective has endeavoured to map relationships between such actors and academia in already existing collaborative arrangements (Hoeijmakers et al., 2012), in a similar way to the programme to reduce health inequities in Montreal (Bernier et al., 2006).

None of these has come up with a magic 'silver bullet' approach that would enable and empower all stakeholders to constructively engage in effective local health policy development, but based on our social network mapping approaches we believe that an interactive, intuitive, and dynamic policy network mapping tool might deliver the information that would put health on the social and policy agendas of all actors. Not incidentally, this also happens to be the stated mission of (at least the European component of) the international Healthy Cities movement (Tsouros, 2009), with which we are also associated.

From opportunistic to strategic policy networks

It will have become clear that our local health policy development inquiry was prominently driven by social network analysis. The fact that we looked, in our research to identify stakeholders, at 'tangible' social network issues (communication, collaborative action, and strategy) was in retrospect perhaps not the wisest option. The result was, as we showed, that inert and stagnant single social networks were described. However, we noticed a certain dynamic undertow when looking at the networks simultaneously, influencing the same process of policy-making. The position and possible (coordinative) activities of actors in the communication network, for instance, would be of interest for taking an influential position in the action or strategic network. With the data from our inquiry we were at the time not yet really able to grasp and underpin this observation, although we were curious how such dynamics could be further stimulated and visualized, especially in order to create better possibilities for community groups to attain positions in policy networks that enable their participation in policy decision-making.

Only when we discussed these findings with policy-makers and put them in the context of the theory that drove our inquiry did it dawn on us that an altogether different approach might well have contributed to policy change. The intent was—as in so much political research—to describe the processes that would lead to change, but to distance ourselves from actual engagement in potential change as 'objective' and 'value-free' researchers. Our policy and practice colleagues, it turned out, were less interested in process descriptions, and much more in tactical process prompts, such as 'So what could we *do* to be more policy-relevant?' It turned out that combining the network perspective with Kingdon's multiple streams theory made for appealing narratives that instantly rang true to those involved in (health) policy networks. Looking back, there may have been more of a need to act ourselves as policy entrepreneurs than we ever anticipated— and our adopting a participatory action research perspective would possibly have had an impact on the local policy games (e.g. Quoss et al., 2000). We also learned an important lesson on choosing and applying theory: adopting hybrid frameworks in which several commensurate and complementary theories are applied may yield important new insights (see, for instance, also Greenhalgh and Stones, 2010).

Based on our theoretical foundations we thus developed IMPolS: the interactive mapping of policy streams tool. In a number of sessions with practitioners, policy-makers, and academics we presented and tested the dummy version, which evolved as a consequence. IMPolS operates, still in its alpha version, on the internet. One of the key considerations in implementation is that its management and operation are essentially driven by the end users themselves, and that very little 'theoretical debris' or 'text ballast' should be present on the site. End users would self-identify as actor-stakeholders in a specific policy domain, either by directly signing up to a specific (self-defined) URL within IMPolS and then nominating network colleagues (the tool will then send e-invites), or by initiating an IMPolS instance during a network meeting (for instance, an annual general meeting), at which a first round of network data is entered.

At this stage, actor-stakeholders also choose a representative icon (categories in Figure 8.5 seen in the shaded box at the bottom of the screen, but fully adaptable to other specific policy domains), and may define and select categories of participants. Actors may continue to be added; the expectation is that from the initiation stage onward actors will regularly access their domain and answer about a dozen questions relating to their position and connection in the network. These data will then be added to the

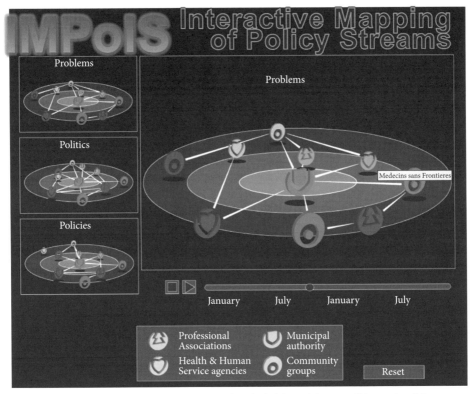

Figure 8.5 IMPoIS main visualization screen with switchable problems, politics and policies networks. Actor-stakeholder descriptions appear when the cursor is hovered over the actor icon (in this case, Medecins Sans Frontieres).

database: first, the network visualization algorithm will recalculate the three network configurations; and second, it will notify other members of the network that an actor has updated their position and connection (thus prompting others to do the same). Over time, with the addition of more data, the network mapping visualizations (and possibly actor behaviour, as discovered in alpha testing results) will gain intricacy, and will allow for a dynamically animated, pulsing set of network configurations. Further sophistication could be added, either by the self-selected network members or by a network manager (see the following section), through the refinement of the timeline with critical events, such as the process described by Kingdon (1995) (elections, climactic events, policy changes, press releases etc.).

In our alpha testing of the IMPoIS tool we have found a number of things: first, a visually attractive and transparent architecture of both the input screens (user identification and network variable entry) and the network screens would increase the likelihood of actors engaging with the tool. This is precisely what the developers of the Gephi software platform (Gephi is an interactive visualization and exploration platform for all kinds of networks and complex systems, dynamic, and hierarchical graphs—see <http://gephi. org>) found: applying visualization principles from the gaming sector enhances the attractiveness of the application (Bastian et al., 2009). Second, and in full accordance with both the propositions by Kingdon and our initial research, virtually all actors in their 'colloquial analysis' of the network outputs focused more on the problem stream than on either of the other streams. They found that problem stream graphic network visualizations provided them with arguments and impulses to reconsider:

◆ the nature of the problem they are engaging with;

◆ their framing of the problem, and how it might link with other actors if reframed (a process Kingdon calls 'alternative specification'); and

◆ how to seek alliances with actors found to be similar (sometimes called 'homophilic network relations', e.g. Monge and Contractor, 2003; Provan and Kenis, 2008), either in their position in the problem network (in terms of connectedness and centrality), or in perceived similarities in mission or vision of the institutional characteristics of the actor.

In their reflections on the problem stream, most alpha testers were also curious about how changes in problem framing and perception would:

◆ affect reconfigurations of the problem network (e.g. would they come closer to central actors?); and possibly as a consequence

◆ affect their capacity and capability to reconfigure the policy and politics streams.

Answers to such questions would be theory-informed but relatively speculative until we have accumulated enough data to develop an algorithm that might suggest such outcomes. Third, we were interested in the question of whether the nodes in our network visualizations should be seen as individuals operating in organizations or as actors representing institutions. Although we feel that this issue can ultimately only be resolved empirically (when, over time, large amounts of data have been input into a range of policy domain IMPolS instances, and changes in policy have been mapped onto the resulting network configurations), our alpha testers felt that the tool would work at both levels: individuals engaging in policy change 'à la Kingdon', but also institutional actors assessing their positions in network configurations.

A final theoretical reflection

For a moment we will return to the research question and our 'inertia' findings in the local health policy study. We set out to find Kingdon's 'policy entrepreneurs' and did not encounter any (Hoeijmakers et al., 2007). Whether or not the policy inertia was a consequence of this absence could not unequivocally be attributed. However, our alpha testing of IMPolS suggested that participants in this policy domain might have been connected and activated to the problems, politics, and policies discourse if they had had insight in their own and others' network positions. The question of whether this would have led to stronger policy entrepreneurial activity, although speculative, seems to have to be answered in the affirmative. Further theoretical thinking about network governance may shed light on this.

Provan and Kenis (2008) and Kenis and Provan (2009) have postulated some interesting theory-based propositions on network performance and effectiveness. This is not the place to reflect comprehensively on their material, but in light of our quest for policy entrepreneurs in networks we find that their views on 'network management' are valuable. Are policy entrepreneurs network managers? And under which circumstances would they be able to break through the inertia we identified? Based on their work, we can suggest theoretical and empirical—and tentative practical—approaches that would enhance the functionality of IMPolS. The two network scholars suggest a typology (see Table 8.1) for predictors of forms of network governance (Provan and Kenis, 2008: 237).

It is useful to bear in mind that the perspective they offer is on whole-network efficiencies, and not on the bilateral or nodal dimensions of networks. This means that for each member of the network there is a continuous trade-off between collaborative action, internal organizational goals and objectives, and network efficiency (the degree to which the network as a whole attains its objectives). How, if at all, that trade-off tips the balance toward network efficiencies is extremely contextual, as they assert, and each unique policy network will establish its unique governance configuration (that is, the institutional arrangements it forms explicitly or allows to form implicitly to manage its work). Four types of variable (trust, the number of participants in the network, goal consensus, and network-level competencies) drive such networks to management and governance forms on a continuum between full shared governance (where all participants have a say in its management) and the creation and maintenance of a network-internal, or external network administrative organization.

In our research we have seen that, for local health policy formulation and implementation, each of these variables is elusive, unstable, ill-defined (or 'wicked'), invisible or

Table 8.1 Provan and Kenis' key predictors of effectiveness of network governance forms

Governance forms	Trust	Number of participants	Goal consensus	Need for network-level competencies
Shared governance	High density	Few	High	Low
Lead organization	Low density, highly centralized	Moderate number	Moderately low	Moderate
Network administrative organization (NAO)	Moderate density, NAO monitored by members	Moderate to many	Moderately high	High

intangible, and sometimes even fully escapes the grasp of the network participant supposedly in control of network governance (i.e. the local government authority and/or its public health service). Network development was here not purposely stimulated to serve local health policy-making—the ultimate goal. Kaashoek et al. (2009) have determined these different consequences as first and second order effects of policy interventions. From this observation it will be clear that we cannot see Kingdon's policy entrepreneur as the network manager, but rather—and at best—as a 'network catalyst'. It is also helpful to bear in mind that, in our view, many health policy networks exist because they *should* exist. That is, actors follow official or statutory rhetoric (e.g. the pervasive 'intersectoral action' incantations since the Alma-Ata Declaration), rather than finding an organizational shape that serves its purpose best. Clearly, 'simple' problems need 'simple' policy responses (de Leeuw, 2012), and the creation of elaborate collaborative systems would not do much good in situations where the solution is straightforward. Earlier, we described conditions under which partnerships and networks are formed. Hueben and de Leeuw (1991), based on Gray (1985), describe the conditions under which partnership work is important and likely:

- when stakeholders are challenged by a multitude of challenging issues;
- when these problems are perceived to be exceeding the problem-solving capacities of individual, autonomous sectoral stakeholders;
- when traditional routines of problem-solving no longer yield results;
- when competing agencies or units start creating unanticipated and dissonant consequences of actions that might still be considered 'routine' responses; and
- when stakeholder agencies or units recognize mutual and often reciprocal temporal and causal interdependencies.

The work by Provan and Kenis adds important parameters to these primal motivations; when these circumstances lead to the creation of networks, they need to start operating, and preferably efficiently, to attain their joint objectives. It seems critical that any organizational network has gone through these considerations in order to attain at least a modicum of trust, some membership, a sense of joint purpose, and a degree of recognition that networking requires new skills and competencies. Capello (2000), in his element of a wider European Healthy Cities evaluation, looked at the value of 'imposed' networking on the perceived outcomes for the European Healthy Cities membership. Networking between cities is one of the key requirements for aspiring European Healthy Cities to be so designated by the WHO Regional Office for Europe, and as the Healthy Cities movement is often accused of being a 'traveling circus of mayors and politicians' it was important to assess whether networking 'works'. Capello showed that it does: more networking leads to more knowledge utilization. What this tells us in more abstract terms is that an informed (not merely invoked) requirement to engage in networking does yield important results.

Our research, then, seems to suggest that policy entrepreneurs can and should play roles of clarification rather than roles in network governance. We have, with Catford

(1998), described these roles as the ability '…to analyse, to envision, to communicate, to empathise, to enthuse, to advocate, to mediate, to enable and to empower…', rather than '…to manage, to organise, to budget, to control, to sanction or to comply' (de Leeuw, 1999: 261). IMPolS would, our alpha testing has demonstrated, provide policy entrepreneurs with the tools and ammunition to support change through enabling strategies. In our earlier paper (Hoeijmakers et al., 2007) we limited our recommendations for policy entrepreneurial action to stating that these activists should engage in network mapping in order to support their efficacy. Based on our newer insights, we could frame some further views. Policy entrepreneurs who want to make an impact should consider:

- the complexity of the policy domain at hand, in terms of problems, policies, and politics streams;
- the identification of actor-stakeholders, their relations and perceptions in these streams;
- the potential for further, bespoke, 'alternative specifications' for bringing in actor-stakeholders from the periphery to the centre of, particularly, the problem stream network;
- the identification and empowerment of as yet disconnected actor-stakeholders to connect to the policy discourse (cf. de Leeuw and Clavier, 2011);
- the identification (and possibly 'naming and shaming') of actor-stakeholders who sustain policies and politics streams inertia, thereby pointing to issues of trust, network membership, and joint purpose;
- the analysis and description of critical agents in network governance; and
- the identification and enabling of new skills and competencies required for network governance.

It will be clear that such roles, objectives, and techniques require a certain degree of mastery of the theoretical foundations for network mapping, management, and operations, as quite tentatively outlined. The professionals and activists engaging in these entrepreneurial roles will also have to possess great skills and knowledge around issues of knowledge utilization (de Leeuw et al., 2008), and it will help if they can speak with a certain authority on health (equity) issues not only to those that are affected (i.e. communities) but also, certainly, to those that hold the key or potential (ownership) to making critical changes to problems, policies, and politics. We acknowledge, of course, that much of the inertia that we and others have identified in the health policy game may be attributed to stagnant, hierarchical, and inflexible statutory contexts. Change will thus not be easy. The theory, however, strongly suggests that much can be done practically to reconfigure policy networks to make them ready for change (e.g. Breton and de Leeuw, 2011).

Conclusion

The dynamics in policies for health development processes can be better understood by applying different theoretical lenses, and by the use of interactive techniques in analysing network development and its efficiency as first order effects. Furthermore, techniques such as IMPolS provide participants in the network with necessary insights to further aim their actions and strengthen their position to communicate, collaborate, and make (joint) decisions in making policies for health. This is of utmost importance for community groups to better integrate in health policy networks. Network development then needs the explicit attention of stakeholders in health policy-making. Policy entrepreneurs should be active in raising this attention and awareness.

References

Bastian, M., Heymann, S. and Jacomy, M. (2009). *Gephi: an Open Source Software for Exploring and Manipulating Networks*. International AAAI Conference on Weblogs and Social Media.

Bernier, J., Rock, M., Roy, M., Bujold, R. and Potvin, L. (2006). Structuring an inter-sector research project. A negotiated zone. *Sozial- und Präventivmedizin/Social and Preventive Medicine*, **51**, 335–44.

Blackman, T., Elliott, E., Greene, A., Harrington, B., Hunter, D., Marks, L. and Williams, G. (2006). Performance assessment and wicked problems: the case of health inequalities. *Public Policy and Administration*, **21** (2), 66–80.

Blum, H. L. (1974). *Planning for Health Development and Application of Social Change Theory*. New York: Human Sciences Press.

Börzel, T. A. (1998) Organizing Babylon: on the different conceptions of policy networks. *Public Administration*, **76** (2), 253–73.

Brass, D. J., Galaskiewicz, J., Greve, H. R. and Tsai, W. (2004). Taking stock of networks and organizations: a multilevel perspective. *Academy of Management Journal*, **47**, 795–818.

Breton, E. and de Leeuw, E. (2011). Theories of the policy process in health promotion research: a review. *Health Promotion International, 26* (1), 82–90.

Brugha, R. and Varvasovszky, Z. (2000). Stakeholder analysis: a review. *Health Policy and Planning*, **15**, 239–46.

Capello R. (2000). The city-network paradigm: measuring urban network externalities. *Urban Studies*, **37**, 1925–45.

Catford, J. (1998). Social entrepreneurs are vital for health promotion—but they need supportive environments too. Editorial. *Health Promotion International*, **13** (2), 95–8.

Chapman, S. and Wakefield, M. (2001). Tobacco control advocacy in Australia: reflections on 30 years of progress. *Health Education & Behavior*, **28** (3), 274–89.

Commers M. J. (2002). *Determinants of Health: Theory, Understanding, Portrayal, Policy*. Dordrecht: Kluwer Academic Publishers.

Commers, M. J., Visser, G. and de Leeuw, E. (2000). Representations of preconditions for and determinants of health in the Dutch Press. *Health Promotion International*, **15** (4), 321–32.

CSDH (2008). *Closing the gap in a generation. Health Equity through Action on the Social Determinants of Health. Final Report of the Commission on Social Determinants of Health*. Geneva: World Health Organization.

de Goede, J., Putters, K. and van Oers, H. A. M. (2012). Utilization of epidemiological research during the development of local public health policy in the Netherlands: a Case Study Approach. *Social Science & Medicine*, **74**, 707–714.

de Goede, J., Putters, K., van der Grinten, T. and van Oers, H. A. M. (2010). Knowledge in process? Exploring barriers between epidemiological research and local health policy development. *Health Research Policy and Systems*, **8**, 26.

de Leeuw, E. (1989). Concepts in health promotion: the notion of relativism. *Social Science & Medicine*, **29** (11), 1281–8.

de Leeuw, E. (1999). Healthy Cities: urban social entrepreneurship for health. *Health Promotion International*, **14** (3), 261–9.

de Leeuw, E. (2007). Policies for health. The effectiveness of their development, adoption, and implementation, in: **D. McQueen** and **C. M. Jones** (eds.) *Global Perspectives on Health Promotion Effectiveness*, pp. 51–66, New York: Springer.

de Leeuw, E. (2012). Do Healthy Cities work? A logic of method for assessing impact and outcome of Healthy Cities. *Journal of Urban Health,* **89** (2), 217–31.

de Leeuw, E. and Clavier, C. (2011). Healthy public in all policies. The Ottawa Charter for Health Promotion 25 years on. The move towards a new public health continues. *Health Promotion International*, **26** (Suppl. 2), ii237–ii244.

de Leeuw, E. and Polman, L. (1995). Health policy making: the Dutch experience. *Social Science & Medicine*, **40** (3), 331–8.

de Leeuw, E., Abbema, E., and Commers, M. (1998). *Healthy Cities Policy Evaluation—Final Report*. Maastricht /EU DG V, Luxembourg: WHO Collaborating Centre for Research on Healthy Cities.

de Leeuw, E., McNess, A., Crisp, B., and Stagnitti, K. (2008). Theoretical reflections on the nexus between research, policy and practice. *Critical Public Health*, **18** (1), 5–20.

Department of Human Services (2001). *Environments for Health, Promoting Health and Wellbeing through the Built, Social, Economic and Natural Environments, Municipal Public Health Planning Framework*. Victoria, Melbourne: DHS.

Gray, B. (1985). Conditions facilitating interorganizational collaboration. *Human Relations*, **38** (10), 911–36.

Greenhalgh, T. and Stones, R. (2010). Theorising big IT programmes in healthcare: strong structuration theory meets actor-network theory. *Social Science & Medicine*, **70**, 1285–94.

Gusfield, J. (1981). *The Culture of Public Problems: Drinking-Driving and the Symbolic Order*. Chicago, IL: University of Chicago Press.

Hancock, T. (1985). Beyond health care: from public health policy to healthy public policy. *Canadian Journal of Public Health*, **76** (Suppl. 1), 9–11.

Harting, J., Kunst, A. E., Kwan, A., and Stronks, K. (2011). A 'health broker' role as a catalyst of change to promote health: an experiment in deprived Dutch neighbourhoods. *Health Promotion International*, **26** (1), 65–81.

Hasselaar, E. (2006). *Health Performance of Housing*. Delft: Delft University Press.

Hill, M. and Hupe, P. (2006). Analysing policy processes as multiple governance: accountability in social policy. *Policy & Politics*, **34** (3), 557–73.

Hoeijmakers, M., Raab, J., and Jansen, M. (2012). Academische werkplaatsen ter versterking van kennisontwikkeling en kennisuitwisseling in de publieke gezondheidszorg. Resultaten van netwerkanalyses in de Limburgse werkplaats. *Tijdschrift voor Gezondheidswetenschappen,* **90** (7), 442–52.

Hoeijmakers, M., de Leeuw, E., Kenis, P., and de Vries, N. K. (2007). Local health policy development processes in the Netherlands: an expanded toolbox for health promotion. *Health Promotion International*, **22** (2), 112–21.

Howlett, M. (2002). Do networks matter? Linking policy network structure to policy outcomes: evidence from four Canadian policy sectors 1990–2000. *Canadian Journal of Political Science,* **35** (2), 235–67.

Hueben, F. and de Leeuw, E. (1991). Intersectorale samenwerking: de theorie en de praktijk, in E. de Leeuw (ed.) *Gezonde Steden. Lokale gezondheidsbevordering in theorie, politiek en praktijk*, pp. 87–108, Assen/Maastricht: Van Gorcum.

International Conference on Primary Health Care (1978). *Declaration of Alma-Ata*. Geneva: World Health Organization.

Jansen, M. W. J., van Oers, H. A. M., Kok, G., and de Vries, N. K. (2010). Public health: disconnections between policy, practice and research. *Health Research Policy and Systems*, **8**, 37–49.

Kaashoek, B., Ongena, G., and Raab, J. (2009). Netwerken die werken? Netwerkanalyse als instrument voor beleidsevaluatie. *Bestuurswetenschappen*, **1**, 55–72.

Kenis, P. and Provan, K.G. (2009). Towards an exogenous theory of public network performance. *Public Administration*, **87** (3), 440–56.

Kenis, P. and Raab, J. (2003). Wanted: a good network theory of policy making. *National Public Management Conference, Proceedings*. Washington, DC.

Kickbusch, I. (2010). Health in All Policies: the evolution of the concept of horizontal health governance, in: **I. Kickbusch** and **K. Buckett** (eds.), *Implementing Health in All Policies*, pp. 11–23, Adelaide: Government of South Australia.

Kingdon, J. W. (1995). *Agendas, Alternatives, and Public Policies*. New York: Longman.

Laframboise, H. L. (1973). Health policy: breaking the problem down into more manageable segments. *Canadian Medical Association Journal*, **108**, 388–93.

Lalonde, M. (1974). *Nouvelle perspective sur la santé des Canadiens/A new perspective on the health of Canadians*. Ottawa: Gouvernement du Canada.

Lasswell, H. D. (1936). *Politics: Who Gets What, When, How*. New York: McGraw-Hill

Laumann, E. O. and Knoke, D. (1987). *The Organizational State. Social Choice in National Policy*. Madison, WI: University of Wisconsin Press.

Laumann, E. O., Marsden, P. V., and Prensky, D. (1989). The boundary specification problem in network analysis, in **L. C. Freeman**, **D. R. White**, and **A. K. Romney** (eds.) *Research Methods in Social Network Analysis*, pp. 61–87, Fairfax: George Mason University Press.

Lemstra, W. C. (1996). *Gemeentelijk Gezondheidsbeleid. Beter op zijn Plaats.* [Municipal Health Policy. Better placed]. Den Haag: Commissie Versterking Collectieve Preventie [Committee Reinforcement Collective Prevention].

Löfgren, H., Leahy, M. and de Leeuw, E. (2011). Participation and democratization in health and health care, in **H. Löfgren, E. de Leeuw**, and **M. Leahy** (eds.) *Democratising Health: Consumer Groups in the Policy Process*, pp. 1–14, Cheltenham: Edward Elgar Publishing.

Mazmanian, D. A. and Sabatier, P. A. (1989). *Implementation and Public Policy* (2nd edn.). Lanham, New York and London: University Press of America.

Milio, N. (1981). *Promoting Health through Public Policy*. Philadelphia: Davis.

Ministerie van VWS (Volksgezondheid Welzijn en Sport) (2000). *Spelen op de Winst. Een Visie op de Openbare Gezondheidszorg [Go for Victory. A Vision on Public Health]*. Den Haag: Ministerie van Volksgezondheid, Welzijn en Sport [Ministry of Health, Welfare and Sports].

Ministerie van VWS (Volksgezondheid Welzijn en Sport) [Ministry of Health, Welfare and Sports], GGD Nederland [Association of Dutch Public Health Services], VNG [Association of Dutch Municipalities], and Ministerie van Binnenlandse Zaken [Ministry of Home Affairs] (2001). *Nationaal Contract Openbare Gezondheidszorg [National Public Health Contract]*. Leiden: Platform Openbare Gezondheidszorg [Public Health Council].

Monge, P. R. and Contractor, N. S. (2003). *Theories of Communication Networks*. New York: Oxford University Press.

Navarro, V. (1986). *Crisis, Health, and Medicine: a Social Critique*. New York: Tavistock.

Provan, K. G. and Kenis, P. (2008). Modes of network governance: structure, management, and effectiveness. *Journal of Public Administration Research and Theory*, **18** (2), 229–52.

Putland, C., Baum, F. E., and Ziersch, A. M. (2011). From causes to solutions—insights from lay knowledge about health inequalities. *BMC Public Health*, **11**, 67.

Quoss, B., Cooney, M., and Longhurst, T. (2000). Academics and advocates: using participatory action research to influence welfare policy. *Journal of Consumer Affairs*, **34** (1), 47–61.

Sabatier, P. A. (ed.) (2007). *Theories of the Policy Process* (2nd edn.) Boulder, CO: Westview Press.

Salganik, M. J. and Heckathorn, D. D. (2004). Sampling and estimation in hidden populations using respondent-driven sampling. *Sociological Methodology*, **34**, 193–239.

Scott, J. (2000). *Social Network Analysis. A Handbook.* London; New Delhi: Sage Publications.

Skok, J. E. (1995). Policy issue networks and the public policy cycle: A structural-functional framework for public administration. *Public Administration Review*, **55** (4), 325–32.

Tsouros, A. (2009) City leadership for health and sustainable development: the World Health Organization European Healthy Cities Network. *Health Promotion International*, **24** (Suppl. 1), i4–i10.

van Bon-Martens, M. J. H., Achterberg, P. W., van de Goor, I. A. M., and van Oers, H. A. M. (2011). Towards quality criteria for regional public health reporting: concept mapping with Dutch experts. *European Journal of Public Health*, **22** (3), 337–42.

Waddell, S. (1995). Lessons from the Healthy Cities movement for social indicator development. *Social Indicators Research*, **34** (2), 213–35.

WHO (1986). *First International Conference on Health Promotion. The Ottawa Charter for Health Promotion.* Geneva: World Health Organization.

Winslow, C. E.-A. (1920). The untilled fields of public health. *Science*, **51** (3106), 23–33.

Chapter 9

Action theory and policy analysis: the ADEPT model

Alfred Rütten, Peter Gelius, and Karim Abu-Omar

Introduction

This chapter presents ADEPT (analysis of determinants of policy impact), an approach to policy analysis in health promotion that is easy to use, parsimonious, and empirically tested. ADEPT can make an important contribution to current discussions on theory development in health promotion, in particular with regard to theories of structure and agency, and theories of the policy process. To introduce the approach and position it vis-à-vis other theoretical approaches to health promotion policy analysis, we will first present a model of the determinants of individual action and then adapt this model to policy analysis. Second, we will discuss the specific contributions of the ADEPT model to empirical research and practical policy development. Third, we will consider potential links to other theoretical frameworks for the policy process: the institutional rational choice theory (IRC), the multiple streams theory, and the Advocacy Coalition Framework (ACF). Finally, we will illustrate how ADEPT, while rooted in action theory, can be linked to comprehensive theoretical frameworks of the interplay of structure and agency in health promotion.

The ADEPT model

In an attempt to explain the basic mechanisms underlying individual human behaviour, Georg Henrik von Wright developed a theory to explain the factors that determine human action and the logic that underlies the interaction of these factors (von Wright, 1976). He identified four 'determinants' that influence an individual's intention to act: wants, duties, abilities, and opportunities. Central to the theory is the interplay between these four determinants—what von Wright calls the *logic of events*: 'As the situations change, creating new opportunities for action, intentions articulate under the already existing wants and duties and within the frame of given abilities' (von Wright, 1976: 432). In addition, every action creates new situations (i.e. opportunities), which may, in turn, trigger subsequent events.

The ADEPT model is an adaptation of von Wright's original theory to the field of health promotion policy (Rütten et al., 2000a; 2000b; 2003a; 2003b). To apply von Wright's approach to the organizational/policy level, the determinants have to be 'translated' from the individual to the collective level (Rütten et al., 2000a). One must now, for example, consider not only the personal wants of policy-makers, but also the wants of their organizations (e.g. parties, ministries, municipal authorities, and non-governmental organizations (NGOs)). Consequently, ADEPT employs the term 'goals' rather than 'wants'. Similarly, duties become obligations, which encompass both policy-makers' professional duties and regulations governing the policy system. Abilities become resources in the ADEPT model, reflecting policy-makers' individual abilities as well as the capacities of their organizations (e.g. personnel and finances). Finally, ADEPT distinguishes between three different subtypes of opportunity: organizational opportunities, which arise from internal changes in organizations (e.g. new decision structures or actors); political opportunities, which arise from external changes in political and interorganizational settings (e.g. changes in the responsibilities of different political levels); and public opportunities, which emerge from external changes in public awareness, engagement by the population, or mass media interest.

The different elements and phases of the policy process can be conceived of as 'dependent variables' in the ADEPT model. In particular, the model has been designed to explain the potential policy impact. This impact comprises both the policy output (i.e. the actions taken on the policy level) and the policy outcome (i.e. the health effects on the population level). Figure 9.1 gives a schematic representation of the full ADEPT model.

Empirical research based on ADEPT

The ADEPT model aims to bridge the gaps between theory, research, and practice in health promotion. To achieve this, it provides an operationalization of the four determinants. It has developed a quantitative questionnaire consisting of 20 items, each scored with a 5-point Likert scale, along with a shorter 14-item version. There is also an interview guide for conducting semi-structured qualitative interviews.

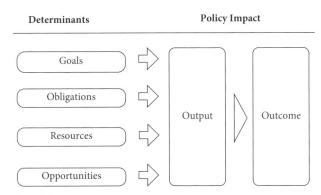

Figure 9.1 ADEPT model.
Reproduced from Rütten, A. et al., Policy development and implementation in health promotion—from theory to practice: the ADEPT model, *Health Promotion International*, Volume 26, Issue 3, Copyright © The Author 2010, by permission of Oxford University Press.

ADEPT has been empirically tested and applied in a number of policy analysis and policy development projects. The MAREPS project (methodology for the analysis of rationality and effectiveness of prevention and health promotion strategies) tested the model using data from interviews based on the written questionnaire with 719 policy-makers from six European nations. The four determinants of goals, obligations, resources, and opportunities served as independent variables, while the dependent variable was health policy impact, as measured by the policy-makers' self-assessment of three items related to policy outcome and one item related to policy output. The correlation coefficient analysis showed that obligations toward the health of the population, personal/professional commitment, and organizational opportunities (e.g. improved cooperation within organizations) were determinants of policy output. The outcome of policies was determined by the concreteness of goals and by the availability of sufficient resources and public opportunities, such as increasing support from the population and the media (Rütten et al., 2003b).

The EUNAAPA project (European network for action on ageing and physical activity) used ADEPT to assess existing policies in the area of physical activity promotion among older people. It carried out 248 interviews with policy-makers in 15 European nations using the 14-item abbreviated version of the original quantitative questionnaire. The researchers found pronounced differences in the perceptions of policy-makers from different sectors and nations in terms of goals, resources, obligations, and opportunities for physical activity promotion among older people (Rütten et al., 2012). For example, policy-makers from the sport sector rated the availability of resources for physical activity promotion among older persons most favourably. By contrast, policy-makers from the health sector rated such resources least favourably, while at the same time reporting high obligations to act on physical activity promotion among older people.

The PASEO project (physical activity among sedentary older people) used ADEPT to assess existing policy capacities and to guide a planning process for capacity building. A total of 234 policy-makers were questioned in semi-structured qualitative interviews based on the ADEPT determinants model. Project partners in 15 participating nations then set up national alliances for the promotion of physical activity among sedentary older people. The work of these alliances was directly based on the results of the qualitative interviews (Rütten and Gelius, 2013).

The ADEPT approach has also been adopted to prospectively assess the readiness of organizations to implement health promotion programmes. The BIG project (German acronym for 'movement as an investment for health') carried out 21 qualitative in-depth interviews with representatives of governmental organizations and NGOs. These interviews assessed goals, resources, obligations, and opportunities for physical activity promotion among women in difficult life situations (e.g. ethnic minority or low socioeconomic status), as perceived by these representatives. In subsequent phases of the project, the researchers attempted to engage these organizations in efforts to promote physical activity among this target group. In general, the evaluation confirmed that, in most organizations, the determinants were not favourable for policy action aimed at promoting physical activity among women in difficult life situations. However, organizations with a more favourable constellation of determinants—that is, at least some degree of specified goals, allocated resources, and perceived opportunities—were more likely to get involved in policy development/implementation (Rütten et al., 2009).

Policy development based on ADEPT

The ADEPT approach has been used for policy development in the context of several research and development projects. Using the model in this context builds, to a large degree, on insights into the interactive processes of policy analysis and development derived from empirical research with ADEPT. For example, in the EUNAAPA project, the results of the policy-maker survey were subsequently used to initiate a discourse between policy-makers from different sectors, experts, and practitioners on physical activity promotion for older people. This was achieved by presenting the results to policy-makers and experts at national workshop meetings and promoting work on the 'least developed' determinants (Rütten et al., 2012).

ADEPT was also used to guide policy development and build policy capacities for physical activity promotion among older people in PASEO, a project funded by the Health Programme of the European Union from 2009 to early 2011 (Rütten and Gelius, 2013). The goal of this project was to build capacities for health promotion in 15 European nations, thereby contributing to improved physical activity promotion for older people. The overall design of PASEO involved the setting up of national or regional alliances in all participating countries. The alliances brought together relevant organizations in physical activity promotion for older people from the sport, health care, social care, and other sectors. Using the terminology for policy process frameworks discussed earlier, one could say the project was attempting to build new 'advocacy coalitions' for physical activity and ageing in the countries involved. The main element of policy development was a 4-phase collaborative process to develop capacity-building measures based on the concept of cooperative planning (Rütten, 2001). The planning process was informed by qualitative phone interviews, at the beginning of the project, with representatives of the organizations participating in the planning process. The results were then reported back to the planning groups, which were advised to work on the determinants 'most in need' of improvement in their respective countries.

The design of the project consisted of qualitative interviews based on ADEPT at the start of the project to measure existing capacities among participating organizations and to inform the planning process. To assess the build-up of capacities during and after the end of the process, a mix of additional methods, including meeting minutes and observational notes and, most importantly, two online surveys (post test and six-month follow-up) were employed. The data thus gathered suggested a clear increase of policy capacities as conceptualized by ADEPT. Across the 15 nations taking part in the project, PASEO involved more than 130 organizations from all sectors, including national and regional ministries from Bavaria, Extremadura, Finland, Flanders, France, and

Vienna. A total of 114 specific measures were developed. These targeted both the collective choice level of policy-making for physical activity promotion for older people (e.g. in the form of networking activities, dissemination of alliance results, and staff training) and the operational level of directly increasing physical activity levels in older people (e.g. by improving infrastructures or through campaigns, pilot projects, or new sport programmes). An in-depth analysis of the German experience (Rütten and Gelius, 2013) shows that the PASEO alliance was particularly helpful in providing new *opportunities*, especially in the form of new contacts to other important actors in the field, as well as additional *resources* to many organizations, via the concept of cooperative planning and the time devoted to the project by the researchers and their main project partners.

Linking the ADEPT model to theoretical frameworks of the policy process

Health promotion researchers have recently begun to incorporate theories of the policy process into their work. Examples include studies that investigate policy networks in health promotion policy (de Leeuw, 2010; Hoeijmakers et al., 2007), analyses of media coverage (Breton et al., 2008) and agenda-setting on certain health promotion policy issues (Bryant, 2010), and investigations of policy windows and the behaviour of policy entrepreneurs in public health (Guldbrandsson and Fossum, 2009).

Various theories of the policy process have been developed by political scientists in recent decades (Sabatier, 2007). Among the most prominent are ACF (Sabatier and Jenkins-Smith, 1988; 1993; Sabatier, 2007), the multiple streams theory (Kingdon, 1984), and the institutional analysis and development (IAD) framework (Kiser and Ostrom, 1982; Sabatier, 2007). While the ADEPT model is not inextricably linked to any of these frameworks, we believe it shares a number of similarities in terms of fundamental components with these other frameworks.

To start with, the ADEPT model and IRC, along with the related IAD framework (Kiser and Ostrom, 1982; Ostrom, 2005; 2007), both assume a certain degree of rationality and predictability in actions, and both allow for actors to be either individual or collective. Moreover, the central categories of these frameworks, while not always absolutely congruent, do show considerable overlap. First, a key component of IRC (as specified in the IAD framework) is 'institutional arrangements' or 'rules-in-use'. Here 'rules' are 'enforced prescriptions about what actions (. . .) are required, prohibited, or permitted' (Ostrom, 2007: 36). Thus, there is a connection between this component of IRC/IAD and the component of 'obligations' in the ADEPT model. Second, fundamental assumptions about the 'attributes of the individual decision maker', as outlined in early IRC, refer to 'motives' and 'valued outcomes': 'individuals must have some notion of how actions link up with outcomes and how values are realized by selecting among alternative actions' (Kiser and Ostrom, 1982: 184). Such assumptions are at least partly covered by the component of 'goals' in ADEPT. Third, 'resources' are a critical component of both ADEPT and IRC/IAD. Within the latter framework, the notion of resources refers to both 'attributes of states of the world' (in terms of physical/material conditions) and 'attributes of the community' (social distribution of resources) (Ostrom, 2007). In addition, early IRC theory (Kiser and Ostrom, 1982) explicitly includes 'capabilities' as 'attributes of the individual decision maker'. Finally, although 'opportunities' play a minor role in IRC/IAD theory, at least certain aspects of the 'attributes of the community', such as the importance of 'common understanding' (Ostrom, 2007) can be related to the subcomponent of 'organizational opportunities' in ADEPT.

Of course, there are also important differences between IRC/IAD and ADEPT. While IRC/IAD is a highly developed theoretical model that is accepted as one of the major theoretical frameworks of the policy process, ADEPT is a rather simple model derived from individual action theory. However, a 'grand theory' like IRC/IAD has a number of limitations with respect to its practical applicability. First, due to its very character as a framework and to its greater emphasis on structures (namely, action arenas), many IRC/IAD concepts must, naturally, remain comparatively general and unspecific, making it somewhat difficult for practitioners to apply and operationalize them. Second, while it is a very powerful approach for policy analysis, it does not lend itself easily to being used for policy development. The IAD framework puts somewhat less emphasis on the dynamics of the policy-making process than do the other approaches. ADEPT addresses this problem by giving specific value to the determinant 'opportunities'. In addition to 'organizational opportunities', as mentioned above, ADEPT pays particular attention to 'public opportunities' like public support and media interest, and to political opportunities like the political climate, cooperation between the different political sectors and levels, and public–private partnerships.

In this regard, the ADEPT model overlaps somewhat with a second major framework of the policy process, the multiple streams theory (Kingdon, 1984; Zahariadis, 2007). Key issues of this framework, such as explanations for the setting and changing of policy agendas—'what makes an idea's time come' (Kingdon, 1984: 1)—are related to the concept of the 'policy window', which is defined as 'an opportunity for advocates of proposals to push their pet solutions, or to push attention to their special problems' (Kingdon, 1984: 165). The emergence of such opportunities can be conceptualized as times when the problem stream, the politics stream, and the policy stream are coupled, and 'policy entrepreneurs', for example, are able to change a policy agenda. In the multiple streams theory, opportunities refer to 'problem windows' and 'political windows'. In particular, the latter overlap with two opportunity components of the ADEPT model: 'political opportunities' like a change of administration, and 'public opportunities'—what Kingdon calls 'the national mood', which includes changes in public opinion, broad social movements, and comments in the media (Kingdon, 1984). Besides this most striking overlap with regard to 'opportunities' in ADEPT, there is a second major connection between these two models, related to the concept of resources. In the multiple streams theory, the concept of resources refers to the 'skills', 'time', and 'energy' of policy entrepreneurs, and is an important variable determining success (Zahariadis, 2007). This part of the concept overlaps with the 'individual abilities' of policy-makers as part of resources in ADEPT.

On the other hand, the multiple streams theory differs from ADEPT in that it puts an explicit focus on the agenda-setting and decision-making phases of the policy process, while ADEPT may potentially be applied to the entire policy cycle, but especially focuses on policy impact. The two concepts also differ with respect to their epistemological approach: while ADEPT is particularly useful for ascertaining *why* policies are shaped the way they are, the multiple streams theory is mainly concerned with *when* decisions are made and *how* this happens. A third difference is that the multiple streams theory regards 'an entire system' as its primary unit of analysis (Zahariadis, 2007), while ADEPT focuses on individual organizations and their representatives. The advantage of the former is the ability to build complex explanations with a strong focus on interaction effects between actors; the advantage of the latter is its parsimony and the ability to actually *measure* the specific determinants of actors.

Finally, there are several links between ADEPT and ACF (Sabatier and Jenkins-Smith, 1988; Sabatier, 2007). The first pertains to ACF's core conceptualization of the policy subsystem and how coalitions within this subsystem interact. While 'policy beliefs' is one of the key components of ACF's policy subsystem design, they are only rudimentarily covered by ADEPT. 'Resources' constitute the second key component of ACF, and they are one of the ADEPT key determinants as well. It should be noted, however, that the concept of resources in ACF (Sabatier, 2007) is more comprehensive than in ADEPT: it includes not only 'skilful leadership' and 'financial resources', but also 'public opinion' and 'formal legal authority'—elements that are related to different determinants like public opportunities and obligations in ADEPT.

The course of action as depicted in ACF's policy subsystem is similar, in some respects, to the logic of events in ADEPT. Both ACF and ADEPT perceive collective actors to be coalitions with particular orientations (policy beliefs, goals, and obligations) and resources to be the driving force of policy processes, both consider the importance of stimulation by 'external events' (opportunities), and both ultimately relate the course of action to policy output and policy impact (Sabatier, 2007). The third link between the theoretical models of ADEPT and ACF is this consideration of external events, including changes in public opinion, policy decisions, and impacts from other subsystems. These events are deemed to be crucial dynamic factors that determine policy-making within the subsystem. The opportunities category of ADEPT focuses precisely on these factors. However, 'opportunity' has a different connotation in ACF: while Sabatier employs the term 'opportunity structures' to 'refer to relatively enduring features of a polity that affect the resources and constraints of subsystem actors' (2007: 200), ADEPT follows von Wright's 'logic of events' by relating 'opportunities' to permanent situational changes in the policy environment.

In addition to these links between the theoretical models of ADEPT and ACF, there is a parallel in terms of policy development. In ACF, one path to policy change is negotiated agreements. Sabatier (2007) lists nine propositions for how to successfully conduct negotiations toward policy change. We consider most of these propositions in our own policy development projects: we employ a cooperative planning process that is based on the analysis of policy determinants following the ADEPT model and addresses issues of coalition building (see Rütten and Gelius, 2013).

Beyond these differences in meaning with regard to notions such as resources and opportunities, there are also some major conceptual differences between ACF and ADEPT. At least two of them should be mentioned here. The first is ACF's distinction between three levels of assumption in the model: the macro level, which deals with factors of the external 'political and socioeconomic system'; the micro level, which focuses on the individual policy-maker; and the meso level, which concerns 'a multiplicity of actors in a subsystem' (Sabatier, 2007). While ADEPT also considers micro- and macro-level assumptions, it is rather weak in conceptualizing the meso level. In particular, the ADEPT model may be less appropriate when dealing with interactive policy processes, such as within or between advocacy coalitions, as conceptualized by ACF. The other conceptual difference between the two models is the concept of policy change. While in ACF policy changes are highly dependent on changes in policy beliefs—caused either by 'external perturbation' or 'policy-oriented learning' (Sabatier, 2007)—ADEPT, like the multiple streams theory, includes the crucial role of 'opportunities' as triggers for policy changes.

ADEPT and structure versus agency

In the social sciences, there has been a long-standing dispute between proponents of structural approaches versus advocates of action theory. More recently, this debate has also arisen in the field of public health and health promotion, as in the discourse on the 'inequality paradox', which some believe to be caused by certain kinds of structural approaches in health promotion. For example, a population approach focusing on changes in environmental conditions in order to either decrease health risks or increase opportunities (e.g. new sport facilities) may lead to increased health inequalities because vulnerable groups may profit less from such changes than wealthier groups (Allebeck, 2008; Frohlich and Potvin, 2008; 2010; McLaren et al., 2010). Contributions to this issue have made reference to the duality of structure and agency—that is, the inter-relationship between structures and the human ability to act—and to the way in which these two aspects reinforce each other in social practice. With regard to health promotion, this discussion underlines the importance of participatory and enabling strategies that integrate 'agentic' and 'structural' perspectives in order to contribute simultaneously to health and social equity in a population (Frohlich and Potvin, 2008; 2010; Rütten and Gelius, 2011).

The most prominent work in this area is undoubtedly Anthony Giddens's structuration theory (1984). Although Giddens's work is not chiefly concerned with policy-making, it does provide useful insights for the study of policy-making processes. In a recent contribution (Rütten and Gelius, 2011), we introduced a multilevel model that relates structure and agency to both the 'operational' level (including the everyday life of individuals) and the 'collective choice' level (including policy-making). Our work not only looked at policy-making in general but also focused specifically on policy-making in health promotion. It demonstrated how fundamental domains in health promotion action like creating supportive environments and building healthy public policies have to be linked to the domains of developing personal skills and community action.

As it is based on a theory of individual action, the main focus of ADEPT is on the agentic aspects of policy-making. However, an examination of determinants suggests an important potential link to structural perspectives on the policy-making process. To explore further potential links between ADEPT and theories on structure and agency, we will first show how ADEPT links to structuration theory and to related sociological approaches. We will then position ADEPT within a multilevel model of the interplay of structure and agency in health promotion.

Giddens's original approach to conceptualizing 'the duality of structure and agency' emphasizes the interconnectedness of the two components. For example, agency refers to the 'capabilities' of actors—that is, how they are able 'to make a difference' (Giddens, 1984: 14). Thus, agency is closely related to Giddens's concept of power as 'transformative capacity' and of 'resources' as 'media through which power is exercised' (Giddens, 1984: 16). Resources are also one of the two subcategories of the second component, structure. In ADEPT, both structure and agency are considered in the concept of resources. On the one hand, resources in ADEPT are characterized as the capacities of individual policy-makers (e.g. qualifications of staff) and of the organization. These subcategories overlap with agency/capabilities in the structuration theory approach. On the other hand, resources in ADEPT also include material/financial resources or organizational support, which are subcategories that overlap with structure/resources in structuration theory. Moreover, one could also conceive of a second ADEPT determinant, namely obligations, as 'structure' in the sense used by Giddens. This ADEPT category can be linked to 'rules', the second subcategory of structure according to Giddens (see also the links between obligations and rules with regard to IRC/IAD).

As authors such as Sewell (1992) and Archer (1995) have argued, one of the major drawbacks of Giddens's work is that it does not properly recognize the potential for structural change. Archer criticizes the 'central conflation' in structuration theory, and presents a 'morphogenetic approach' to structure and agency that attempts to cover the full 'timescale through which structure and agency themselves emerge, intertwine and redefine one another' (Archer, 1995: 76). Likewise, Sewell introduces different constructs to explain how the interaction of structure and agency can lead to structural change. For example, the 'multiplicity' and the 'intersection of structures' confronted by actors imply certain options for structural change, particularly when combined with a third construct: the ability of actors, in new situations, to draw on patterns of action they have already acquired from other settings—'transposability of schemas' (Sewell, 1992). These approaches to integrating the concept of structural change into the structure–agency interplay connect, at least to a certain extent, to the logic of events in the ADEPT model. In particular, ADEPT explicitly refers to structural changes with its key determinant of 'opportunities', both as inputs for actual policy-making and as outcomes of previous policy-making. For example, organizational opportunities are internal changes in organizations, political opportunities arise from external changes in political and interorganizational settings, and public opportunities arise from external changes in public awareness, engagement of the population, or mass media interest.

In his consideration of the 'forms of institutions', Giddens introduces a classification of institutional orders, including political institutions. However, he has reservations about making clear-cut distinctions between the different institutional spheres, and thus remains rather vague on this point. He therefore does not provide a solid starting point for a concrete operationalization of the interplay between structure and agency in policy-making. Ostrom's IAD framework provides a potential way of integrating the policy dimension into concepts of structure and agency. A crucial aspect of the IAD framework is the concept of different levels of action: (1) the operational level, which encompasses the everyday life of individuals and the working level of organizations; (2) the collective choice level, which includes more formal settings like legislatures, regulatory agencies, and courts, as well as informal arenas like gatherings, appropriation teams, and private associations; and (3) the constitutional level (Ostrom, 2007). Of particular interest to the context of health promotion are the collective choice level, where health promotion policy is formulated, and the operational level, where individual health behaviour occurs. In Ostrom's view, the different levels build upon each other, with more basic levels influencing structures and actions at more specific levels by determining how their rules can be altered. In addition, individual actors usually take part in multiple action arenas, both at the operational level (e.g. within family, school, or work) and at the collective choice level (e.g. as voters in an election).

The ADEPT model places a strong emphasis on the collective choice level because this model was explicitly designed to assess the determinants of outputs and outcomes of policy-making in health promotion. At the same time, however, it takes into account the fact that the major actors involved in policy-making (e.g. ministries, agencies, and NGOs) are, themselves, collective in nature. All of these organizations are composed of individuals, and there is always an operational level within organizations at the policy-making level. ADEPT makes this clear on several occasions; for example, via the subcategory of 'obligations', which assesses to what degree individuals within an organization who deal directly with a certain policy issue are committed to that issue. In addition, ADEPT may also be combined with von Wright's original theory of individual action to take into account other operational levels, such as individual physical activity behaviour. In the MAREPS project, which developed and tested the original version of ADEPT, the determinants of action at the policy-making level were assessed using ADEPT, while health behaviour in the population was conceptualized using the original von Wright categories (Rütten et al., 2003a; 2003b). As part of this project, more than 700 policy-makers in six European nations were interviewed with standardized questionnaires. At the population level, more than 3,300 interviews were conducted. The correlation coefficient analysis (Pearson coefficients, $p < 0.01$) showed that obligations toward the health of the population, personal/professional commitment, and organizational opportunities (e.g. improvement of cooperation within organizations) were determinants of policy output. The outcome of policies was determined by the concreteness of goals, the availability of sufficient resources, and public opportunities such as increasing support from the population and the media.

We have elsewhere (Rütten and Gelius, 2011) proposed a multilevel model of structure and agency that uses the general framework provided by Giddens but includes additions by Sewell and Ostrom. As discussed, such an approach shows great potential for further integration with ADEPT, as there are important links both to Giddens's original work and to Sewell's concept of change and Ostrom's notion of levels. An interesting endeavour would be to combine this advanced model of structure and agency with ADEPT. This could also help to expand the scope of ADEPT, transforming it from a simple and easy-to-use, but focused and somewhat restricted, model into a broader framework for policy analysis that takes into account a multitude of factors that influence the policy-making process, and that deals explicitly with both the operational and the collective choice levels of health promotion.

Conclusions: the ADEPT model and its implications for health promotion theory research and policy

The ADEPT model was originally designed with an eye to analysing the 'inputs' (determinants) and 'impacts' of the policy process, not as a framework for analysing the policy process per se. Nevertheless, we are confident that this chapter has shown that it can be applied to policy processes in a number of different ways. First, ADEPT can easily be linked to major frameworks of the policy process that are especially focused on process (e.g. ACF). One potential advantage here is that the model has a high degree of 'theoretical flexibility': it is linked to several frameworks without being bound exclusively to any of them, allowing it to be used with various general approaches to policy-making. Second, as ADEPT is derived from von Wright's action theory, it is based on fundamental assumptions about 'the logic of events', which, in von Wright's words, 'constitutes the cogwheels of the "machinery" which keeps history moving' (1976: 432). Thus, the theoretical framework of ADEPT may, in the future, be used to build a more explicit concept of 'process' into the model, which would allow us to consider policy-making as a chronological sequence and as an 'interplay' of action situations and actors. As shown above, the model is also compatible with theories of structure and agency, above all with Giddens's seminal approach. While retaining simplicity and parsimony through its actor-centred focus, the inclusion of determinants allows ADEPT to include structural considerations in health promotion policy-making. Finally, our previous research on policy development has demonstrated that practical approaches to policy development like cooperative planning processes can be based on the analysis of policy determinants following the ADEPT model, and, at the same time, may address issues such as coalition building, which are primarily process-oriented. Such research may also lead to further improvement of ADEPT's policy process-related components.

We are aware that ADEPT, in its current form, still has a number of limitations and shortcomings. For example, it does not reflect networking as comprehensively as does the ACF framework. The same applies to other important aspects of the policy-making process. However, certain limitations are the price to pay for the great parsimony of ADEPT, which makes the model so easy to operationalize and apply. In addition, we want to stress again that ADEPT is explicitly conceptualized as a model, not as a full-fledged framework of the policy process. It therefore does not aim to compete with the very comprehensive (yet difficult-to-measure) frameworks discussed above. At the same time, this chapter has shown that that there may be ways of developing the model into a broader framework.

We believe that ADEPT, despite its limitations, constitutes a valuable contribution to improving policy analysis and policy development in health promotion in various theoretical and also practical ways. ADEPT is theory-driven, yet at the same time it is more than just a theoretical aid to help us conceptualize reality in our minds. Rather, its operationalization, both quantitative and qualitative, allows us to measure determinants and to test the model as a whole. Empirical analysis and application have shown that ADEPT actually works. Another advantage of the model is its parsimony. Limiting the determinants to just four components ensures that the model is easy to use and can be applied not only by scientists but also by practitioners. In addition, due to its simplicity, ADEPT can be used for cross-national comparisons or development efforts, as the four determinants can be assumed to operate under a broad range of political and societal environments. It can be used both for policy analysis ('retrospectively') and for policy development ('prospectively'). Potentially, ADEPT could also be coupled with various methods of community development (Rifkin et al., 2000), with capacity building (NSW Health Department, 2001), and with cooperative planning processes (Rütten and Gelius, 2013).

References

Allebeck, P. (2008). The prevention paradox or the inequality paradox? *European Journal of Public Health*, **18** (3), 115.

Archer, M. S. (1995). *Realist Social Theory: The Morphogenetic Approach*. Cambridge: Cambridge University Press.

Breton, E., Richard, L., Gagnon, F., Jacques, M., and Bergeron, P. (2008). Health promotion research and practice require sound policy analysis models: the case of Québec's Tobacco Act. *Social Science & Medicine*, **67** (11), 1679–89.

Bryant, T. (2010). The influence of politics and political ideology on social and health spending, in D. Raphael, T. Bryant, and M. Rioux (eds.) *Staying Alive: Critical Perspectives on Health, Illness, and Health Care* (2nd edn.), pp. 239–63, Toronto: Canadian Scholars' Press.

de Leeuw, E. (2010). *Online tool for network participants, stakeholders, social and policy entrepreneurs to map policy networks*. Available at: <http://www.evelynedeleeuw.net/Home/for-my-colleagues--or-th ose-who-believe-they-are/multiple-streams-multiple-networks/lookheremultiplestreamsandmulti-plenetworks> (accessed 16 June 2010).

Frohlich, K. and Potvin, L. (2008). The inequality paradox: the population approach and vulnerable populations. *American Journal of Public Health*, **98** (2), 216–21.

Frohlich, K. and Potvin, L. (2010). Commentary: structure or agency? The importance of both for addressing social inequalities in health. *International Journal of Epidemiology, 39*, 378–9.

Giddens, A. (1984). *The Constitution of Society: Outline of the Theory of Structuration.* Berkeley and Los Angeles, CA: University of California Press.

Guldbrandsson, K. and Fossum, B. (2009). An exploration of the theoretical concepts policy windows and policy entrepreneurs at the Swedish public health arena. *Health Promotion International, 24* (4), 434–44.

Hoeijmakers, M., De Leeuw, E., Kenis P., and de Vries, N. K. (2007). Local health policy development processes in the Netherlands: an expanded toolbox for health promotion. *Health Promotion International, 22* (2), 112–21.

Kingdon, J. (1984) *Agendas, Alternatives, and Public Policies.* Boston, MA: Little, Brown & Co.

Kiser, L. and Ostrom, E. (1982). The three worlds of action: a metatheoretical synthesis of institutional approaches, in E. Ostrom (ed.) *Strategies of Political Inquiry,* pp. 179–222, Beverly Hills, CA: Sage.

McLaren, L., McIntyre, L., and Kirkpatrick, S. (2010). Rose's population strategy of prevention need not increase social inequalities in health. *International Journal of Epidemiology, 39*, 372–37.

NSW Health Department (2001). *A Framework for Building Capacity to Improve Health.* Gladesville, NSW: Better Health Centre–Publications Warehouse.

Ostrom, E. (2005). *Understanding Institutional Diversity.* Princeton, NJ: Princeton University Press.

Ostrom, E. (2007). Institutional rational choice: an assessment of the institutional analysis and development framework, in P. A. Sabatier (ed.) *Theories of the Policy Process,* pp. 21–64, Boulder, CO: Westview Press.

Rifkin, S. B., Lewando-Hundt, G., and Draper, A. K. (2000). *Participatory Approaches in Health Promotion and Health Planning. A Literature Review.* London: Health Development Agency.

Rütten, A. (2001). Evaluating healthy public policies in community and regional contexts, in I. Rootman, M. Goodstadt, B. Hyndman, D. McQueen, L. Potvin, J. Springett, and E. Ziglio (eds.) *Evaluation in Health Promotion. Principles and Perspectives*, pp. 341–63, Copenhagen: WHO Regional Office for Europe.

Rütten, A. and Gelius, P. (2011). The interplay of structure and agency in health promotion: integrating a concept of structural change and the policy dimension into a multi-level model and applying it to health promotion principles and practice. *Social Science & Medicine, 73* (7), 953–9.

Rütten A. and Gelius P. (2013). Building policy capacities: an interactive approach to knowledge translation in health promotion. *Health Promotion International*, Advance Access published 6 March 2013, doi: 10.1093/heapro/dat006.

Rütten, A., Gelius, P., and Abu-Omar, K. (2010). Policy development and implementation in health promotion—from theory to practice: the ADEPT model. *Health Promotion International, 26*, 322–9.

Rütten, A., Röger, U., Abu-Omar, K., and Frahsa, A. (2009). Assessment of organizational readiness for health promotion policy implementation: test of a theoretical model. *Health Promotion International, 24*, 243–51.

Rütten, A., Abu-Omar, K., Gelius, P., Dinan-Young, S., Frändin, K., Hopman-Rock, M., and Young, A. (2012). Policy assessment and policy development for physical activity promotion: results of an exploratory intervention study in 15 European nations. *Health Research Policy and Systems, 10*,14.

Rütten, A., Lüschen, G., von Lengerke, T. Abel, T., Kannas, L., Rodríguez Díaz, J. A., Vinck, J., and van der Zee, J. (2000a). *Health Promotion Policy in Europe. Rationality, Impact, and Evaluation.* München: Oldenbourg.

Rütten, A., Lüschen, G., von Lengerke, T., Abel, T., Kannas, L., Rodríguez Díaz, J. A., Vinck, J., and van der Zee, J. (2003a). Determinants of health policy impact: a theoretical framework for policy analysis. *Sozial- und Präventivmedizin/Social and Preventive Medicine, 48*, 293–300.

Rütten, A., Lüschen, G., von Lengerke, T., Abel, T., Kannas, L., Rodríguez Díaz, J. A., Vinck, J., and van der Zee, J. (2003b). Determinants of health policy impact: comparative results of a European policymaker study. *Sozial- und Präventivmedizin/Social and Preventive Medicine*, **48**, 379–391.

Rütten, A., von Lengerke, T., Abel, T., Kannas, L., Lüschen, G., Rodríguez Díaz, J. A., Vinck, J., and van der Zee, J. (2000b). Policy, competence and participation: empirical evidence for a multilevel health promotion model. *Health Promotion International*, **15**, 35–47.

Sabatier, P. A. (ed.) (2007). *Theories of the Policy Process* (2nd edn.) Boulder, CO: Westview Press.

Sabatier, P. A. and Jenkins-Smith, H. C. (eds.) (1988). Special issue: policy change and policy-oriented learning: exploring and advocacy coalition approach, *Policy Sciences*, **21**, 123–272.

Sabatier, P. A. and Jenkins-Smith, H. C. (1993). *Policy Change and Learning: an Advocacy Coalition Approach*. Boulder, CO: Westview.

Sewell, W. (1992). A theory of structure: duality, agency, and transformation. *American Journal of Sociology*, **98** (1), 1–29.

von Wright, G. H. (1976). Determinism and the study of man, in J. Manninen and R. Tuomela (eds.) *Essays on Explanation and Understanding*, pp. 415–35, Dordrecht: Deidel.

Zahariadis, N. (2007). The multiple streams framework: structure, limitations, prospects, in P. A. Sabatier (ed.) *Theories of the Policy Process* (2nd edn.), pp. 65–92, Boulder, CO: Westview Press.

Chapter 10

Health in All Policies from international ideas to local implementation: policies, systems, and organizations

Fran Baum, Angela Lawless, and Carmel Williams

Introduction

This chapter examines the concept of Health in All Policies (HiAP) as a mechanism to promote population health, and discusses the implementation of the idea in the Australian state of South Australia between 2007 and 2012. In this chapter we draw on three main bodies of theory. First we use the work of Kingdon (2011) on the ways in which policy is developed and how evidence, politics, and context intersect to create the opportunity for new policies. We also use theory regarding organizational change (Kaluzny and Hernadez, 1988) to consider the organizational factors that support the implementation of HiAP within complex bureaucracies. We draw on systems theory and its application to health systems (de Savigny and Adam, 2009), and use this to examine HiAP's implementation in the context of complex systems and the requirement for system actors to develop ways of thinking compatible with working in complex and adaptive systems. Finally, we make a critical assessment of the institutionalization of HiAP in South Australia.

In this chapter, we reflect theoretically on a policy that all three of us have followed closely in recent years. First, we have all been involved in the evaluation of this policy in our respective roles as academics and practitioner working with the South Australian Department of Health and Ageing (DHA). Second, as manager of this unit, Williams has also been involved in the implementation of HiAP from its beginnings. Third, Baum wrote the original proposal to the South Australian Government for Kickbusch's term as Thinker in Residence,while Lawless and Williams were both policy advisers to this residency.

Theory used in this chapter

The HiAP approach draws together a number of areas of knowledge, theory, and policy. HiAP is an approach to health promotion which reflects the World Health Organization's (WHO) growing critique of health promotion based on behaviourism and an increased focus on approaches aimed at changing the environments in which people live. HiAP rests on the values and understanding of the social determinants of health as laid out in the report of the Commission on Social Determinants of Health (CSDH, 2008). From this base it aims to promote health across all sectors through policy change. Consequently, understanding the ways in which the policy world works is vital to understanding the effectiveness of HiAP.

Before describing our policy and organizational theories we pay attention to one aspect of HiAP that needs some theoretical explanation—that of 'health'. Often this term is taken to mean absence of disease, whereas it implies much more. The broader meaning of health was enshrined in the WHO (1948) Constitution, which defined health as 'a state of complete physical, mental, and social well-being and not merely the absence of disease or infirmity'. This definition stresses the positive aspects of health and has been developed further through the theory of 'salutogenesis' (Antonovsky, 1996; Kickbusch, 1996). Antonovsky calls for health promotion to go beyond disease and risk factor prevention, to see health as a positive state of well-being. Salutogenesis is concerned with the roots of health and how it is created. HiAP can be conceptualized as a means of implementing a salutogenic perspective at a population level.

Kingdon (2011) examined policy-making processes in relation to health care services and transportation in the US federal government; on that basis, he developed the idea of streams of influence that need to come together in order for policy ideas to be adopted and implemented. His argument is that convergence or coupling of the separate policy streams—problems, proposals, and politics—creates a window of opportunity for an issue to be elevated to the public policy agenda. He also demonstrated that coupling of the policy streams can be assisted by policy entrepreneurs who advance the innovative policy.

Kingdon's agenda-setting can be conceived of as a first stage in the policy process. Organizational theory provides frameworks to examine how innovative proposals move through stages of implementation. Kaluzny and Hernandez (1988) describe four stages in the adoption of change: awareness, adoption, implementation, and institutionalization. Context and structure are important factors in the change process. Butterfoss et al. (2008) see that a suite of complementary strategies operating at multiple organizational levels and responsive to internal and external environments is required to bring about changes.

We have also found it useful to use complex systems thinking to examine the ways in which the various organizations involved in HiAP interact synergistically. The value of systems thinking in relation to health systems has been stressed by WHO:

> Systems thinking works to reveal the underlying characteristics and relationships of systems. Work in fields as diverse as engineering, economics and ecology shows systems to be constantly changing, with components that are tightly connected and highly sensitive to change elsewhere in the system. They are non-linear, unpredictable and resistant to change, with seemingly obvious solutions sometimes worsening a problem.

> (de Savigny and Adam, 2009: 19)

Increasingly, literature on health promotion recognizes that much health promotion action happens as part of a 'complex adaptive system'—one that self-organizes, adapts and evolves with time (Hawe et al., 2009a; Hawe et al., 2009b). 'Complexity' arises from a system's interconnected parts, and 'adaptivity' from its ability to communicate and change, based on experience. Systems thinking is an approach to problem-solving that views 'problems' as part of a wider, dynamic system (de Savigny and Adam, 2009). HiAP is clearly implemented as part of a complex system that involves different organizations and Kingdon's three streams of influence.

Table 10.1 summarizes common system characteristics and demonstrates the complexity of systems that evaluation designs need to take into account if they are to be capable of assessing interventions within their system context. Of particular relevance to HiAP is the need to understand and manage system networks, which comprise the web of all stakeholders and actors, individual and institutional, in the system (de Savigny and Adam, 2009: 45) in order to be an effective actor within the network. Systems thinking requires a different set of skills from those which focus on particular organizations (see Table 10.2). The use of these skills will be discussed in the section on implementation.

Table 10.1 Common systems characteristics

Systems characteristics	Description
Self-organizing	Systems dynamics arise spontaneously from internal structure
Constantly changing	Systems adjust and readjust at many interactive time scales and change is a constant in all sustainable systems
Tightly linked	The high degree of connectivity means that change in one subsystem affects the others
Governed by feedback	A positive or negative response may alter the intervention or expected effects
Non-linear	Relationships within a system cannot be arranged along a simple input–output line and the system is unpredictable
History dependent	Short-term effects of intervening may differ from long-term effects so evaluations have to take a long-term perspective
Counterintuitive	Cause and effect are often distant in time and space, defying solutions that pit causes close to the effects they seek to address, which means a systems view needs to inform evaluations
Resistant to change	Seemingly obvious solutions may fail or worsen the situation—system characteristics can render the system 'policy resistant'

Table 10.2 Skills of systems thinking

Usual approach	Systems thinking approach
Static thinking: focusing on particular events	Dynamic thinking: framing a problem in terms of a pattern of behaviour over time
System-as-effect thinking: viewing behaviour generated by a system as driven by external forces	System-as-cause thinking: placing responsibility for a behaviour on internal actors who manage the policies and 'plumbing' of the system
Tree-by-tree thinking: believing that really knowing something means focusing on the details	Forest thinking: believing that to know something requires understanding the context of relationships
Factors thinking: listing factors that influence or correlate with some result	Operational thinking: concentrating on causality and understanding how a behaviour is generated
Straight-line thinking: viewing causality as running in one direction, ignoring (either deliberately or not) the interdependence and interaction between and among the causes	Loop thinking: viewing causality as an ongoing process, not a one-time event, with effects feeding back to influence the causes and the causes affecting each other

Reproduced with permission from de Savigny, D. and Adam, T (eds.), *Systems Thinking for Health Systems Strengthening*, Alliance for Health Policy and Systems Research, Geneva, Copyright © World Health Organization 2009. Originally modified from Richmond B., *The 'Thinking' in Systems: Seven Essential Skills*, Pegasus Communications, Massachusetts, USA, Copyright © 2000.

History of the HiAP idea

HiAP rests on the notion that health is created predominantly outside the health sector. This view has been recognized in many different times and contexts. In the 14th century the republican city states of Florence and Venice introduced boards of public health and established fountains, baths, and sewers. They also introduced lay health committees during epidemic crisis (Lewis, 2003: xv). The birth of the modern public health movement in the 19th century saw widespread acknowledgement that living and working conditions had a massive impact on health (Baum, 2008). In England the 1848 Public Health Act gave local authorities the power to remedy unsanitary conditions and to require adequate drainage and sanitation in towns (Kearns, 1988). In Europe both Engels and Virchow recognized that disease affected the poor more than the rich, and that social conditions were vital in this relationship (Engels, 1993[1845]; Virchow, 1848). McKeown (1979) developed the thesis that rising living standards, rather than improvements in medical technology, were responsible for the decline in mortality from the mid-19th to the mid-20th century. Srezter (1988) expanded on McKeown's thesis to argue that economic growth itself did not guarantee improved health; rather, it was intervention from governments in terms of improved sanitation, urban planning, and education that was able to translate the fruits of economic growth into improved health. Srezter argues that these gains were hard-fought and resulted from a 'rich history of political, ideological, scientific and legal conflicts and battles at both national and local levels' (1988: 35). Civil society played a vital role in advocating these health-improving investments. Thus,

19th-century history highlights the essentially political nature of public health and how civil and political actions combine to lead to healthy public policy (Baum, 2008).

In most Organisation for Economic Co-operation and Development (OECD) countries the period following the Second World War through to the 1970s witnessed the establishment of welfare states, in which nations took increased responsibility for the health and welfare of their citizens. This period saw access to many of the vital social determinants of health extended to whole populations in a period of high employment and a growing consensus of the importance of universal education, welfare, and health services. It was also a period in which inequities tended to decline (Stilwell, 1993). This picture changed with the oil crisis of the 1970s and the ensuing period of neo-liberal economic policies.

Neo-liberalism led to questioning of the role of the State in the provision of health, education, housing, and other services, and the ensuing three decades have seen economic inequities increase. It is from this context that the idea of HiAP has emerged, perhaps as one mechanism to reassert the role of the State.

The health promotion movement and HiAP

The notion of health promotion was born in the 1970s and, at that time, had a focus on lifestyles and behavioural change to reduce disease risk factors drawing on psychological theories. It was the recognition that these approaches met with very limited success in the absence of more structural changes to the conditions that shaped people's health in their everyday lives (see Baum, 2008: 456–75) that led to increasing interest in the role played in creating or detracting from health by different parts of the social and economic system. From then to the present, WHO has played a crucial role in advancing and developing this idea, and it is in these developments that the HiAP initiative has its roots.

The Health for All strategy noted that primary health care:

> involves, in addition to the health sector, all related sectors and aspects of national and community development, in particular agriculture, animal husbandry, food, industry, education, housing, public works, communications and other sector; and demands the co-ordinated efforts of all those sectors.
>
> (International Conference on Primary Health Care, 1978: 4)

This policy direction was seen primarily as directed at middle- and low-income countries, and so did not attract much attention in OCED countries. By contrast, the Ottawa Charter for Health Promotion (WHO, 1986) was taken up with enthusiasm by many health promoters in rich countries, and was welcomed for its focus on the environments that affect health and its emphasis on healthy public policy and community involvement. The subsequent conference in Adelaide led to the Adelaide Recommendations on Healthy Public Policy (WHO, 1988), which developed this concept and provided an international mandate that eventually led to the adoption of the HiAP approach as a mechanism to realize healthy public policy. The Ottawa Charter has been very influential in shaping the nature of HiAP. It influenced the emerging Healthy Cities movement, which Ashton and Seymour (1988: 154) said took the Health for All strategy 'off the shelves and into the streets of Europe'.

WHO took up the Healthy Cities idea and its *Twenty Steps for Developing a Healthy Cities Project* (WHO, 1995) included setting up a city-wide intersectoral committee and taking a range of intersectoral action. The Healthy Cities movement did much to promote the importance of the social determinants of health at the local level, and to highlight the role of all sectors of city government in promoting health. Throughout the 1990s WHO organized further global health promotion conferences, each of which reinforced the notion that the social, economic, and environmental determinants were crucial to good population health and health equity (see Catford, 2011).

These ideas were reinforced by significant national-level academic work on the social determinants of health equity. Perhaps most significantly, the Black Report (Townsend and Davidson, 1982) put the strong argument that health inequities were best explained by the material differences in people's lives that were structured by social class and access to income, education, housing, and clean environments. This report was ignored by the incoming Thatcher Government, but had a large impact around the world in making the case for the social determinants of health inequity and the need for policies in many sectors beyond health to address them.

In the past decade the intensity of advocacy for HiAP has increased. Two crucial initiatives have been from the European Union (EU) and WHO once again. During the Finnish EU Presidency in 2006, HiAP was the main theme in the area of health. This was based on Article 152 of the Amsterdam Treaty (corresponding closely to Article 168 of the recently ratified Lisbon Treaty (Council of the European Union, 2012)), which states that a 'high level of human health protection shall be ensured in the definition and implementation of all Union policies and activities' (Ollila, 2011: 12). The CSDH's 2008 report presented a strong evidence-based case for the importance of action on social determinants of health in order to promote health equitably. It argued for improving the conditions of everyday life and for attention to be paid to issues of power, money, and resources at the global and national levels. It put a strong case for the importance of health equity in all policies, arguing that health equity impact assessment 'must happen as a matter of course' (CSDH, 2008: 190), and noting that evidence suggests that the benefits of health equity impact assessment far exceeds the costs. In 2009 the World Health Assembly in its resolution WHA62.14 on reducing health inequities through action on social determinants of health urged the international community, WHO, and its member states, as well as other relevant actors, to take various actions towards reducing health inequities. This resolution was followed up by the World Conference on Social Determinants of Health, held in Rio de Janeiro in October 2001. The background paper for this conference presented HiAP as a mechanism to encourage government action on the social determinants of health (WHO, 2011).

We see HiAP as one expression of the Ottawa Charter's healthy public policy, which has been implemented in many different settings dealing with many different policy issues including tobacco use, road safety, alcohol and other drug control, and healthy food supply. In Chapter 2, de Leeuw and Breton provide a fuller discussion of healthy public policy. Literature on the implementation of HiAP is in its infancy. Shankardass et al. (2011) provide a realist review, which details 16 countries in which there is evidence of some HiAP activity. Our rapid assessment of the related literature only found six instances where any theory had been applied to HiAP. Details are provided in Box 10.1.

Genesis of HiAP in South Australia

In Australia from the 1970s there were movements, government reports, and research, which put the case for the social determinants of health. The Aboriginal Community Controlled Health Movement (Foley, 1982; Hunter, 1999), the women's health movement (Broom, 1991), and the community health movement (Baum et al., 1992) all argued strongly for a social perspective in health from the 1970s, and created an alternative voice to the medical model of health and behavioural forms of health promotion. The most striking example of government documents putting forward a social determinants of health perspective was the South Australian Social Health Strategy (South Australian Health Commission, 1988). This strategy argued for health to be a consideration in all policy areas. At the same time, the South Australian Labor Government established a Human Service Sub-Committee of Cabinet, which gave rise to a number of cross-department initiatives. A number of the policy actors who are active in the South Australian HiAP initiative worked in the health system at the time of both of these innovations, and so cut their practice and/or policy teeth at a time these strategies were current.

We also note the strong history of social innovation in South Australia established in the 19th century and still evident. Adelaide Thinker in Residence and Head of the UK Young Foundation, Geoff Mulgan, notes: 'Social innovation remains an enduring feature of South Australian society' (Mulgan, 2008: 13). Examples of innovation in the past decade have been the establishment of a social inclusion unit and board (see Baum, Newman et al., 2010) and a Thinker in Residence scheme, which included Ilona Kickbusch, whose recommendations included adoption of an HiAP approach. Collectively, these international, national, and state developments created a history of ideas that all are likely to have made some impact on the readiness of South Australia to adopt the HiAP idea.

Establishing HiAP on the political and policy agenda

The list of ideas that make it to the policy agenda is limited, and of those that do make it, many fail to maintain support and are eventually discarded. Drawing on Kingdon's work and that of other policy analysts we consider the conditions and forces acting on the social determinants of health as a public issue and HiAP as a policy response. Kingdon's framework has been applied in a range of policy domains including in relation to HiAP (e.g. Sihto et al., 2006; Ollila, 2011; Mannheimer et al., 2007).

Box 10.1 Using theory to explain HiAP: a brief global review

Finland

Ollila (2011) uses an adaption of the Kingdon model to analyse policy and make suggestions about what is needed to strengthen the HiAP approach. She discusses the need to identify and create windows of opportunity for HiAP by promoting health issues on policy agendas, proposing solutions, and creating professional and public constituencies that support HiAP.

Sweden

Mannheimer et al. (2007) describe an analysis of HiAP's progress in Sweden, which used the Kingdon framework to assess progress. The analysis of the three streams of influence showed that political support for HiAP was not strong at the national level, and that this had impeded progress with the implementation of HiAP. Locally and nationally specific plans for implementation of HiAP were weak, which also impeded effective implementation.

The Netherlands

Steenbakkers et al. (2012) describe a coaching programme provided by the regional public health agency for actors in municipal goverments charged with implementing HiAP relating to obesity. They found that within municipalities HiAP proposals are not given a high priority, either at the strategic or tactical levels. The coaching was driven by a systems understanding that considered vertical and horizontal collaboration across the embedded systems domains of strategic, tactical, and operational. The authors argue that in order to create intersectoral collaboration, the usual communication in a vertical, hierarchical direction needs to be supplemented with communication horizontally between these different policy domains. Policy capacity relates to available human resources in terms of time, competence, and capability—i.e. the ability to adapt to change, to generate new knowledge, and continuously to improve performance with colleagues in other policy domains. At the operational level knowledge, attitudes, perceived social and outcome expectations, and self-efficacy were seen to be important personal determinants of both judging one's own policy frame of reference and of entering another policy domain.

Wales

Warner and Gould (2009) examine the detailed processes of how organizations need to work in order for the interorganizational working at the heart of HiAP to be effective. They maintain that 'multisectoral arrangements are inherently messy and that

(Continued)

Box 10.1 (Continued)

networked activity across organizations needs governance' (Warner and Gould, 2009: 147). They draw on network and organizational culture theory to examine the structural, procedural, financial, professional, and status and legitimacy barriers to organizational integration. They also use network theory to consider the formation and emergence, structure, and governance of networks. They provide a detailed assessment of the skills needed for 'boundary spanning' and virtual coordination of networks. They propose the utility of 'neutral white space' as a means of 'creative network activity'. These theoretical ideas are applied to a Welsh case study of HiAP.

EU as a whole

Koivusalo (2010) provides a commentary on the progress in the EU towards achieving HiAP. The paper provides a critical account of what the author sees as a lack of action. She concludes: 'A substantial amount of knowledge and strategies in HiAP are based on mutual, joint and cooperative action, yet perhaps we might need to think about how strategies move with reluctant partners and conflicting interests and how to preserve policy space for health' (Koivusalo, 2010: 502).

Fictional nation

Use the theory of salutogenesis and a Quality of Life model to envision what public policy would look like it if it were driven by this theory, using a constructed country 'Nation' as a case study.

Gaining the attention of policy-makers

Gaining attention is a key element in agenda-setting theories. The problem stream in Kingdon's framework refers to how problems come to the attention of policy-makers and how they are responded to. Conditions or issues only become 'problems' when there is a will to change the condition (Kingdon, 2011). Green-Pedersen and Wilkersen (2006) note that some issues possess agenda-setting attributes that mean they gain the attention of policy-makers. Health care issues have many agenda-setting attributes, resulting in considerable political attention with a focus on finding solutions rather than debating the problem. On the other hand, social determinants of health and health inequities have been described as sometimes invisible to policy-makers (Dahlgren and Whitehead, 2006). Exworthy (2008: 321) suggests that their complexity as 'multi-faceted phenomena with multiple causes' has frustrated their elevation onto political agendas. So while 'health' in terms of disease and health care has high visibility and is high on governmental agendas (Kingdon, 2011), the determinants of health largely remain as 'conditions' rather than 'problems' gaining serious policy attention.

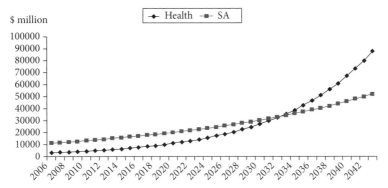

Figure 10.1 South Australia health spending.

Reproduced from Health in All Policies Unit, *The South Australian Approach to Health in All Policies: Background and Practical Guide: Version 2*, Government of South Australia, p.9, Copyright © Department of Health, Government of South Australia, 2011, with permission from the Department of Health and Ageing, Government of South Australia, Copyright © 2013. Data from Department of the Premier and Cabinet, South Australia.

This means that the increasing volume of research on social determinants of health and health inequities will not necessarily constitute identification of a problem. Kingdon notes that problems are often not self-evident and require a 'little push' to attract attention. A focusing event may provide the push, and this may come in the guise of a 'powerful symbol that catches on' (Kingdon, 2011: 95). Hajer (1995) draws attention to the use of storylines in creating opportunities for change. In South Australia the 'health budget crisis' has emerged as such a key storyline. The South Australian HiAP unit uses data developed by the state's Treasury that shows that on current trends health care spending will account for the whole of the state's budget by 2030 (Figure 10.1). This storyline has been oft repeated by health bureaucrats in intersectoral fora. The spectre of health budget blow-out has been picked up and exploited by policy entrepreneurs to reframe the health budget and as a means of containing it as a storyline to attract the attention of other sectors. Since this information was first reported the threat of escalating health budgets has only increased, and so it remains a strong policy driver for HiAP. It forms the main justification for SA Health investing in HiAP: to control, slow down, and even arrest the growing health sector budget. Other sectors appear to accept the argument that an investment in HiAP is a mechanism to reduce health care spending in the future.

Another narrative employed in promoting an HiAP approach is that of population health underpinning productivity and economic development. This case was argued in the report of the Commission on Macroeconomics and Health: 'Although health is widely understood to be both a central goal and an important outcome of development, the importance of investing in health to promote economic development and poverty reduction has been much less appreciated' (2001: vii). The positive contribution of health was also a strong theme in Kickbusch's Thinker in Residence report: 'Health is a productive force in the economy. It is a determinant of growth and productivity, wealth and quality of life' (Kickbusch, 2008: 15).

Hajer notes that a 'weak' policy field, in this case the social determinants of health, can gain traction by linking its discourse to that of a 'strong' field such as economic development. This convergence of discourses can be seen in this quotation from a bureaucrat within the South Australian Economic Development Agency:

> An economic development agency can no longer just think about economic outcomes....It's true now that over the last 5 or 10 years that the environmental, social and economic issues have really converged...we can't achieve our economic outcomes without addressing the other two.
>
> (1995: 108)

Despite such supportive statements there was a level of scepticism among policy actors from both within health and across government about the HiAP concept. However, there was also a preparedness 'to give it a try', as other strategies were not seen to be succeeding.

Linking HiAP to the potential reduction of health care costs and to economic development was important in opening a window of opportunity that could then be exploited by policy entrepreneurs, as we see below.

Advancing HiAP as a policy proposal

The policy stream accounts for the ways in which policy proposals are generated and circulated, adopted and discarded. As discussed earlier, intersectoral action for health has a long history and South Australia has at times figured at the forefront of calls for the development of healthy public policy. New ideas do not suddenly appear out of nowhere: they can be usefully considered as products of evolution where various old elements are recombined in some new way (Kingdon, 2011). HiAP can be considered a recombination of elements present in various ways in earlier iterations of intersectoral action and healthy public policy proposals. Various policy entrepreneurs from inside and outside the policy community have continued to introduce and push such proposals—a process of 'softening up' the policy community. This preliminary work is important in ensuring that any proposal gains serious consideration when an opportunity for change does occur. The social determinants of health and HiAP gained increased visibility in South Australia through the appointment of Fran Baum (Flinders University) to the CSDH. Other advocates were in key positions within the public health and health promotion areas of DHA, and pursued opportunities to advocate and implement intersectoral action for health where possible.

An opportunity to promote the social determinants of health and HiAP to the government agenda arose when Professor Ilona Kickbusch was appointed as Adelaide Thinker in Residence. The Adelaide Thinkers in Residence programme draws international experts to the state, bringing new ideas and translating them into practical solutions to improve the lives of the people who live here. These residencies have looked at subjects including health, education, water, technology, climate change, transport, design, and road safety. The programme sets out to generate new thinking; inspire momentum; provoke change; and activate results for the people of South Australia. The Thinkers in Residence programme was set up in 2003 and was a personal initiative of the then Premier. The strong support of the Premier for the programme gave the work and recommendations of Thinkers, including those of Ilona Kickbusch regarding HiAP, considerable status and momentum. There have been 22 residencies to date; Professor Kickbusch's was the 13th, in 2007. Her appointment was a product of the efforts of academic and bureaucratic policy entrepreneurs to advance the case for healthy public policy. This position provided her with a 'claim to a hearing' and access to high-level decision-makers in the political and policy streams—the Premier, Cabinet, Health Department and other bureaucrats.

The Kickbusch residency also brought together partner agencies—local governments, universities, the Department of the Premier and Cabinet (DPC), the Department of Health, the Department of Education and Children's Services, workers' compensation and road safety and injury agencies, regional health services, and a Healthy City initiative. This mustered existing advocates of intersectoral action and exposed others to its possibilities. Overlapping with the Kickbusch residency was that of Dr Fraser Mustard, whose residency focused on investing in the early years of life. The discourse associated with Dr Mustard's residency reinforced the call for integrated, whole-of-government responses.

HiAP as a policy proposal faces particular challenges because it is seeking to capture the attention and endorsement of the whole of government rather than a single policy community. In South Australia the proposal to implement an HiAP approach used an existing overarching government policy framework—South Australia's Strategic Plan (SASP)—to argue its relevance across government (Government of South Australia, 2011). The SASP sets out a vision for South Australia and a set of targets, many of which require intersectoral action to be achieved. It represented a platform for health advocates to link population health issues with the business of sectors not usually related to health (Tryens, 2008). Individual chief executives of government departments are held directly accountable to the Premier for the achievement of the targets allocated to their department, which creates a very significant incentive for them to be involved in HiAP. Having received in-principle support, however, there was still a need to establish the feasibility of an HiAP approach in terms of the political stream and this is discussed in the section below.

The political stream

The political stream exists largely independently of the problem and policy streams; it is where political and administrative changes, portfolio reshuffles, bureaucratic staff turnover, lobbying, and public opinion can influence which issues make it to the political agenda (Kingdon, 2011). In South Australia the incumbent Labor administration is in its third four-year term of government, which has provided a stable and receptive political climate for adoption of an HiAP approach. The HiAP initiative has survived a change of Premier and appears to have bipartisan support, with the Shadow Minister for Health promoting the need for policy-makers to incorporate considerations of health into their policies (South Australian House of Assembly, 2010).

Kingdon's original work is based on research at the national level in the US. Work undertaken by Liu et al. suggests that building consensus and coalitions assumes greater importance in the political stream at a more local level: they describe consensus building as 'a process to mobilize similar interests and settle conflicts that involve multiple parties' (2010: 83). The following description of the early implementation of the HiAP approach in South Australia outlines a deliberate strategy of consensus building using the SASP as a framework of mutual interest and the adoption of a win-win approach to HiAP work.

In this section we have used Kingdon's framework to examine how and why HiAP as a policy proposal made its way onto the government agenda. The next section details how the HiAP moves from the policy agenda into operation.

Implementation of HiAP

After gaining in-principle government support for the adoption of an HiAP approach, there remained the challenge of translating the policy intention into practice. We use Kaluzny and Hernandez's (1988) framework of the four stages in the adoption of change (awareness, adoption, implementation, and institutionalization). We also consider each stage through the lens of complex systems thinking as outlined in the earlier sections and in Tables 10.1 and 10.2. In this section we examine the implementation of HiAP from its very early days to March 2012.

Awareness

Gaining the attention of policy-makers regarding HiAP built on significant advocacy and developmental work over a prolonged period. Real momentum was gained through Professor Kickbusch's term as Thinker in Residence. With the endorsement of the heads of DHA and DPC, staff within these departments were able to explore mechanisms to develop an HiAP approach in South Australia. This required key actors in DHA and DPC to accept that health is more than the absence of disease, results from complex interactions in a range of different systems, and is created primarily outside the health sector; and thus, that addressing the social determinants of health requires action on the part of sectors that traditionally do not see health as part of their remit. It required them to appreciate the nature of complex systems and develop the ability to think constructively about how to bring about change in those systems—systems thinking as displayed in Table 10.2. Even within the health sector, action on the social determinants of health remains a largely peripheral concern, and awareness cannot be taken for granted. Practically, this means that HiAP advocates need to engage with, and convince, a wide range of policy actors across sectors with differing organizational cultures, languages, and priorities. It requires the development of explicit statements about the connections between the public policy area of interest, the social determinants of health, and health impact, as policy actors outside of health often find it difficult to see the linkages between their policy area and health and well-being. Our study of the HiAP processes indicates that awareness is not something that happens prior to other stages of change in a linear manner; rather, awareness needs to be built continually as new actors enter the stage and new policy areas are considered. This conception of awareness as part of the dynamic and loop thinking typical of systems thinking is an important element of implementation.

Adoption

The task of developing effective mechanisms for policy integration—the incorporation of health considerations into policies of other sectors—faces significant challenges. Ross and Dovers observe that 'any policy integration task "cuts against the grain" of the specialized hierarchical public administrative system' (2008: 246). Add this to the fact that social determinants of health do not have high political visibility and it is evident that moving to the stage of having HiAP adopted as a programme of a state government across a complex system required considerable skills from the public servants seeking to bring about the change. Each of these challenges needed to be negotiated in the implementation of HiAP.

The most vital factors were the endorsement from the Premier and Health Minister and the championing of HiAP by DPC. SA Health and DPC worked in collaboration to develop strategies, processes, and structures that were robust enough to be adapted to the changing and dynamic world of policy. The adoption required considerable relational work and 'forest thinking' to engage and mobilize other stakeholders. Gaining commitment from senior decision-makers in other sectors to trial the process was a critical step. The HiAP team found it necessary to engage in dynamic processes that required them to raise awareness while developing and fine-tuning a process robust enough to work in the complexity required of policy analysis and change across government departments. Assessment of the ways in which the HiAP team worked over this period shows their systems thinking abilities: a sophisticated understanding of the machinery of government, existing policies and structures, and points of influence (forest thinking); engagement of policy actors with significant influence across government (system-as-cause); and an iterative, reflexive approach to developing relationships and strategies to progress intersectoral work (loop thinking). They were well aware of the policy networks and appeared able to 'work' these networks for the advantage of HiAP in the way de Leeuw et al. (see Chapter 8 in this volume) suggest is necessary for local intersectoral policy development.

In 2007 three interconnected strategies were implemented (see Williams et al., 2008):

1. a desk-top application of a 'health lens' to a sample of SASP targets;

2. the development of case studies on selected SASP targets engaging policy actors from across government; and

3. the coordination of an HiAP state conference.

Linking the HiAP approach to the SASP provided an important entry point to the engagement of other sectors. While accountability is tied to a particular department, many of the targets require the involvement of multiple sectors to achieve the best outcome. To demonstrate the applicability of an HiAP approach to the SASP, DPC undertook a desk-top analysis of the plan, examining the connections between a sample of targets and their health impacts. For example, for a SASP target aimed at increasing the proportion of the population with access to digital technology, the desk-top analysis assessed the impact on health and well-being of having or not having digital access. This work identified both that people from disadvantaged backgrounds had less access to digital technology and that without public policy that aimed to overcome the disadvantage these inequities were likely to persist and possibly grow.

The notion of a 'health lens' was developed as the analysis focused on a policy or programme in terms of its positive and negative health impacts. Figure 10.2 shows the health lens analysis (HLA) process, which has much in common with health impact assessments and certainly demonstrates such elements, as outlined in the Gothenburg Consensus (WHO, 1999). We note that the definition of health impact assessments is not straightforward, and in practice they take many different forms (Harris-Roxas and Harris, 2011). One characteristic of the HiAP work in South Australia has been proactive engagement with other sectors even prior to a particular policy proposal or policy change being put forward. In some HLAs the process began essentially with conversations about possible points of overlap between the concerns of health and the core

South Australia's Health in All Policies (HiAP) Model

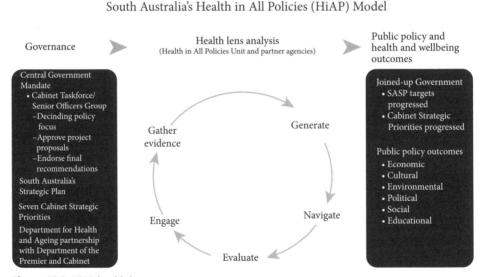

Figure 10.2 HiAP health lens process.

Reproduced from Health in All Policies Unit, Copyright © Department of Health, Government of South Australia, 2013, with permission from the Department of Health and Ageing, Government of South Australia, Copyright © 2013.

business of the other sector. The starting point was identification of an issue of policy importance rather than a specific proposal. This initial and sometimes lengthy dialogue identified an area of focus and stimulated policy action. HLAs are essentially a within-government method forming part of the policy-making process.

Building on the health lens work, HiAP project staff organized workshops involving stakeholders from a range of government departments to examine seven SASP targets (see Williams et al., 2008). Workshops provided input from population health experts, and were informed by a discussion paper that examined interactions between the particular policy area and health. Thinking about health in terms of determinants rather than disease and care challenged many participants, and discussion in the workshops frequently returned to individual health and health care services. This suggests that the salutogenic view of health, which is at the heart of HiAP, is not widely understood. The workshops sought to identify win-win solutions, where both improved health outcomes and progress towards the SASP target relevant to non-health departments could be achieved. This process represented the beginning of the HLA as an interactive process rather than a desk-top exercise.

The lessons from the desk-top analysis and the workshops were brought together at a state HiAP conference co-convened by DHA and DPC. The conference promoted a broad understanding of health and its determinants, and explored interactions and synergies between health, the economy, and the achievement of SASP targets. Over 150 senior public servants participated. The conference identified future opportunities for action and agreed on a set of ten HiAP principles, which would underpin action in South Australia (see Box 10.2). These principles reflect an understanding that contemporary policy is implemented in a very complex environment and, again, demonstrate systems thinking.

These activities provided opportunities for stakeholders from other sectors to be involved in the developmental phase of HiAP in South Australia. Following the 2007 conference policy actors from three government departments indicated their interest in HiAP, leading to the first three health lens projects. These receptive policy actors and their willingness to innovate allowed HiAP to establish proof of concept. Based on these early successes, policy actors from other government departments were invited to apply a health lens to their SASP targets and public policies. This period saw significant investment in relationship building with key stakeholders from a range of government departments and the HiAP unit.

Implementation: structures and processes

The developmental processes resulted in a South Australian HiAP model (see Figure 10.3), which sees the HLA forming one cornerstone of the HiAP approach in South Australia. A small HiAP unit was established within SA Health, with a mandate to drive the adoption of HiAP across government. Centralized governance structures, the other cornerstone of the approach, have been developed and provide cross-sectoral oversight of both HiAP and SASP. Until early 2012 this occurred through the Executive

Box 10.2 South Australian HiAP principles

A HiAP approach reflects health as a shared goal of all government. In particular it:

1. Recognises the value of health for the wellbeing of all citizens and for the over-all social and economic development of South Australia—health is a human right, a vital resource for everyday life and a key factor of sustainability.

2. Recognises that health is an outcome of a wide range of factors—such as changes to the natural and built environments and to social and work environments—many of which lie outside the activities of the health sector and require a shared responsibility and an integrated and sustained policy response across Government.

3. Acknowledges that all Government policies can have positive or negative impacts on the determinants of health and such impacts are reflected both in the health status of the South Australian population today and in the health prospects of future generations.

4. Recognises that the impacts of health determinants are not equally distributed among population groups in South Australia and aims at closing the health gap, in particular for the Aboriginal peoples.

5. Recognises that health is central to achieving the objectives of the South Australian Strategic Plan (SASP)—it requires both the identification of potential health impacts and the recognition that good health can contribute to achieving SASP targets.

6. Acknowledges that efforts to improve the health of all South Australians will require sustainable mechanisms that support Government agencies to work collaboratively to develop integrated solutions to both current and future policy challenges.

7. Acknowledges that many of the most pressing health problems of the population require long-term policy and budgetary commitment as well as innovative budgetary approaches.

8. Recognises that indicators of success will be equally long-term and that regular monitoring and intermediate measures of progress will need to be established and reported back to South Australian citizens.

9. Recognises the need to regularly consult with citizens to link policy changes with wider social and cultural changes around health and wellbeing.

10. Recognises the potential of partnerships for policy implementation between Government levels, science and academia, business, professional organisations and non-governmental organisations to bring about sustained change.

Health in All Policies Horizontal and Vertical Governance

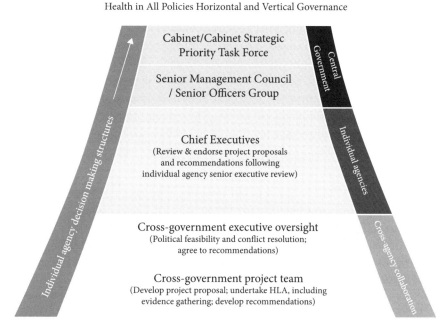

Figure 10.3 South Australian HiAP governance overview.
Reproduced from Health in All Policies Unit, Copyright © Department of Health, Government of South Australia, 2013, with permission from the Department of Health and Ageing, Government of South Australia, Copyright © 2013.

Sub-Committee of Cabinet—known locally as ExComm—which provides a mandate for the application of HiAP to SASP and the work of non-health agencies. This mandate is coordinated by the Cabinet Office in the DPC. Obtaining central government leadership of the HiAP process has been an essential step. It has provided a clear statement of commitment that HiAP will be supported by the whole government, not just the health sector, and has given other sectors the impetus to 'engage' in HiAP.

A new Premier took office in late 2011 and introduced seven Cabinet Strategic Priorities linked to the SASP targets. Seven sub-committees of cabinet (supported by senior officers' groups) have been established to oversee the implementation of the priorities across government including HiAP. When the HiAP health lens does not directly relate to one of the seven Cabinet Strategic Priorities, oversight is provided by senior management council and finally cabinet itself. It is significant that, despite key political and administrative leadership changes, the demise of the ExComm and the introduction of new governance arrangements, HiAP has maintained its relevance and acceptance as a way of working across government to obtain improved public policy and health outcomes. The adaptation of HiAP core staff to their new bureaucratic environment is another example of their skills in systems thinking.

Implementation: health lens initiatives

The early stages of implementing HiAP required considerable awareness-raising and the establishment of processes to engage the non-health sectors by showing the relevance of HiAP to their own agendas and to the over-riding goals of the SASP. Fourteen health lens projects were set up between 2007 and early 2012: these have been completed or are ongoing under the HiAP banner (see Box 10.3). They have covered a variety of topics and involved many state government departments. The outcomes of the health lens projects have not been systematically evaluated thus far but will be the subject of a 5-year evaluation starting in mid-2012.

Institutionalization

The final step from organizational change theory is institutionalization of change. This step is obviously crucial. Kingdon (2011) points out that policy windows do not stay open forever, and some may close rapidly. This means that the innovations resulting from the opening of policy windows have to be embedded as routine governance processes in order to survive further change in the system. Governance has been defined as 'sustaining coordination and coherence among a wide variety of actors with different purposes and objectives' (Pierre, 2000: 3–4). Obviously, one of the most important factors in determining the sustainability of HiAP will be if it is seen to have been successful as a governance mechanism for achieving societal goals. In the case of South Australia this translates to achieving the SASP targets and advancing the Cabinet Strategic Priorities. We have assessed the implementation of HiAP in its first years of operation against steps for successful implementation of intersectional action developed by the Public Health Agency of Canada (2007) and WHO (2011), and added two of our own—skills in systems thinking and use of developmental and outcome evaluation. Table 10.3 lists the

---

Box 10.3 South Australian health lens projects in progress as of April 2012

Water Sustainability HLA focused on the potential health impacts associated with increasing use of alternative water sources—rainwater, stormwater, and greywater.

Regional Migrant Settlement HLA examined the interplay between the social, economic, and health factors impacting on migrant settlement in three regional areas of South Australia.

Digital Technology HLA supported increased use of digital technology among low socioeconomic status groups in ways that promote health.

Transit-Oriented Development HLA explored the complex links between health and planning, with a particular focus on the potential health impacts (both positive

(Continued)

Box 10.3 (Continued)

and negative) of more condensed, walkable, sustainable urban development. The project resulted in the 'Healthy TOD Principles', designed to guide policy-makers and planners.

Healthy Weight Desk-top Analysis examined opportunities to strengthen healthy weight action by facilitating cross-government collaboration between DHA and other government departments.

Castle Plaza Transit-Oriented Development, City of Marion aimed to improve how urban environments support health and well-being at the Castle Plaza site and to test the applicability of the 'Healthy TOD Principles' as a guide in a local government development assessment process.

International Students Health and Well-being HLA identified the health and well-being needs of international students, the structures and services available to address these needs, and the barriers to access and opportunities to improve student information and support.

Active Transport undertook a targeted policy review to strengthen economic arguments for investment in cycling and walking infrastructure.

***Aboriginal Road Safety HLA** identified ways of increasing Aboriginal healthy life expectancy by improving road safety through increasing safe mobility options. It examined the impact of the drivers' licensing system and court diversionary programmes on Aboriginal peoples' ability to obtain and retain their drivers' licences.

***Parental Engagement in Children's Literacy HLA** aimed to raise parental engagement with literacy to improve literacy outcomes for children in the early years of schooling, and ultimately improve their health.

***Healthy Sustainable Regional Communities HLA** identified mechanisms and strategies to enable communities in the Upper Spencer Gulf Region of South Australia to capitalize on emerging regional development opportunities in the mining sector and the rollout of the National Broadband Network, leading to improved health, sustainability and economic positioning of these communities.

***Promoting active ageing through supporting workforce participation HLA** used desk-top analysis to consider the determinants of active ageing, with a particular focus on assisting older people in rural South Australia to remain in the workforce.

***Learning or earning HLA** aimed to improve the successful transition of young people aged 15–24 years of age from education to employment and re-engage young people in learning or earning.

***The South Australian Cycling Strategy HLA** aimed to facilitate engagement and cross-government ownership through applying an HiAP approach.

* Indicates that those health lens projects are still active as of November 2012.

Source: Data from Health Lens Analysis, Government of Southern Australia, available from: <http://www.sahealth.sa.gov.au/wps/wcm/connect/public+content/sa+health+internet/health+reform/health+in+all+policies/health+lens+analysis>.

Table 10.3 Measuring South Australia's HiAP against steps for successful implementation of intersectoral action

Steps	South Australian HiAP performance
FRAMEWORKS	
Create a policy framework and an approach to health that are conducive to intersectoral action	The SASP provided this frameworkThe new Public Health Act (2011) gives a mandate for continued implementation of HiAP
Develop practical models, tools, and mechanisms to support the implementation of intersectoral action	The health lens has been developed
Ensure appropriate horizontal linking across sectors as well as vertical linking of levels within sectors	The Executive Sub-Committee of Cabinet used as mechanism to link across sectors
Ensure systems thinking drives the initiative and actors have relevant skills	Evidence that the key actors in HiAP's implementation are able to think dynamically, taking into account a whole-system perspective that appreciates the non-linear nature of policy and systems dynamics
Undertake a developmental and outcomes evaluation of the intersectoral action	An evaluation partnership has been developed with HiAP and researchers at Flinders University and had led to a successful 5-year National Health and Medical Research Council grant application
BUILDING AND MAINTAINING SUPPORT	
Ensure political support, build on positive factors in the policy environment	Political support from the South Australian Premier was won and the initiative was led from DPCThe Thinkers in Residence programme helped to open the policy window
Emphasize shared values, interests, and objectives among partners and potential partners	HiAP Principles were established (see 1) The health lens process was explicitly based on a win-win strategy
Invest in the alliance-building process by working towards consensus at the planning stage	Achieving consensus is one of the key features of the health lens process
Focus on concrete objectives and visible results	The aim of the HLA is to identify areas in which results can be gained
ENGAGING PEOPLE	
Ensure that leadership, accountability, and rewards are shared among partners	Leadership is shared between SA Health and DPC. Actors from other sectors are encouraged to report on the HLAs and credit is shared between partners
Build stable teams of people who work well together, with appropriate support systems	An HiAP unit has been established in SA Health

(Continued)

Table 10.3 (Continued)

Steps	South Australian HiAP performance
Ensure public participation: educate the public and raise awareness about health determinants and intersectoral action	More development is needed in this area

Adapted with permission from World Health Organization, *Closing the Gap: Policy into Practice on Social Determinants of Health—Discussion Paper*, World Health Organization, p. 15, Copyright © World Health Organization 2011 and WHO and Government of South Australia, *Adelaide Statement on Health in All Policies: Moving Towards a Shared Governance for Health and Well-being*, World Health Organization and Government of South Australia, Copyright © World Health Organization 2010.

steps and a brief summary of our assessment of HiAP's performance against them. We have grouped the steps in to three—frameworks, building and maintaining support, and engaging people—and discuss each below. In each case we also discuss some of the difficulties and challenges HiAP has faced in South Australia.

Frameworks

A crucial framework for HiAP has been the SASP, which provides an overarching scaffold. Evaluation of individual HLAs has reinforced the importance of governance structures as proof of high-level support for the process, providing clear decision-making pathways and giving weight and impetus to recommendations emerging from the projects.

Clear governance structures and commitment to the process are critical when conflict arises. The transit-oriented development HLA encountered difficulties when the evidence to inform the process was contested. This HLA took place in a politically charged environment, with considerable media focus on the government's commitment to transit-oriented development and a controversy over a related land deal in the midst of an election campaign.

Much debate arose over the use of the evidence to inform design criteria for healthy transit-oriented developments. SA Health staff led the evidence-gathering process. The design principles of various transit-oriented developments can vary, and as much of the literature came from overseas its applicability to Australia was contested. The partners from the planning, development, and transport sectors considered that the evidence gathered by their health colleagues overstated the associated risks and did not adequately describe their health-promoting potential, as documented in the HLA process evaluation and shown by this quotation from the report:

> it came down to very much a clash of professional cultures. The methodology—it made me realise—it dawned on me that they are essentially using—they were using a risk analysis approach…because it was written by a non-planner or a non-designer, it didn't really get to the right level of understanding.
>
> (Lawless and Hurley, 2010)

Such debates over the use of evidence are not unusual in public health decision-making, as Petticrew and Roberts record: 'The research findings to help answer the question may well exist, but locating that research, assessing its evidential "weight" and relevance, and incorporating it with other existing information is often difficult' (2003: 527). Although there was a pause in the project while contested issues were resolved, commitment remained high. The HiAP team worked to maintain relationships with all stakeholders, problem-solve and engage senior levels of the participating sectors in resolving the impasse. Involvement of agency directors was seen as a positive step in resolving the direction the project would take, particularly given the political context.

We have noted that salutogenic thinking about health does not come easily and many policy actors see 'health' as being about health care. For example, links between digital technology and health and well-being and health equity were difficult for that HLA project group to detail, but following commissioned research on digital technology and equity (Golder et al., 2010) the links were made explicit and the project group accepted the new evidence. It is a little more difficult to build health equity into HiAP. Equity has not always been explicit in the health lens thinking, although it does feature in most of the 14 HLAs conducted to date. Some of the exercises have put equity to the forefront— for example, the broadband exercise—but the HiAP staff report that doing so remains a challenge because people in other sectors do not automatically think about the health equity implications of their work. Equity can be a 'slippery' concept and its meaning contested, as this quotation from a participant in the evaluation of the transit-oriented development HLA illustrates:

> When you talk about putting on an equity lens, first SA Health has to explain the problem. What is the problem?…if the problem is around long commuting times, access to job and access to services, the planning solution is to make sure there's access to services on the outer, not to try and provide million dollar homes for—houses that cost a million dollars to build in Bowden. So, I think the stuff that we build when you can touch and see it is much easier to explain to people. Equity—it needs more explaining.
>
> (Lawless and Hurley, 2010)

It remains a task for future health lens exercises to incorporate health equity more centrally.

Studying the implementation of HiAP has raised the question of where HiAP begins and ends. The traditional roles of the public health sector in addressing areas such as health protection through regulation and legislation remain important. A new Public Health Act was approved by the South Australian Parliament in June 2011. The Act was based on major review of the previous Public and Environmental Health Act, and represents a significant change to legislation in order to respond to 21st century health needs. It also provides an ideal framework for HiAP.

While the South Australian HiAP model details the health lens process, many initiatives could be positioned under the HiAP banner, where it is considered 'effective and systematic action for the improvement of population health, using genuinely all available measures in all policy fields' (Ståhl et al., 2006: xvi). Two examples demonstrate this point. The HiAP unit and the Health Promotion Branch of SA Health have undertaken a desk-top analysis that considers the core business and policy directions of 44 state government departments and agencies in terms of actions that contribute to or detract from obesity (the reduction of which features in the SASP). The findings have been used to develop cross-government policy commitments that address the factors driving obesity.

In a similar vein, 'Health in Planning' is a project funded by the South Australia Health Promotion Branch, which aims to embed health considerations in the policy, planning, and practices of the Department of Planning and Local Government. SA Health has funded a full-time position within this Department, enabling substantial input to the 30-Year Plan for Greater Adelaide—the document that will guide planning and development in Adelaide and shape urban form and land use. Embedding health considerations into the 30-year plan will lead to cascading effects as local policy development and implementation plans must address the broader goals of the overarching plan. The project also intersected with the HLA on transit-oriented development and played an important role in advocating targets for affordable housing in developments—an important equity outcome.

The role of the mainstream health sector in HiAP

Our early evaluation also raises issues about the role of the mainstream health sector in HiAP. The South Australian HiAP initiative has focused its efforts on forging links with sectors outside health, but this raises the question of how HiAP can be made relevant more broadly within the health sector. Primary health care services have had a mandate to undertake intersectoral work since the days of the WHO Alma-Ata Declaration (International Conference on Primary Health Care, 1978). In South Australia the community health sector has conducted some innovative cross-sectoral work over the last 25 years (see Baum, 1995). In the past five years this work appears to have been less evident, with a focus on primary health care and behavioural chronic disease prevention becoming more evident. HiAP could assist in creating a policy window for primary health care services to re-engage in cross-sectoral work that aims to tackle the social determinants of chronic disease. In recognition of this, an initiative started in early 2102 between the HiAP unit and the country's health services will build the capacity of the primary health care service providers to re-engage with other sectors, using a 'learning by doing' approach.

Building and maintaining support

Interviews with key stakeholders in the early days of the initiative revealed that high-level support was seen as critical to the success of the initiative. Political support from the South Australian Premier was won and the initiative led from DPC. The Thinkers in Residence programme helped open the policy window. The continued leadership, advocacy, and energy of the HiAP unit maintain the visibility and momentum of the initiative as well. Our analysis suggests that the international profile of the work—for instance, the WHO background paper for the World Conference on Social Determinants of Health, which features the South Australian work and includes a quotation from the then

Premier Mike Rann (WHO, 2011: 15)—will assist this process. Partner agencies and sectors have been encouraged to present their projects at conferences and intersectoral for a, and 'champions' for the process are emerging from outside the health sector.

Given the positioning of the HLA as a win-win or cooperation strategy, this is particularly important in order for the health sector to continue its role in shaping public policy where common ground is less easily found. Ollila (2011) suggests that the cooperation strategy may need to remain separate from areas of conflict in order to protect the underpinning cooperation. The HLA does just that through its pragmatic scoping out of issues that are not politically feasible to address, or that would fail to gain buy-in from other sectors. One example was around the issue of water security, where the state government had committed to building a desalination plant at the height of the drought. There was some vocal community opposition to this plant on ecological grounds, and consequently the water security HLA excluded consideration of the desirability or otherwise of the plant on the grounds that the political decision had been made. It is clear, however, that action to achieve improved health and increased health equity may sometimes be at odds with the core concerns of other sectors. One example is that while the State has a commitment to population growth, an HLA might suggest this policy has adverse health implications because of the impact of population growth on sustainability. A further example is that a significant proportion of South Australia's revenue is derived from poker machines, but an HLA of poker machines would highlight the increase in problem gambling and its health impact, especially on low-income communities. In such cases a cooperation strategy is unlikely to bring about intersectoral action for health. Dealing with such situations remains a challenge for HiAP.

The South Australian HiAP from the start has engaged outside evaluation from Flinders University. This has provided valuable feedback on the process of implementation. This evaluation partnership has resulted in a successful application to the Australian National Health and Medical Research Council for a 5-year grant to conduct a more formal evaluation, which will happen from mid-2012 to 2016. Our initial analysis has shown that HiAP in South Australia has been a high-profile project relying on strong political support, which has given it legitimacy. This makes its evaluation particularly challenging. Some early work we have conducted examining the different requirements of policy-makers and researchers has confirmed the literature (Denis and Lomas, 2003; Mitton et al., 2007), which highlights the differences in perspectives. Policy-makers have an obvious stake in seeing their policy 'babies' favourably evaluated and in protecting their political leaders. These considerations have to be weighed against the importance of working on the basis of the evidence that evaluative research can produce. Researchers, on the other hand, want to produce insightful evaluations that contain appropriate critiques and can make a valuable contribution to the peer-reviewed literature.

Engaging people

The discussion above shows that both political and policy actors have been engaged in HiAP. The catalyst unit in SA Health has paid careful attention to engaging those in other sectors, and the support from the Premier and DPC has ensured buy-in from senior public servants. HiAP has been less successful in involving the broader community. To date, the South Australian HiAP initiative has relied on policy cooperation between government departments, and there has been little emphasis on involving communities in the policy process. The setting of the SASP targets (which as we have seen is an important driver for HiAP itself) has involved an extensive process of community consultation. There is scope for this participatory approach to be extended to the HLAs and the subsequent implementation of HiAP initiatives. Increased community involvement may be one means of keeping the policy window open for HiAP by gaining broader community support for the approach.

The future: sustainability of HiAP beyond the innovation stage

HiAP in South Australia has been sustained so far by its early successes through the HLAs and its ability to cope with complex policy issues, as well as the fact it has enjoyed high-level political support, has received international recognition, and has been supported by a Thinkers in Residence programme. Kingdon (2011) warns that policy windows can close as quickly as they open and this could potentially happen to HiAP. True sustainability over the long term probably relies on HiAP becoming institutionalized as a way of doing core business for the departments involved. While the present and future cost pressures within the health sectors have, to date, operated in favour of HiAP, in the future these pressures might come to mean that the health portfolio resorts to seeing its core business solely in terms of the provision of health care services. Consequently, we suggest that ongoing work needs to be done to keep the policy window open for activities that focus on population health and disease prevention and health promotion. The new South Australian Public Health Act is likely to be crucial to ensuring this happens. Sustainability will also require creative revitalization of HiAP, as suggested by the change management literature (Senge, 1992). We hope our planned evaluation (2012–2016) will assist in pinpointing areas in need of revitalization and will provide data to fine-tune and improve the implementation and population health outcomes of HiAP. At the end of 2011 the South Australian Premier who first supported HiAP retired and the new Premier, Hon. Jay Weatherall, while continuing the SASP, established within this framework seven strategic priorities for his government. The HiAP unit immediately responded to this new environment and in mid-late 2012 are conducting HLAs on each of these priorities. Again, this adaptability is likely to be crucial to the survival of HiAP.

Conclusion

We have shown that HiAP in South Australia evolved from a unique combination of historical, political and policy opportunities. Kingdon's theory was useful in understanding the processes by which HiAP was able to move to a central position on the policy agenda in the state. Increasingly, responding to policy issues demands an understanding of the complex systems to which they are required to respond. We found that HiAP has been implemented in a manner that takes account of and permits a response to these complexities. HiAP has followed the stages of awareness, adoption, and implementation: the next few years will determine whether it becomes institutionalized.

References

Antonovsky, A. (1996). The salutogenic model as a theory to guide health promotion. *Health Promotion International*, **11** (1), 11–18.

Ashton, J. and Seymour, H. (1988). *The New Public Health.* Milton Keynes: Open University Press.

Baum, F. (ed.) (1995). *Health for All: the South Australian Experience.* Kent Town, SA: Wakefield Press.

Baum, F. (2008). *The New Public Health,* (3rd edn.). Melbourne: Oxford University Press.

Baum, F., Fry, D., and Lennie, I. (eds.) (1992). *Community Health Policy and Practice in Australia.* Sydney: Pluto Press, Australian Community Health Association.

Baum, F., Newman, L., Biedrzycki, K., and Patterson, J. (2010). Can a regional government's social inclusion initiative contribute to the quest for health equity? *Health Promotion International,* **25** (4), 474–82.

Broom, D. H. (1991). *Damned if We Do. Contradictions in Women's Health Care.* St. Leonards, NSW: Allen & Unwin.

Butterfoss, F. D., Kegler, M. C., and Francisco, F. D. (2008). Mobilizing organizations for health promotion: theories of organizational change, in: K. Glanz, B. K. Rimer, and K. Viswanath (eds.) *Health Behavior and Health Education: Theory, Research and Practice,* (4th edn.), pp. 335–61, San Francisco, CA: Jossey-Bass.

Catford, J. (2011). Health promotion: origins, obstacles and opportunities, in H. Keleher and C. MacDougall (eds.) *Understanding Health* (3rd edn.), pp. 134–51, Melbourne: Oxford University Press.

Commission on Macroeconomics and Health (2001). *Macroeconomics and Health: Investing in Health for Economic Development Report of the Commission on Macroeconomics and Health.* Geneva: World Health Organization.

Council of the European Union (2012). *Consolidated Versions of the Treaty on European Union and the Treaty on the Functioning of the European Union and the Charter of Fundamental Rights of the European Union.* Brussels: Council of the European Union.

CSDH (2008). *Closing the Gap in a Generation. Health Equity through Action on the Social Determinants of Health.* Geneva: World Health Organization.

Dahlgren, G. and Whitehead, M. (2006). *A discussion paper on European strategies for tacking social inequities in health: Levelling up (Part 2),* Copenhagen: WHO Regional Office for Europe.

Denis, J.-L. and Lomas, J. (2003). Convergent evolution: the academic and policy roots of collaborative research. *Health Services Research & Policy,* **8**, 1–6.

de Savigny, D. and Adam, T. (eds.) (2009). *Systems Thinking for Health Systems Strengthening.* Geneva: Alliance for Health Policy and Systems Research, World Health Organization.

Engels, F. (1993[1845]). *The Conditions of the Working Class in England.* New York: Oxford University Press.

Exworthy, M. (2008). Policy to tackle the social determinants of health: using conceptual models to understand the policy process. *Health Policy and Planning,* **23** (5), 318–27.

Foley, G. (1982). Aboriginal community controlled health services: a short history. *Aboriginal Health Project Information Bulletin,* **2**, 13–15.

Golder, W., Newman, L., Biedrzycki, K., and Baum, F. (2010). Digital technology access and use as 21st century determinants of health: impact of social and economic disadvantage, in I. Kickbusch and

K. Buckett (eds.), *Implementing Health in All Policies: The South Australian Experience*, pp. 133–43, Adelaide: Government of South Australia.

Government of South Australia (2011). *South Australia's Strategic Plan*. Adelaide: Government of South Australia.

Green-Pedersen, C. and Wilkerson, J. (2006). How agenda-setting attributes shape politics: basic dilemmas, problem attention and health politics developments in Denmark and the US. *Journal of European Public Policy,* **13** (7), 1039–52.

Hajer, M. (1995). *The Politics of Environmental Discourse: Ecological Modernization and the Policy Process.* Oxford: Clarendon Press.

Harris-Roxas, B. and Harris E. (2011). Differing forms, differing purposes: a typology of health impact assessment. *Environmental Impact Assessment Review,* **31** (4), 396–403

Hawe, P., Bond, L., and Butler, H. (2009a). Knowledge theories can inform evaluation practice: what can a complexity lens add? *New Directions for Evaluation,* **124**, 89–100.

Hawe, P., Shiell, A., and Riley, T. (2009b). Theorising interventions as events in systems. *American Journal of Community Psychology,* **43** (3–4), 267–76.

Health in All Policies Unit (2011). *The South Australian Approach to Health in All Policies: Background and Practical Guide: Version 2.* Adelaide: Government of South Australia.

Hunter, P. (1999). The National Aboriginal Community Controlled Health Organisation. *New Doctor,* **70**, 11–12.

International Conference on Primary Health Care (1978). *Declaration of Alma-Ata.* Geneva: World Health Organization.

Kaluzny, A. D. and Hernandez, S. R. (1988). Organizational change and innovation, in **S. M. Shortell** and **A. D. Kaluzny** (eds.) *Health Care Management: A Text in Organization Theory and Behavior,* pp. 379–417, New York: Wiley.

Kearns, G. (1988). Private property and public health reform in England 1830–70. *Social Science and Medicine,* **26** (1), 187–99.

Kickbusch, I. (1996). Tribute to Aaron Antonovsky—'What creates health?' *Health Promotion International,* **11** (1), 5–6.

Kickbusch, I. (2008). *Healthy Societies: Addressing 21st Century Health Challenges.* Adelaide: Adelaide Thinkers in Residence.

Kingdon, J. (2011). *Agendas, Alternatives and Public Policies.* New York: Addison-Wesley Educational Publishers.

Koivusalo, M. (2010). The state of Health in All Policies (HiAP) in the European Union: potential and pitfalls. *Journal of Epidemiology and Community Health,* **64** (6), 500–3.

Lawless, A. and Hurley, C. (2010). *Applying a Health Lens Analysis to Transit-Oriented Development: A Case Study of a Health in All Policies Approach to Policy Development.* Adelaide: South Australian Community Health Research Unit, Flinders University.

Lewis, M. J. (2003). *The People's Health: Public Health in Australia 1799–1950.* Westport, CT: Preader.

Liu, X., Lindquist, E., Vedlitz, A., and Vincent, K. (2010). Understanding local policymaking: policy elites' perceptions of local agenda setting and alternative policy selection. *Policy Studies Journal,* **38** (1), 69–91.

McKeown, T. (1976). *The Role of Medicine: Dream, Mirage or Nemesis.* London: Nuffield Provincial Hospital Trust.

Mannheimer, L., Lehto, J., and Ostlin, P. (2007). Window of opportunity for intersectoral health policy in Sweden open, half-open or half-shut? *Health Promotion International,* **22** (4), 307–15.

Meadows, D., Richardson, J., and Bruckmann, G. (1982). *Groping in the Dark: the First Decade of Global Modelling.* New York: Wiley.

Mitton, C., Adair, C. E., McKenzie E., Patten S. B., and Waye Perry, B. (2007) Knowledge transfer and exchange: review and synthesis of the literature. *The Milbank Quarterly*, **85** (4), 729–68.

Mulgan, G. (2008). *Innovation in 360 Degrees: Promoting Social Innovation in South Australia.* Adelaide: Department of the Premier and Cabinet.

Ollila, E. (2011). Health in All Policies: from rhetoric to action. *Scandinavian Journal of Public Health*, **39** (Sup. 6), 11–8.

Petticrew, M. and Roberts, H. (2003). Theory and methods: evidence, hierarchies, and typologies: horses for courses. *Journal of Epidemiology and Community Health*, **57** (7), 527–9.

Pierre, J. (2000). *Debating Governance: Authority, Steering and Democracy.* Oxford: Oxford University Press.

Public Health Agency of Canada (2007). *Crossing Sectors—Experiences in intersectoral action, public policy and health.* Ottowa: Public Health Agency of Canada, CSDH Health Systems Knowledge Network, Regional Network for Equity in Health in East and Southern Africa.

Richmond, B. (2000). *The 'Thinking' in Systems Thinking: Seven Essential Skills.* Waltham, MA: Pegasus Communications.

Ross, A. and Dovers, S. (2008). Making the harder yards: environmental policy integration in Australia. *The Australian Journal of Public Administration*, **67** (3), 245–60.

Senge, P. (1992). *The Fifth Discipline. The Art and Practice of the Learning Organisation.* Sydney: Random House.

Shankardass, K., Solar, O., Murphy, K., Freiler, A., Bobbili, S., Bayoumi, A., and O'Campo, P. (2011). *Health in All Policies: A Snapshot for Ontario, Results of a Realist-Informed Scoping Review of the Literature.* Ontario: St Michael's.

Sihto, M., Ollila, E., and Koivusalo, M. (2006). Principles and challenges of Health in All Policies, in T. Ståhl, M. Wismar, E. Ollila, E. Lahtinen, and K. Leppo (eds.) *Health in All Policies: Prospects and Potentials*, pp. 3–20, Finland: European Observatory on Health Systems and Policy.

South Australian Health Commission (1988). *A Social Health Strategy for South Australia.* Adelaide: SAHC.

South Australian House of Assembly (2010). *Hansard, House of Assembly November 24 2010: South Australian Public Health Bill.* Adelaide: Government of South Australia.

Ståhl, T., Wismar, M., Ollila, E., Lahtinen, E., and Leppo, K. (eds.) (2006). *Health in All Policies: Prospects and Potentials.* Finland: European Observatory on Health Systems and Policy.

Steenbakkers, M., Jansen, M., Maarse, H., and de Vries, N. (2012). Challenging Health in All Policies, an action research study in Dutch municipalities. *Health Policy*, **105** (2–3), 288–95.

Sterman, J. D. (2006). Learning from evidence in a complex world. *American Journal of Public Health*, **96** (3), 505–14.

Stilwell, F. (1993). *Economic Inequality.* Leichhardt, NSW: Pluto Press.

Szreter, S. (1988). The importance of social intervention in Britain's mortality decline c. 1850–1914: a reinterpretation of the role of public health. *The Society for the Social History of Medicine*, **1**, 1–37.

Townsend, P. and Davidson, N. (eds.) (1982). *Inequalities in Health: the Black Report.* London: Penguin.

Tryens, J. (2008). A seat at the head of the table. *Public Health Bulletin South Australia*, **5** (1), 27.

Virchow, R. (1848). Der Armenarzt. Die medizinische Reform, 18, 125.

Warner, M. and Gould, N. (2009). Integrating Health in All Policies at the local level: using network governance to create 'virtual reorganization by design', in I. Kickbusch (ed.) *Policy Innovation for Health*, pp. 125–63, New York: Springer.

WHO (1948). *Constitution.* Geneva: World Health Organization.

WHO (1986). *First International Conference on Health Promotion. The Ottawa Charter for Health Promotion.* Geneva: World Health Organization.

WHO (1988). *Conference Statement of the 2nd International Conference on Health Promotion: The Adelaide Recommendations—Healthy Public Policy*. Geneva: World Health Organization.

WHO (1995). *Twenty Steps for Developing a Healthy Cities Project (2nd edn.)*. Copenhagen: WHO Regional Office for Europe.

WHO (1999). *Gothenburg Consensus Paper on Health Impact Assessment*. Brussels: European Centre for Health Policy/WHO Regional Office for Europe.

WHO (2011). *Closing the Gap: Policy into Practice on Social Determinants of Health—Discussion Paper*. Geneva: World Health Organization.

WHO and Government of South Australia (2010). *Adelaide Statement on Health in All Policies: Moving Towards a Shared Governance for Health and Well-being*. Adelaide: World Health Organization and Government of South Australia.

Williams, C., Lawless, A., and Parkes, H. (2008). The South Australian Health in All Policies model: the developmental phase. *Public Health Bulletin South Australia,* **5** (1), 30–4.

Chapter 11

Wrap-up: practise a new health political science

Carole Clavier and Evelyne de Leeuw

We started this book with Lewin's premise that 'Nothing is as practical as a good theory' (1945: 129). But just how are theories on the policy process practical for health promotion research and practice? Our answer is that theories are practical because they help to understand policies, and because they help to make policies. The two sections of our book, 'Understanding Policy' and 'Making Policy', reflect these two aspects. We believe there exists a deep chasm at the interface between the scholarly study of health promotion and the discipline of political science: health promoters seem more inspired by individual behaviour than by organization, system, or institutional behaviour; political scientists seem to regard health as merely an intriguing case study; and never the twain shall meet. In this concluding chapter, we make an evidence-based call to both scholars and practitioners/activists to consider theories on the policy process and to draw on them in their research and practice.

Theories are practical because they help to understand policies. In the book's first section, theories on the policy process provided a lens through which to look at, and make sense of, public policies: their content, how they are made, and how they change. As we stated in our introduction, theories establish relationships between different elements of society in an attempt to explain a phenomenon. Theories on the policy process, therefore, all make certain assumptions about public policies and the factors shaping the policy process. Some theories consider the structure of political institutions to be the most important factor in explaining the content, change, and impact of policies (Hall and Taylor, 1996). In Chapter 4, Bryant presented a theory of the influence of political and market ideology on policy choices in an attempt to explain the Canadian government's lack of commitment to developing policies around the social determinants of health. Political economy theory postulates that political ideology shapes the role of the State, in particular as regards the distribution of economic and social resources to citizens. In her discussion, Bryant highlighted the relationship between the Canadian government's increasing shift to neo-liberalism and its reluctance to address the social determinants of health and reduce their unequal distribution across the population.

By contrast, Breton, Richard, Gagnon, Jacques, and Bergeron in Chapter 3, and Potvin and Clavier in Chapter 5, applied theories that focus on the role of individual and institutional actors in the policy-making process. Breton et al. turned to coalition-building theories to explain how an anti-tobacco law came to be adopted in the Province of Quebec (Canada). Such theories—in particular Sabatier's Advocacy Coalition Framework—contend that public policy choices result from the confrontation of different coalitions of actors, each coalition being united around a particular set of values and ideas about a given policy issue. In this particular case, the anti-tobacco coalition gathered a diverse range of actors whose legitimacy and arguments resonated with public opinion, and found a major ally in the Minister of Health. This theoretical framework effectively explained the influence of this particular coalition of actors on the policy decision, as opposed to other coalitions formed by the tobacco industry, the hospitality industry, and the retail sector. Potvin and Clavier chose actor–network theory to make sense of the implementation of public health programmes by a range of actors from several policy sectors, including public health institutions, education institutions, municipal authorities, and community organizations organized around family or neighbourhood issues. As actor–network theory sees innovations as resulting from collaborative processes between a range of actors with diverse interests, Potvin and Clavier focused on the micro-interactions between different actors, showing how their interactions produced effects greater than the sum of individual actions.

In their study of global health governance, de Leeuw, Townsend, Martin, Jones, and Clavier used three different sets of theories to explain different dimensions of global health governance (Chapter 6). They found that theories on implementation were well-suited to questioning discrepancies in the application of an international convention to small island states. Critical discourse analysis helped to make sense of the efforts of different actors to influence the governance and contents of an international trade agreement on intellectual property rights in relation to access to medicines. Faced with the emergence of national policies seeking to act on health at the global scale, de Leeuw et al. called on theories that conceptualize the formulation and circulation of policy ideas across policy sectors and policy-making levels.

As we can see from the chapters in this book's first section, there is not one theory on the policy process, but rather an array of useful theories. These theories can be divided into categories based on the particular explanatory factor used, such as institutions, ideas, or actors and their interests. Among the theories that consider institutions as the main explanatory factor of public policies, institutional rational choice draws on a series of hypotheses about the behaviour of social actors and builds models to explain human behaviour and policy outcomes. Historical institutionalism investigates how institutions shape public policies and political preferences in an attempt to understand why different societies have developed different policies. For other theories, the main explanation of public policy content, change, and impact lies in the ideas and beliefs of the actors, or groups of actors, involved in the policy process (Campbell, 2002). Among these are the coalition-building theories mentioned above, along with theories on policy networks (Marsh and Rhodes, 1992), epistemic communities (Haas, 1992), and policy elites (Hassenteufel et al., 2010). Kingdon's multiple streams theory also considers, albeit not as the main explanatory factor, the role of policy entrepreneurs in creating connections between the problem, policy, and political streams (de Leeuw et al., Chapter 8 in this volume; Kingdon, 1984).

This list of the theories that have been developed to make sense of the policy process is far from exhaustive. The difficulty faced by analysts is selecting the theory that is most appropriate to the issue they are studying. Elsewhere, one of us has asserted that the proper framing of a social issue leads to the logical formulation of an appropriate research question (de Leeuw, 2009). This question—coupled, of course, with the recognition that all inquiry is value laden—leads to the selection of a logically sound theory or conceptual framework, which in turn dictates an appropriate methodology (or 'logic of methods'). The data collection methods chosen should closely and commensurately match the nature of the issue, the research question, and the methodology. At each stage in this development process, choices need to be made, often in close consultation with clients and communities. This is not easy, and perhaps too often scholars jump to conclusions, applying a tried and tested methodology (e.g. the randomized controlled trial) or an established theory—one that does not lend itself 'naturally' to such an approach. This may lead to type III errors ('answering the wrong question') or, perhaps more insidiously, type IV errors ('doing the right research from the wrong paradigm') (Breton and de Leeuw, 2010; de Leeuw, 2012a).

By making assumptions about how public policy works, theories on the policy process allow for an in-depth critical understanding of these processes. The phrase 'critical theory' is sometimes used to characterize studies that question the legitimacy of policy choices. This theory arose from a school of thought rooted in emancipatory political movements, and its aim was to provide normative-oriented arguments for making (emancipatory) choices (Bohman, 2010). Here, we use the phrase as a broad designation of new theoretical developments in policy studies that move away from the technocratic approach to policy analysis and seek to make sense of contemporary policy issues (Orsini and Smith, 2007). Generally speaking, social theory is a powerful cognitive resource for those seeking to understand and question societal trends or policy choices. This observation also extends our theoretical gaze beyond the strict political sciences; for instance, sociologists like Gusfield, Laumann, and Knoke have advanced propositions on the social order that make policy development possible. Gusfield does so by identifying ownership of public problems as a contested arena (Gusfield, 1981), whereas Laumann and Knoke map that contested arena by measuring and constructing networks of actors (Laumann and Knoke, 1987). None of these authors would consider themselves political scientists, and yet they are framing sets of policy assumptions. In their chapters, Breton et al., Potvin and Clavier, and de Leeuw et al. use theories on the policy process in a similar way: to orient their research questions and hypotheses, and as an interpretive resource to make sense of everyday work situations, like the implementation of intersectoral health promotion programmes or of research data (Frohlich et al., 2004). Bryant also used theory as a critical tool in order to appraise and discuss the different arguments put forward in the policy debate on the social determinants of health, as did de Leeuw et al. in their case study of global health governance.

Theories are also practical because they help to make policy. This was the theme of the book's second section. This statement relates to an ongoing debate in the field of political science. Historically, policy studies developed at the juncture of several disciplines and were dedicated to supporting the policy-making process. Then, within the political science discipline, policy analysts strove to define their work in terms of a 'pure' science—that is, an academic discipline that does not meddle with the murky business of politics (Bernier and Clavier, 2011; Donovan and Larkin, 2006). Among those who regret this development is one of the discipline's founders, who believes that it has made political science 'a theory without practice, a knowledge crippled by a know-how void' (Sartori, 2004). Several of us have already noted the ambivalence of policy studies towards policy and political engagement (Bernier and Clavier, 2011). Yet, despite this ambivalence, and despite the decidedly academic orientation of the field, we argue here that theories developed within policy studies produce knowledge that can be of both instrumental and normative use to health promoters. We explicitly take a position that political research must engage with the murky, 'wicked', and messy business of politics. Elsewhere—for example, in the Healthy Cities initiative—one of us has argued that health promotion must embrace both scholarly activism and activist scholarship (de Leeuw, 2012b). In viewing health promotion as a process, rather than (just) a profession or a discipline, such a perspective becomes inescapable.

In applied research, theory is generally considered practical because the patterns it establishes can help in problem-solving (Bartholomew et al., 2011). Following the principles of theory-based evaluation, using theory in the analysis of programmes or policies produces knowledge on whether these programmes and policies work and, most importantly, how and in what circumstances they work (Birckmayer and Weiss, 2000; Pawson, 2003; Weiss, 1995). In other words, theories help to make pronouncements on how to act. For instance, by making explicit the causal mechanisms behind the circulation of micro-organisms, the germ theory of disease allows us to make pronouncements on how to prevent the spread of infectious diseases. Similarly, Giddens's structuration theory has very practical implications for health promotion interventions, such as those that aim to reduce smoking among young people living in deprived neighbourhoods (Frohlich et al., 2002). Structuration theory posits that neither structure nor agency predominates in determining how society is constituted (Giddens, 1984). The social structures of a neighbourhood—for instance, the number of tobacconists and their distance from schools, and the type of housing where young people live—influence the practices of residents, which in turn shape the neighbourhood. Young people hanging out with their friends on the terraces of the large housing projects where they live are more likely to smoke because they want to 'fit in', and they are also more likely to buy cigarettes on their way to school if they pass a tobacconist. But tobacconists are also more likely to settle in places where they know business will be good. Following Giddens, then, a neighbourhood is best conceptualized not as a 'passive container of resources, but as a relational structure' (Bernard et al., 2007: 1842). Consequently, health promotion interventions may want to address not only the lifestyle of young people in the community but also urban planning and community development. In this example, structuration theory is practical because it shows how an intervention needs to be oriented, based on an understanding of how society is structured.

Similarly, in Chapter 8, de Leeuw, Keizer, and Hoeijmakers showed how a combination of Kingdon's multiple streams theory and network theories can help policy actors to figure out their position within a web of actors who all have an interest in a given policy issue. For example, once farmers have identified their own particular interests relative to those of the municipality, public health institutions, greengrocers, and public markets, they can decide the best type of produce to grow and then how to get it on the market. This framework helps actors to see which other actors they are closest to in terms of interests and values, what are the most contentious issues, and what issues could form the basis of an alliance that could then influence the policy process. To further enhance the capacity of actors to 'see' what such theories highlight, de Leeuw et al. presented a very practical, hands-on software that policy actors can adapt to fit with their unique situation. In essence, the software allows users to visualize network positions.

Hunter, in Chapter 7, used theories on knowledge production and utilization to devise new ways of introducing knowledge about health promotion into the practices of policy-makers and health care practitioners in the United Kingdom. He explained how knowledge utilization is intimately dependent on knowledge production, and so knowledge production needs to include policy-makers and practitioners. His research centre organized knowledge translation workshops based on these principles, and the results of these workshops serve as a reminder that knowledge production cannot be conceived of as a social activity removed from the constraints of other social activities—in particular, the policy-making process. Hunter's experience with the World Health Organization is also a powerful reminder of the inherent political nature of the policy process. The conclusion is not that knowledge in the policy process is useless, but rather that policy-making is a process influenced by knowledge *plus* the result of constraints based on ideology, interests, and institutions. The conclusion, therefore, is that knowledge producers, in particular academics, need to become familiar with the policy process and adjust their strategies of knowledge production and translation accordingly.

In Chapter 9, Rütten, Gelius, and Abu-Omar presented their ADEPT model, a tool designed to assist policy-makers and rooted in a theory of action. They identified a set of determinants that influence the likelihood of a particular policy or programme being adopted by policy-makers: goals, resources, obligations, and constraints. Based on this theory, the authors have devised a simple and parsimonious questionnaire that both analysts and policy-makers can use to assess a policy project. This tool is useful for deciding how to act in a specific case as it focuses on the particular conditions that affect a given policy issue in a specific policy area, and on the behaviour of individual actors with an interest in these policy issues.

Baum, Lawless, and Williams reviewed the process that led the government of South Australia to develop a whole-of-government strategy for health, or the 'Health in All Policies' approach (Chapter 10). In this case, theories of agenda-setting helped to make sense of why the issue emerged in the region of South Australia, while organization theory and system change theories identified the factors influencing the implementation and institutionalization of the policy across policy sectors and over time. They used theories primarily in a retrospective way, to identify milestones in the policy-making process as well as strategies, resources, and obstacles. Such theories may, no doubt, be of use to other governments seeking to engage in the development of Health in All Policies. This is another way that theories can help to make pronouncements on how to act.

Theory helps to systematize how we think about health(y) policy and politics; it helps us to understand and critically assess policy processes, and it helps to make pronouncements on how to act at the policy level. We have demonstrated that the health promotion field would benefit from the application of practical theory to health policy research. We see a new generation of scholars emerging, one that actively pursues the integration of insights from both fields. As we have shown, this is certainly a fertile field. We would hope that scholars from both sides can leave their comfort zones and jointly develop a new 'health political science'.

In our minds, there is no doubt that more integration, not only between academic disciplines like health promotion and political science but also between scholarship and activism (Laverack, 2012), creates vibrant opportunities for more and better health policy development. We trust that this book will serve as a stepping stone toward this goal.

References

Bartholomew, L. K., Parcel, G. S., Kok, G., Gottlieb, N. H., and Fernandez, M. E. (2011). *Planning Health Promotion Programs: An Intervention Mapping Approach,* 3rd edn. San Francisco, CA: Jossey-Bass.

Bernard, P., Charafeddine, R., Frohlich, K. L., Daniel, M., Kestens, Y., and Potvin, L. (2007). Health inequalities and place: a theoretical conception of neighbourhood. *Social Science & Medicine*, **65**, 1839–52.

Bernier, N. F. and Clavier, C. (2011). Public health policy research: making the case for a political science approach. *Health Promotion International*, **26** (1), 109–16.

Birckmayer, J. D. and Weiss, C. H. (2000). Theory-based evaluation in practice: what do we learn? *Evaluation Review*, **24** (4), 407–31.

Bohman, J. (2010). Critical theory, in E. N. Zalta (ed.) *The Stanford Encyclopedia of Philosophy* (Spring 2010 edn.). Available at: <http://plato.stanford.edu/archives/spr2010/entries/critical-theory/>.

Breton, E. and de Leeuw, E. (2010). Multiple streams theory in Sweden: an error III. *Health Promotion International*, **25** (1), 134–5.

Campbell, J. L. (2002). Ideas, politics, and public policy. *Annual Review of Sociology*, **28**, 21–38.

de Leeuw, E. (2009). Evidence for Healthy Cities: reflections on practice, method and theory. *Health Promotion International*, **24**, i19–i36.

de Leeuw, E. (2012a). Do Healthy Cities work? A logic of method for assessing impact and outcome of Healthy Cities. *Journal of Urban Health*, **89** (2), 217–31.

de Leeuw, E. (2012b). Healthy Cities deserve better. *The Lancet*, **380** (9850), 1306–7.

Donovan, C. and Larkin, P. (2006). The problem of political science and practical politics. *Politics*, **26** (1), 11–17.

Frohlich, K. L., Mykhalovskiy, E., Miller, F., and Daniel, M. (2004). Advancing the population health agenda. *Canadian Journal of Public Health/Revue Canadienne de Santé Publique*, **95** (5), 392–5.

Frohlich, K. L., Potvin, L., Chabot, P., and Corin, E. (2002). A theoretical and empirical analysis of context: neighbourhoods, smoking and youth. *Social Science and Medicine*, **54** (9), 1401–17.

Giddens, A. (1984). *The Constitution of Society: Introduction of the Theory of Structuration.* Berkeley, CA: University of California Press.

Gusfield, J. R. (1981). *The Culture of Public Problems: Drinking-driving and the Symbolic Order.* Chicago, IL: University of Chicago Press.

Haas, P. M. (1992). Introduction: epistemic communities and international policy coordination. *International Organization*, **46** (1).

Hall, P. A. and Taylor, R. C. R. (1996). Political science and the three new institutionalisms. *Political Studies*, **44** (4), 936–57.

Hassenteufel, P., Smyrl, M., Genieys, W., and Moreno-Fuentes, F. J. (2010). Programmatic actors and the transformation of European health care states. *Journal of Health Politics, Policy and Law*, **35** (4), 517–38.

Kingdon, J. W. (1984). *Alternatives and Public Policies.* Boston, MA: Little, Brown and Co.

Laumann, E. O. and Knoke, D. (1987). *The Organizational State. Social Choice in National Policy.* Madison, WI: University of Wisconsin Press.

Laverack, G. (2012). Health activism. *Health Promotion International*, **27** (4), 429–34.

Lewin, K. (1945) The Research Center for Group Dynamics at Massachusetts Institute of Technology. *Sociometry*, **8 (2)**, 126–36.

Marsh, D. and Rhodes, R. A. W. (1992). *Policy Networks in British Government.* Oxford: Clarendon Press.

Orsini, M. and Smith, M. (eds.) (2007). *Critical Policy Studies.* Vancouver: UBC Press.

Pawson, R. (2003). Nothing as practical as a good theory. *Evaluation*, **9** (4), 471–90.

Sartori, G. (2004). Where is political science going? *PS: Political Science and Politics*, **37** (4), 785–7.

Weiss, C. H. (1995). Nothing as practical as good theory: exploring theory-based evaluation for comprehensive community initiatives for children and families, in J. L. Connell, A. C. Kubisch, L. B. Schorr, and C. H. Weiss (eds.) *New Approaches to Evaluating Community Initiatives. Concepts, Methods, and Contexts*, pp. 65–92, Washington, DC: The Aspen Institute.

Index